Clinical Orthopedic Tests

Prem P. Gogia, MD, DPT, PhD

Copyright © 1994, 2007, 2013 by Ambience Healthcare, LLC

All rights reserved.

No part of this publication my be reproduced, stored in a retrieval system, or transmitted in any form or by any means, electronic, mechanical, photocopying, recording, or otherwise, without the prior permission of Ambience Healthcare, LLC.

Originally published by Academic Press, 15 E 26th St Fl 15, New York, NY 10010

Library of Congress Cataloging-in-Publication Data

Gogia, Prem P., 1953-
 Clinical Orthopedic Tests / Prem P. Gogia

ISBN-13: 978-1494720940 (CreateSpace-Assigned)
ISBN-10: 1494720949

About the Author

Prem P. Gogia, MD, DPT, PhD, has more than 30 years of experience in physical rehabilitation. He is a clinician, researcher, and educator based in Houston, Texas. Dr. Gogia has published 21 research/special interest papers in professional journals. In addition to contributing a few chapters to books, he is the author of four books titled *Clinical Cardiac Rehabilitation, Clinical Alzheimer Rehabilitation, Clinical Wound Management,* and *Clinical Orthopedic Tests*. Dr. Gogia received his MD degree from All Saints University of Medicine, DPT (Doctor of Physical Therapy) degree from Drexel University, and PhD degree from Texas Woman's University. Dr. Gogia also earned a MBA degree from Southern Illinois University.

Dedication

*This book is dedicated to my late parents,
Mr. & Mrs. J. R. Gogia, with love and respect.*

—Prem P. Gogia, MD, DPT, PhD

Preface

Examination of the musculoskeletal system is an important part of many clinicians' daily practice. Orthopedic special tests are routinely used during the physical examination process in order to help diagnose joint pathologies clinically. As a part of physical examination of the musculoskeletal dysfunction, orthopedic special tests help the clinician identify the pain-generating structures in order to define a specific diagnosis and plan of care. Additionally, in certain cases a valid and reliable clinical test may eliminate the need for costly diagnostic testing procedures.

Compared with diagnostic imaging methods, physical examination tests or orthopedic clinical special tests have historically been an integral part of clinical examinations and are presently used by a variety of medical professionals as a less costly means of information gathering and confirmation of hypotheses.

The number of special tests that have been described over the years is enormous. The purpose of this book is to compile and organize these tests systematically. This book is designed as a reference tool for clinicians of all background who are dealing with musculoskeletal dysfunctions. It will be a valuable reference tool for physical and occupational therapy students as well as medical students.

This book, first published in 1994, contains eleven sections dealing with the extremity joints, the temporomandibular joint, the spine, and the sacroiliac joint. Each section contains the clinical tests of the specific area. Each test is first described, interpreted, and then followed by an illustration to add clarity to the performance of the test.

I hope that this endeavor will help the practitioners with diagnosing the musculoskeletal dysfunctions.

Prem P. Gogia, MD, DPT, PhD

Acknowledgement

I extend my gratitude to all the students who performed their clinical training under my mentorship and encouraged me to put my ideas for a reference in the form of a book. I thank Fred Steinberg for his help in reviewing the manuscript. I would like to recognize Wendy Aldwyn for her illustrations. Last, but certainly not least, I wish to thank my wife Suman and daughters Reena and Ruchi for their patience during the long hours I spent in preparing the manuscript.

Contents

Section 1
    Shoulder 1

Section 2
    Elbow 43

Section 3
    Wrist and Hand 53

Section 4
    Hip 75

Section 5
    Knee 101

Section 6
    Ankle and Foot 157

Section 7
    Temporomandibular 175

Section 8
    Cervical 181

Section 9
    Thoracic 215

Section 10
    Lumbar 221

Section 11
    Sacrum and Pelvis 277

Bibliography 309

Index
    Sectional 311
    Alphabetical 315

Section 1
Shoulder

Glenohumeral Joint Stability Test

Description

The patient lies supine. The examiner grasps the patient's proximal humerus with both hands and pulls and pushes the humeral head anteriorly and posteriorly.

Interpretation

A positive test is one in which the humeral head moves excessively anteriorly and/or posteriorly, indicating unstable glenohumeral joint.

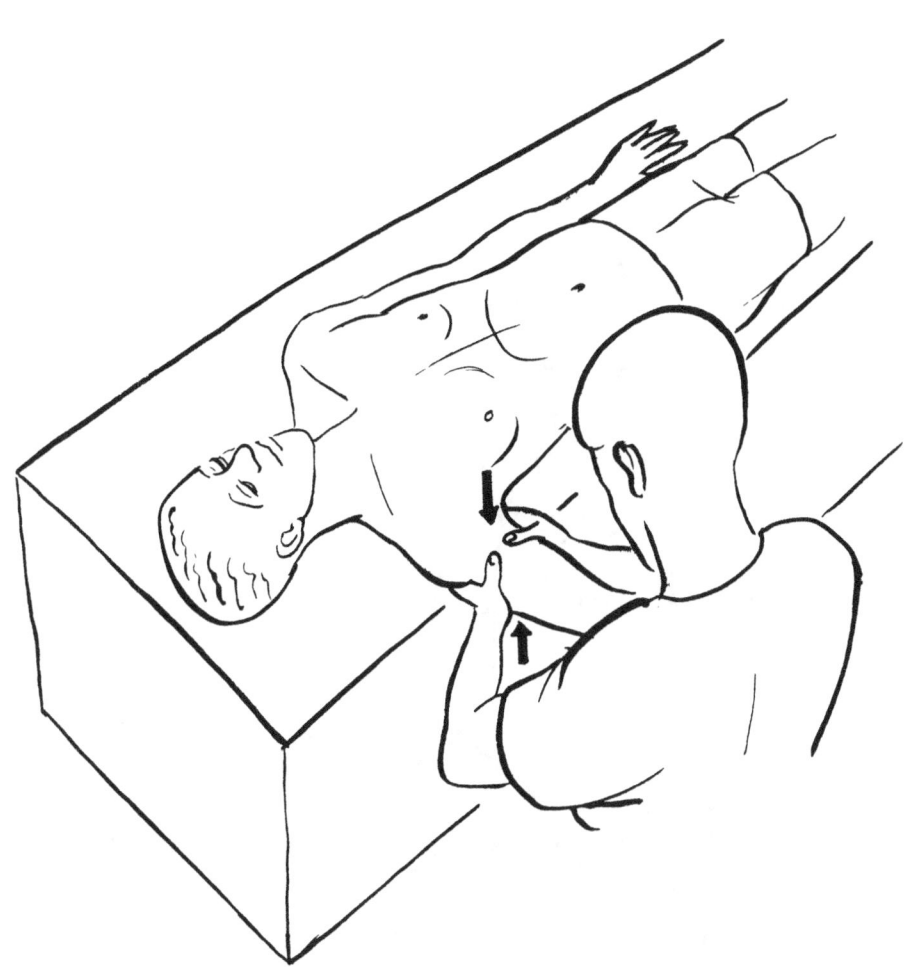

Anterior Apprehension Test

Description
The patient lies supine. The examiner flexes the patient's elbow to 90° and abducts the patient's shoulder to approximately 90°. The examiner holds the patient's forearm distally with one hand and with the other stabilizes the patient's elbow. The examiner then slowly externally rotates the shoulder.

Interpretation
A positive test is one in which the patient has a noticeable look of apprehension or alarm on the face and resists further motion, indicating anterior dislocation of the shoulder.

Comments
It is important that this test be done slowly to avoid dislocation of the shoulder.

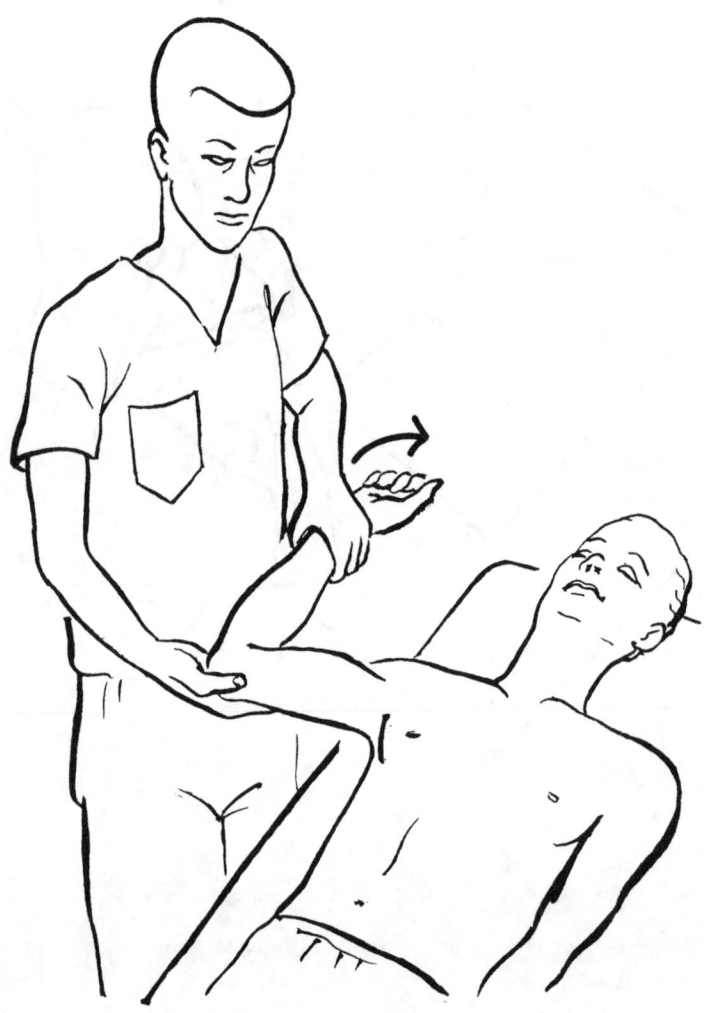

Protzman Test

Description

The patient stands. The examiner abducts the patient's shoulder to approximately 90°. The patient's arm is supported over the examiner's upper arm. The examiner palpates deep in the patient's axilla on the anterior aspect of the head of the humerus with one hand while the fingers of the other hand are placed over the posterior aspect of the head of the humerus. The examiner then pushes the humeral head anteriorly and inferiorly.

Interpretation

A positive test is one which causes pain and abnormal anteroinferior movement, indicating anterior instability of the shoulder.

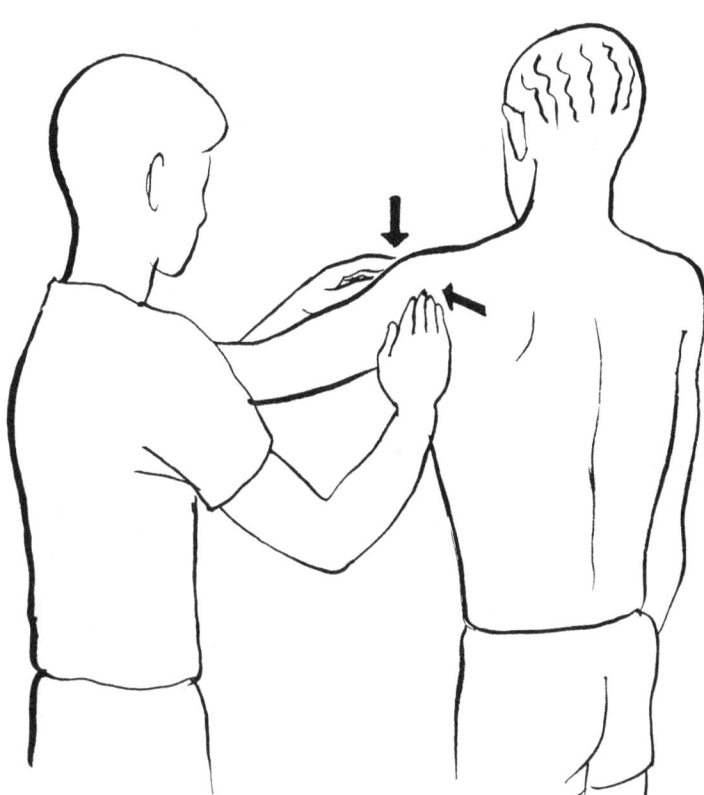

Anterior Instability Test

Description

The patient sits or stands. The examiner stands behind the patient. The examiner places one hand over the involved shoulder so that the index finger is over the humeral head anteriorly and the middle finger is over the coracoid process. The thumb is placed over the humeral head posteriorly. With the other hand the examiner grasps the patient's wrist and abducts and externally rotates the shoulder.

Interpretation

A positive test is one in which the examiner's index finger which is palpating the humeral head anteriorly moves forward as the patient's shoulder is being abducted and externally rotated, indicating anterior instability of the shoulder.

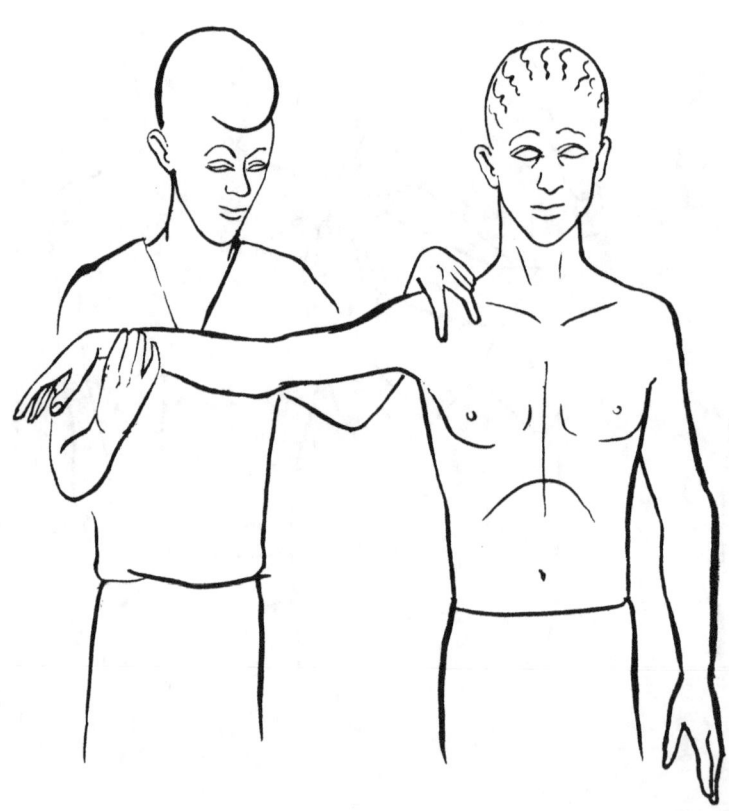

Rockwood Test

Description

The patient sits. The examiner stands behind the patient. The examiner grasps the patient's arms at the wrist and externally rotates the shoulders. The shoulders are brought to neutral position and the examiner first abducts the patient's shoulders to 45° and externally rotates them. This procedure is then repeated at 90° and 120° of the shoulder abduction.

Interpretation

A positive test is one in which pain is elicited in the posterior aspect of the involved shoulder and the patient shows apprehension at 45°, 90°, and 120° of shoulder abduction, indicating anterior instability of the shoulder.

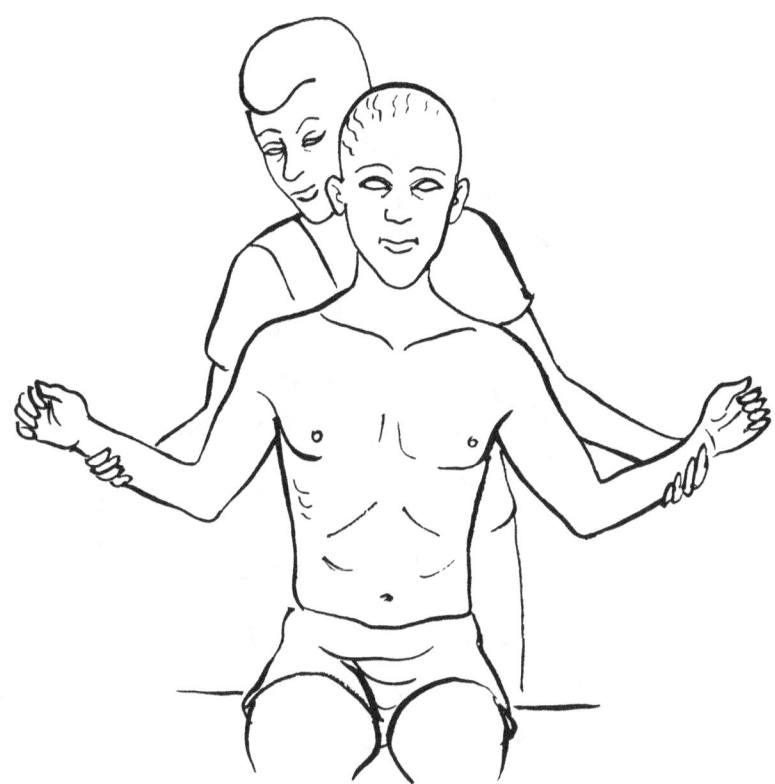

Rowe Test

Description

The patient lies supine. The patient is then instructed to place the hand of the involved side behind his/her head. The examiner places one hand against the patient's posterior humeral head and pushes up while with the other hand slightly extends the patient's shoulder.

Interpretation

A positive test is one in which pain is elicited in the shoulder and the patient shows apprehension, indicating anterior instability of the shoulder.

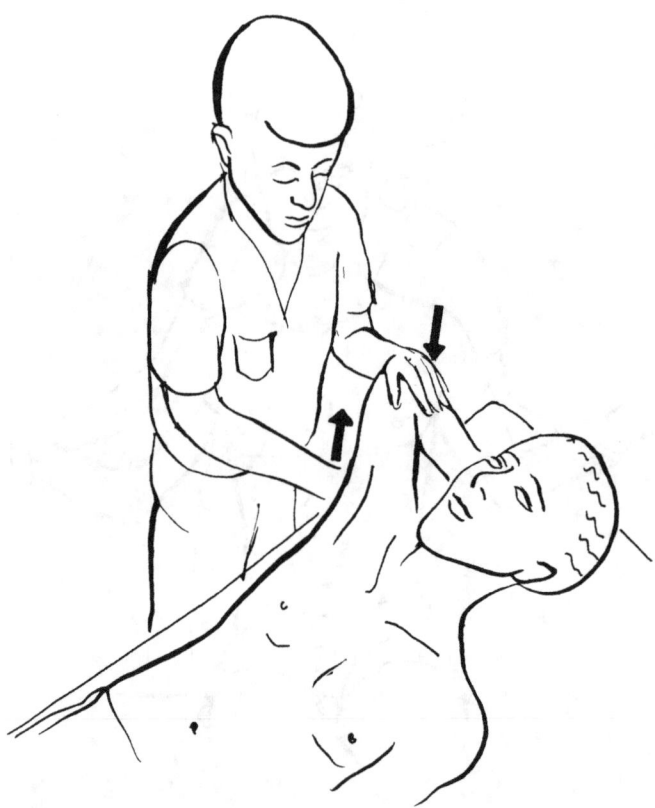

Fulcrum Test

Description

The patient lies supine. The examiner flexes the patient's elbow and abducts the shoulder to 90°. The examiner places one hand under the patient's glenohumeral joint to act as fulcrum and with the other hand holds the patient's wrist. The examiner then gently extends and externally rotates the shoulder over the fulcrum.

Interpretation

A positive test is one in which the patient shows apprehension, indicating anterior instability of the shoulder.

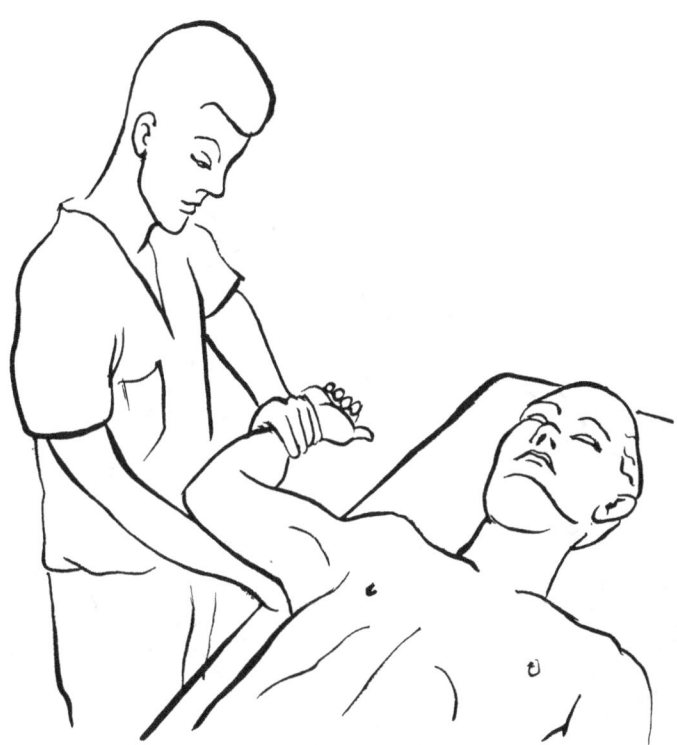

Anterior Drawer Test

Description

The patient lies supine. The examiner abducts the patient's shoulder to approximately 90°. To relax the patient's arm, the examiner places the patient's hand on the involved side in the examiner's axilla. The examiner grasps the patient's proximal humerus with one hand and forward flexes the patient's shoulder to about 20°, and externally rotates it about 20°-30°, while with the other hand stabilizing the patient's scapula. The examiner then pushes the spine of the scapula forward with the index and middle finger of the stabilizing hand and draws the humerus anteriorly with the other hand.

Interpretation

A positive test is one in which the patient shows apprehension and/or a click is felt during movement, indicating anterior instability of the shoulder.

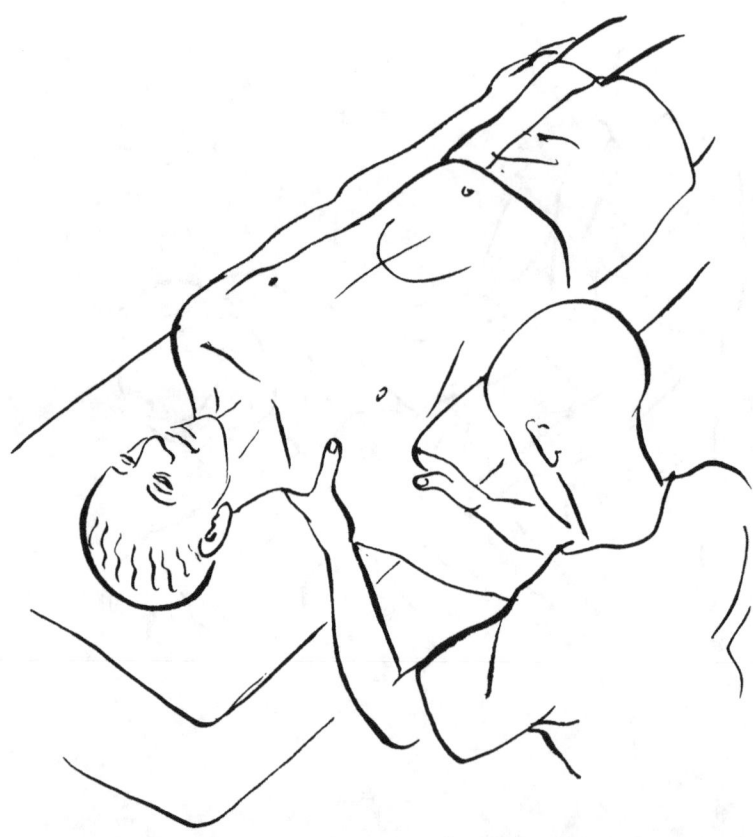

Posterior Apprehension Test

Description

The patient lies supine. The examiner holds the patient's elbow with one hand and stabilizes the shoulder with the other hand. The examiner flexes the patient's shoulder to 90° and internally rotates it, then applies a posterior force on the patient's elbow.

Interpretation

A positive test is one in which the patient has a noticeable look of apprehension or alarm on the face and resists further motion, indicating posterior dislocation of the shoulder.

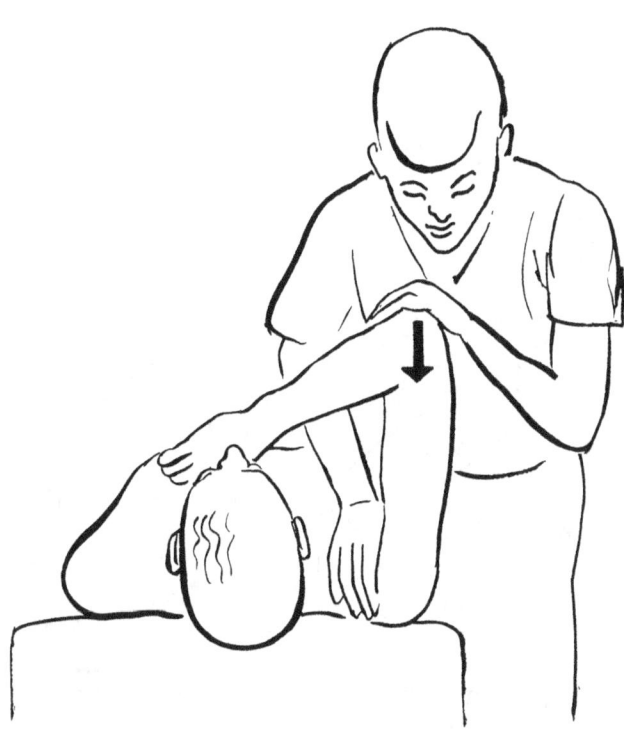

Posterior Drawer Test

Description

The patient lies supine. The examiner grasps the patient's forearm with one hand and flexes the patient's elbow to about 120°, then abducts the shoulder to 80°-120° and forward flexes it 20°-30°. With the other hand the examiner stabilizes the patient's scapula by placing the index and middle fingers on the spine of the scapula and the thumb on the coracoid process. The examiner then internally rotates the shoulder, forward flexes it to 60°-80°, and pushes the head of the humerus posteriorly.

Interpretation

A positive test is one in which the patient shows apprehension, indicating posterior instability of the shoulder.

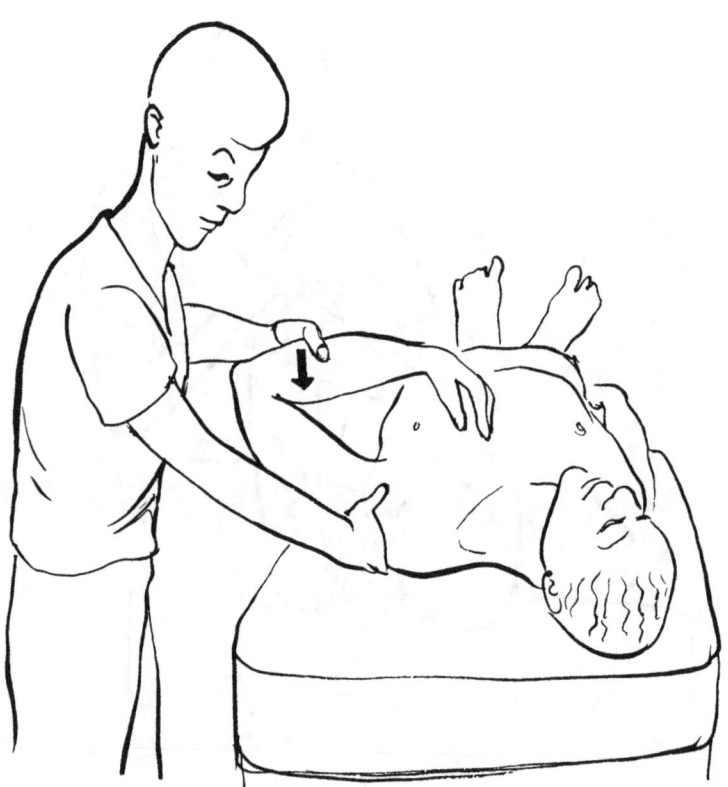

Norwood Test

Description

The patient lies supine. With one hand the examiner externally rotates the patient's shoulder and abducts it to approximately 90°, then flexes the patient's elbow to 90°. The examiner stabilizes the patient's scapula with the other hand. The examiner then moves the patient's shoulder into forward flexion and pushes the forearm posteriorly.

Interpretation

A positive test is one in which the humeral head slips posteriorly relative to the glenoid, indicating posterior instability of the shoulder.

Comments

It is important that this test be done slowly to avoid subluxation or dislocation of the shoulder.

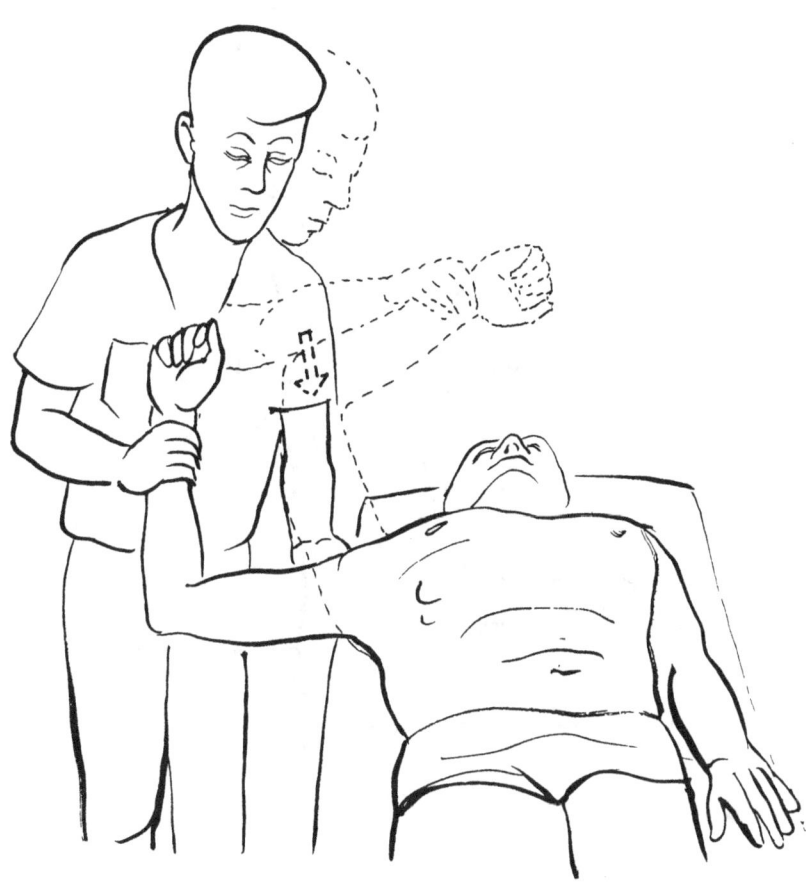

Jerk Test

Description

The patient sits. The examiner flexes the patient's elbow, forward flexes the shoulder to 90°, and internally rotates it. The examiner stabilizes the patient's back with one hand, grasps the patient's elbow with the other hand, and then axially loads the humerus in a proximal direction. The examiner then moves the patient's shoulder horizontally across the body while maintaining the axial loading.

Interpretation

A positive test is one in which the humeral head slides off the back of the glenoid with a sudden jerk, indicating recurrent posterior instability of the shoulder.

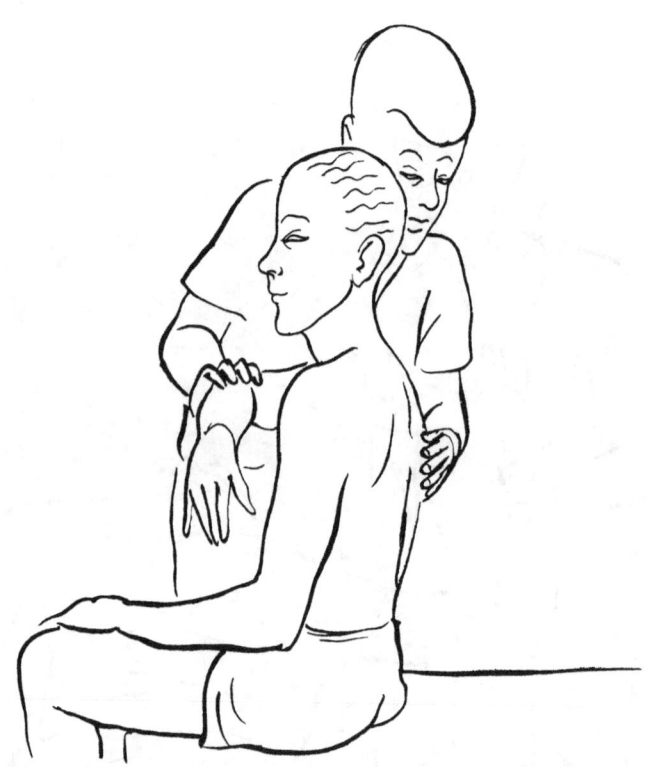

Push-Pull Test

Description

The patient lies supine. The examiner holds the patient's arm at the wrist with one hand. The examiner abducts the patient's shoulder to approximately 90° and forward flexes it about 30°. With the other hand the examiner grasps the patient's proximal humerus close to the humeral head. The examiner then pulls the patient's arm at the wrist and pushes the humerus posteriorly.

Interpretation

A positive test is one in which more than 50% posterior translation occurs or the patient shows apprehension, indicating posterior instability of the shoulder.

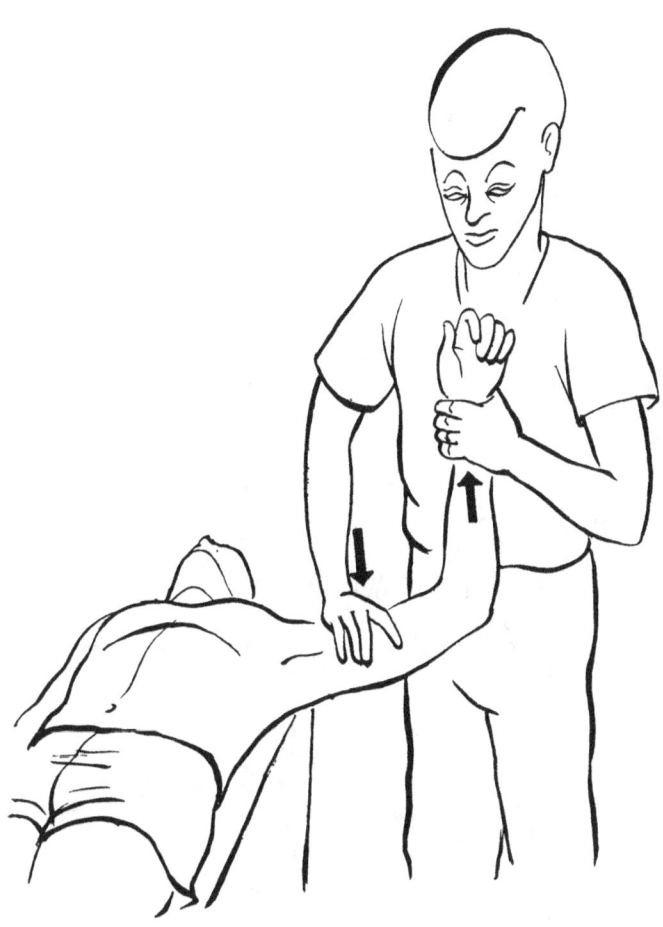

Sulcus Test

Description

The patient sits with the arm by the side. The examiner grasps the patient's wrist with one hand and with the other hand holds the forearm below the elbow. The examiner then pushes the arm distally, applying a longitudinal traction.

Interpretation

A positive test is one which produces a sulcus sign, indicating inferior instability of the shoulder.

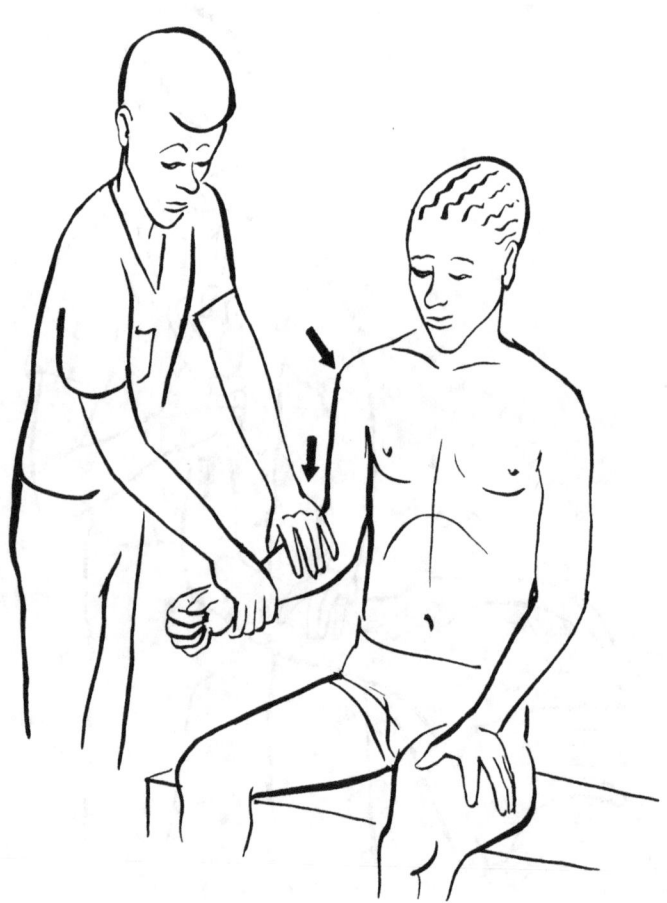

Feagin Test

Description

The patient stands. The examiner abducts the patient's shoulder to 90° and rests it on the examiner's shoulder with the elbow in the extended position. The examiner grasps the patient's proximal humerus with both hands and then the examiner pushes the humerus inferiorly and anteriorly.

Interpretation

A positive test is one in which the patient shows apprehension, indicating anteroinferior instability of the shoulder.

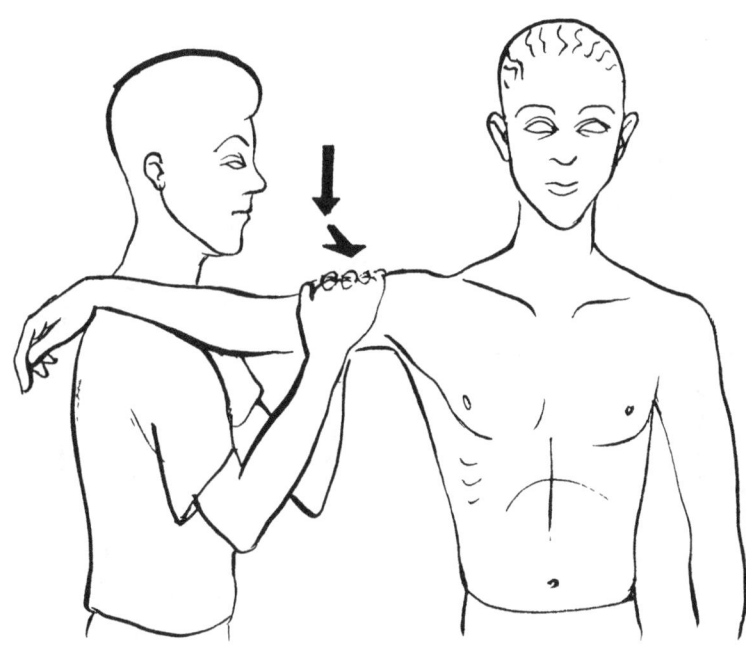

Capsular Laxity Test

Description

The patient stands. The examiner places one hand over the glenohumeral joint and then instructs the patient to flex the shoulder to horizontal position.

Interpretation

A positive test is one in which the glenohumeral joint clicks back into place with some discomfort at about 80° of flexion, indicating a capsular laxity of the glenohumeral joint.

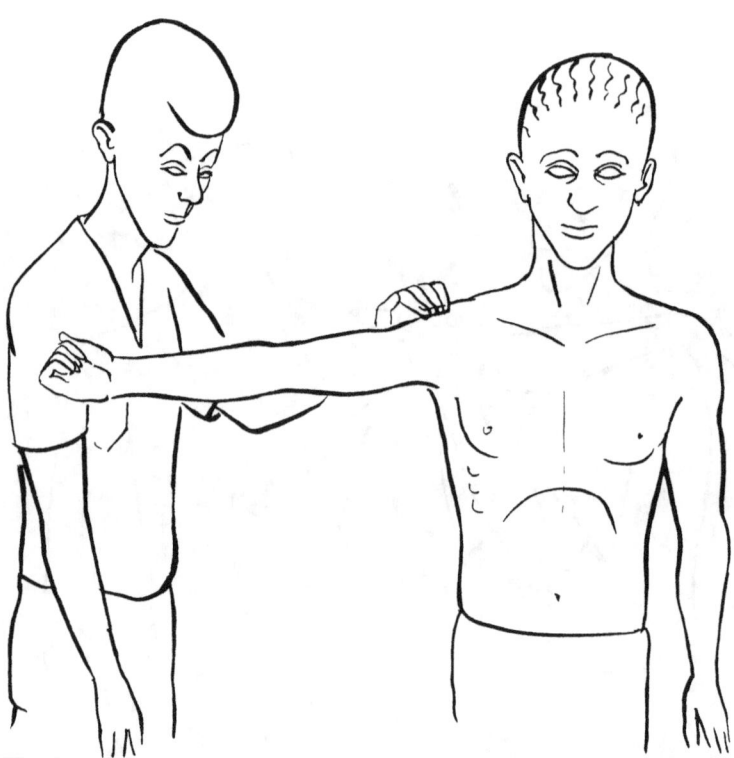

Clunk Test

Description

The patient lies supine. The examiner places one hand posteriorly on the humeral head and with the other hand holds the patient's humerus distally. The examiner fully abducts the patient's shoulder while forcing the humerus anteriorly and externally rotating the shoulder. The examiner then repositions the humeral head by lifting the arm into horizontal adduction.

Interpretation

A positive test is one in which a clunk sensation is felt during relocation, indicating a tear of the glenoidal labrum.

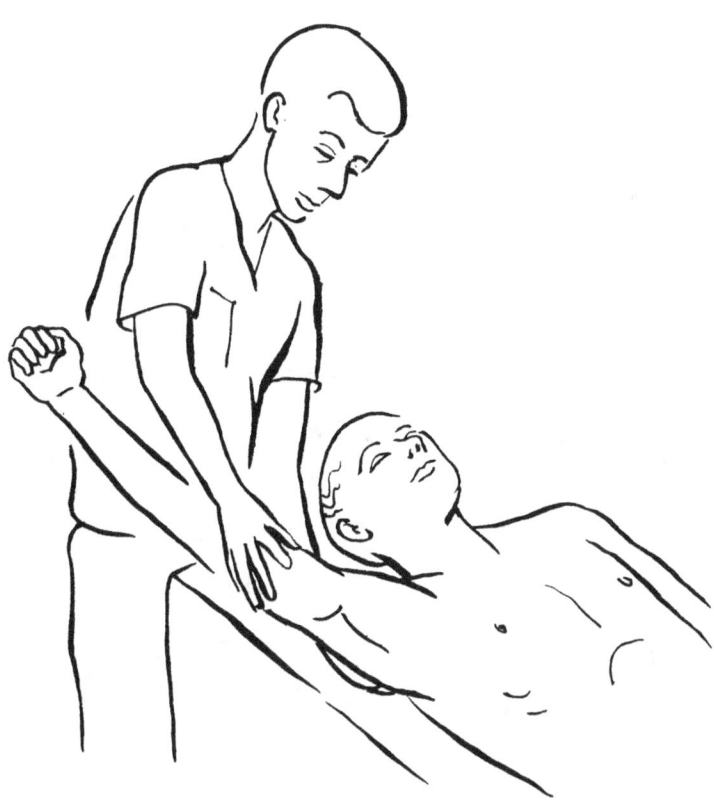

Supraspinatus Tendonitis Test

Description

The patient sits or stands. The examiner holds the patient's forearm and abducts the patient's shoulder to horizontal position. The patient is then instructed to abduct the arm while the examiner applies resistance to it.

Interpretation

A positive test is one in which pain is elicited over the insertion of the supraspinatus tendon, indicating a tendonitis of the supraspinatus tendon.

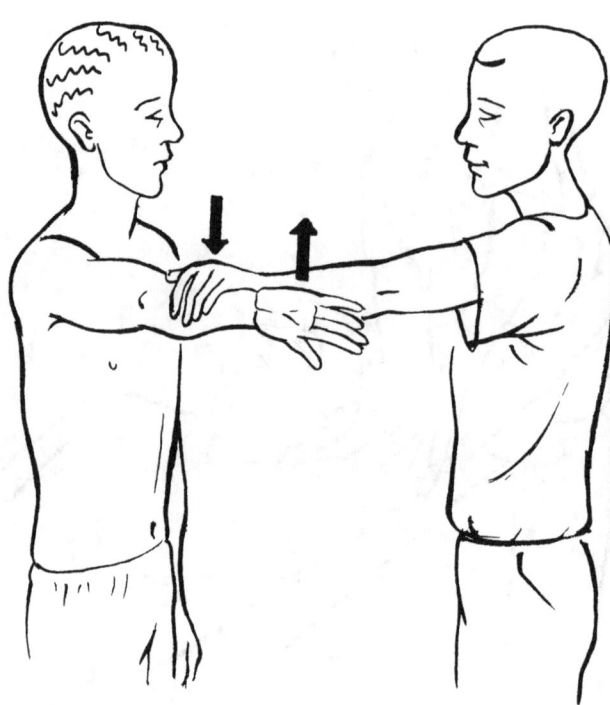

Drop Arm Test

Description

The patient stands. The examiner abducts the patient's shoulder to 90° while keeping the elbow fully extended. The patient is then instructed to slowly lower the arm to the side.

Interpretation

A positive test is one in which the arm drops to the side from a position of about 90° abduction, indicating a rotator cuff tear especially in the supraspinatus muscle.

Comments

If the patient is able to hold the arm in abduction, a gentle tap on the forearm will cause the arm to fall to the side if there is a tear in the rotator cuff.

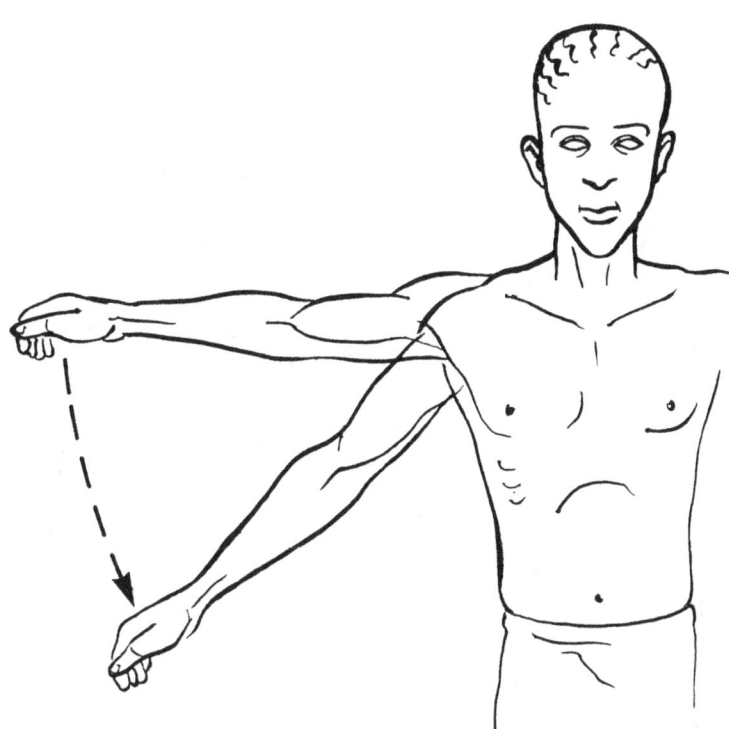

Impingement Test

Description

The patient sits or stands. The examiner holds the patient's forearm and passively abducts the patient's shoulder to about 90°, and then horizontally adducts the arm across the chest while internally rotating the arm and maintaining about 90° of flexion.

Interpretation

A positive test is one which causes pain, indicating impingement of the rotator cuff against the anterior surface of the acromion process.

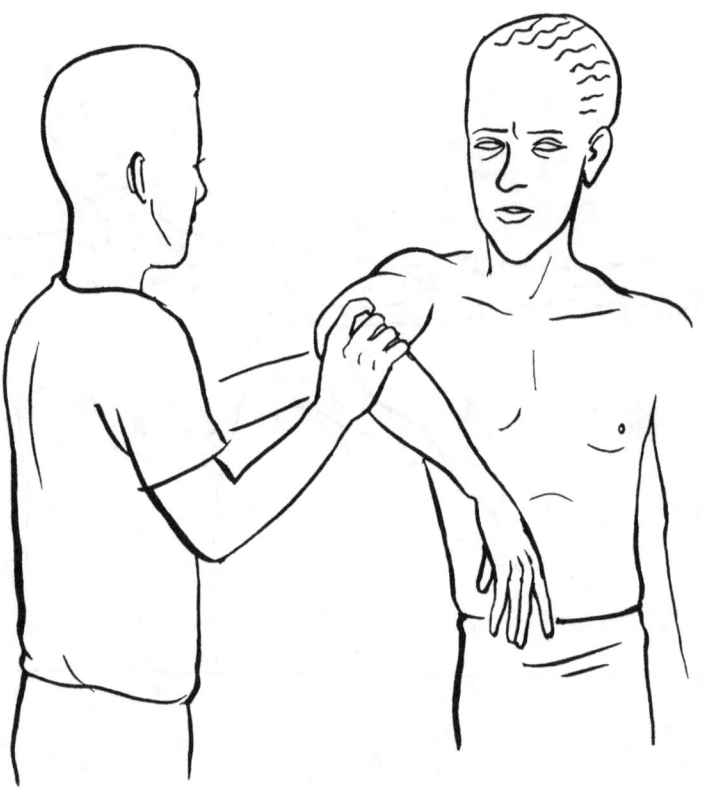

Painful Arc Test

Description

The patient sits or stands. The examiner places a finger at the inferior angle of the scapula. The patient is then instructed to actively abduct the shoulder overhead.

Interpretation

A positive test is one in which the patient hikes the shoulder and the arm falters momentarily, usually at about 90° of shoulder abduction, and then abducts smoothly, indicating impingement syndrome.

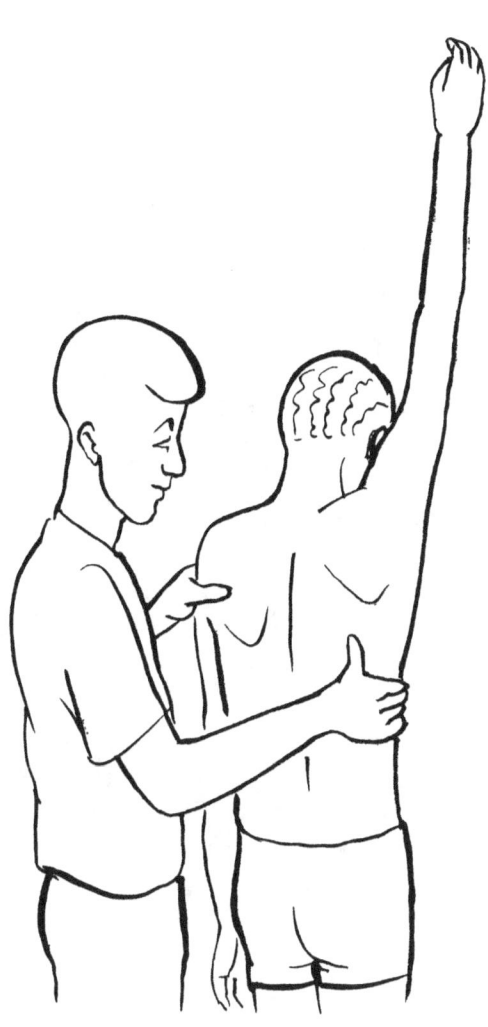

Dugas Test

Description

The patient sits. The patient is instructed to touch the opposite shoulder and then to lower the elbow onto the chest.

Interpretation

A positive test is one in which pain is increased and the patient is unable to lower the arm close to the body, indicating impingement syndrome.

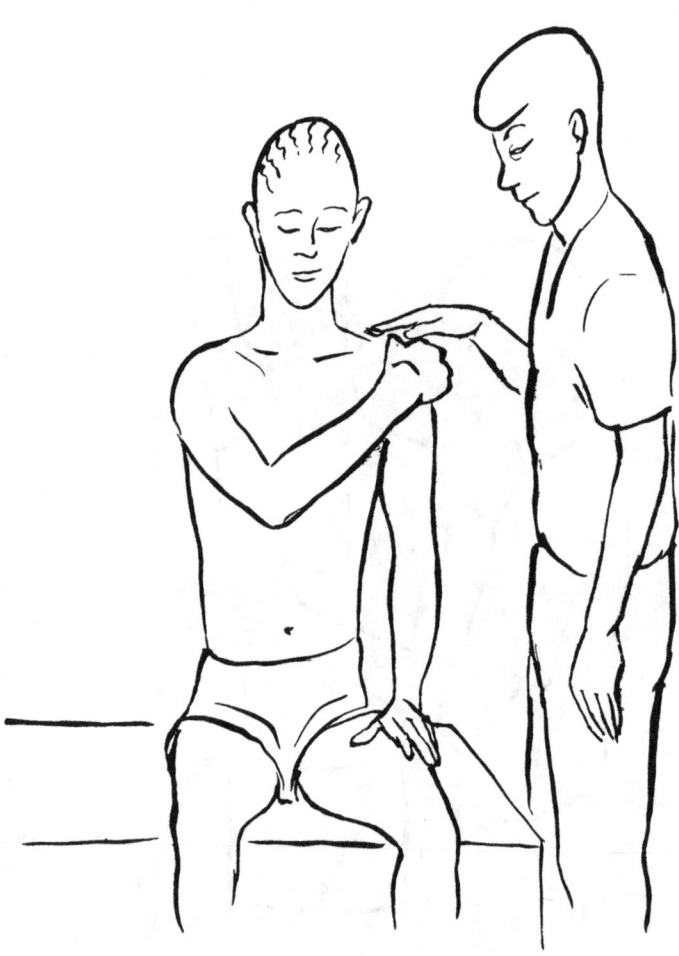

Subacromial Bursitis Test

Description

The patient sits. The examiner stands behind the patient and with the index and middle fingers of one hand applies pressure just below the acromion process.

Interpretation

A positive test is one in which a localized pain and/or tenderness is elicited, indicating a subacromial bursitis.

Comments

Perform Dawbarn Test to further confirm the subacromial bursitis.

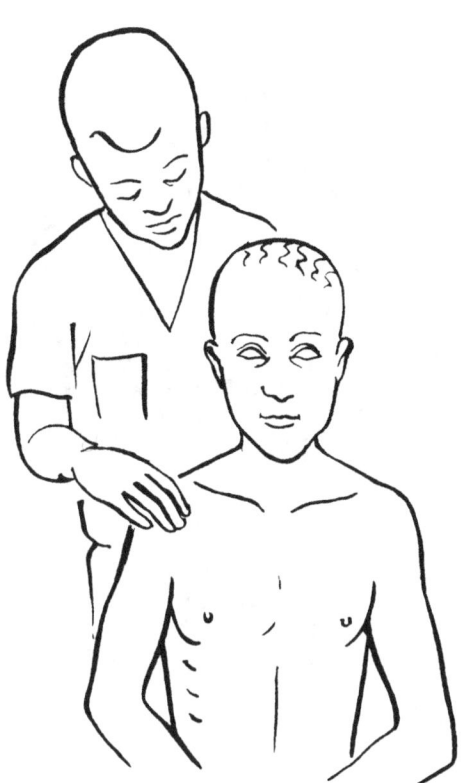

Dawbarn Test

Description

The patient sits. The examiner stands behind the patient and with the index and middle fingers of one hand applies pressure just below the acromion process. If any pain and/or tenderness is observed, the examiner holds the patient's distal forearm and passively abducts the patient's shoulder past 90° while maintaining the pressure just below the acromion process.

Interpretation

A positive test is one in which pain and/or tenderness is decreased as the shoulder reaches 90° of abduction, indicating a subacromial bursitis.

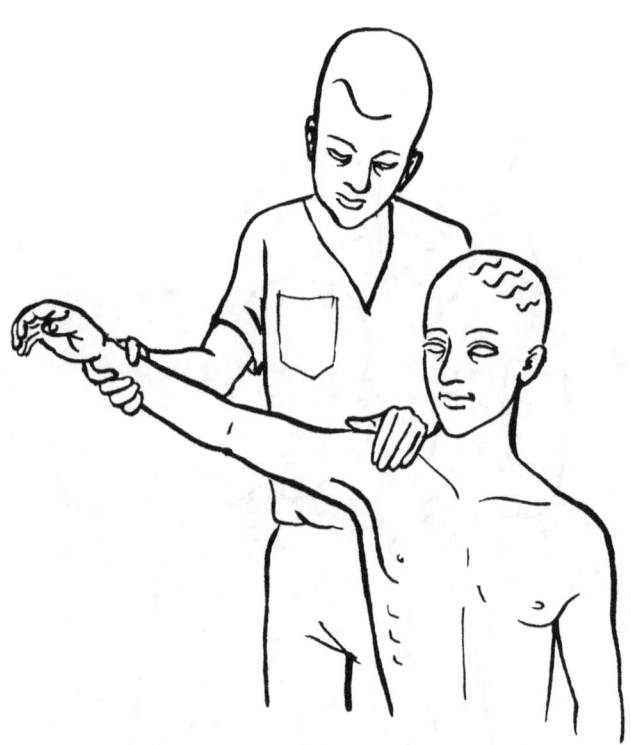

Transverse Humeral Ligament Test

Description

The patient sits. The examiner places fingers of one hand along the bicipital groove and with the other hand holds the patient's distal forearm and abducts the shoulder and externally rotates it. The examiner then internally rotates the patient's shoulder.

Interpretation

A positive test is one in which the tendon snaps in and out of the bicipital groove, indicating ruptured transverse humeral ligament.

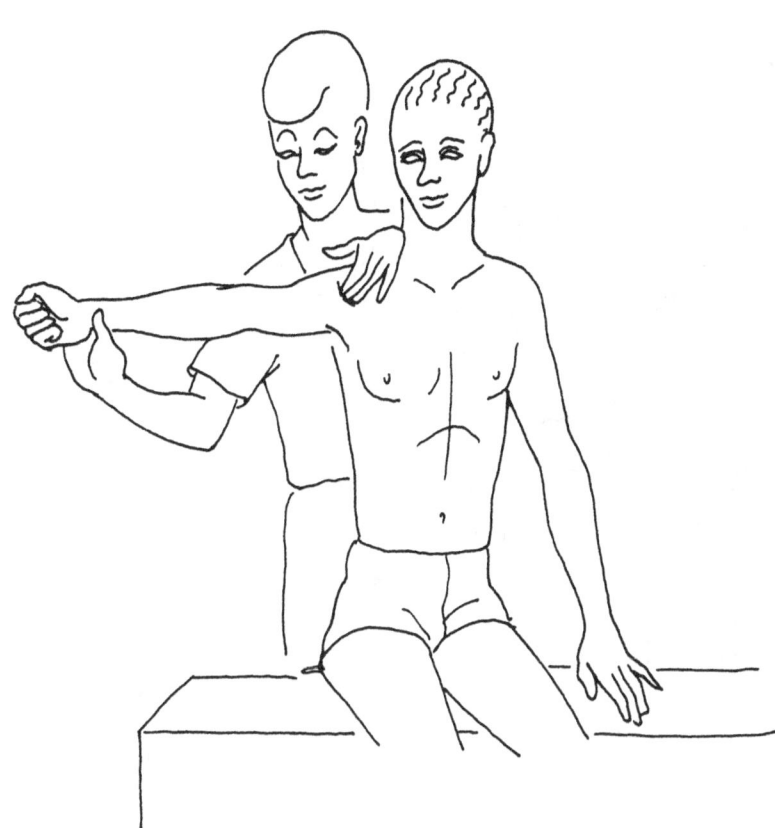

Bicipital Tendonitis Test

Description

The patient lies supine with shoulder abducted to 90° and held in neutral position. The examiner stabilizes the patient's scapula with one hand and with the other hand flexes the patient's elbow to 90°. The examiner first internally rotates the shoulder to about 15° and then externally rotates it.

Interpretation

A positive test is one in which pain is elicited in the bicipital groove, indicating inflammation of the long head of biceps.

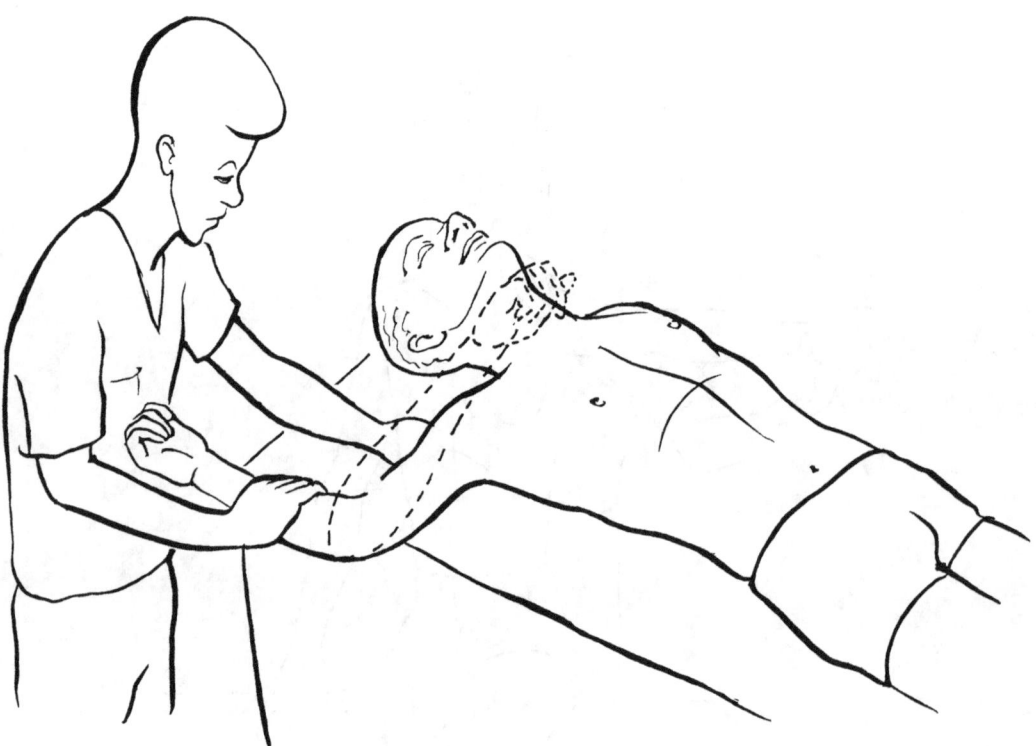

Yergason Test

Description

The patient sits or stands with elbow flexed to 90° and the forearm pronated. The examiner holds the patient's flexed elbow in one hand while holding the patient's wrist with the other hand. The examiner then supinates the forearm while the patient resists the motion.

Interpretation

A positive test is one in which pain is elicited and the biceps tendon pops out of the bicipital groove, indicating biceps tendonitis or instability of the long head of the biceps tendon.

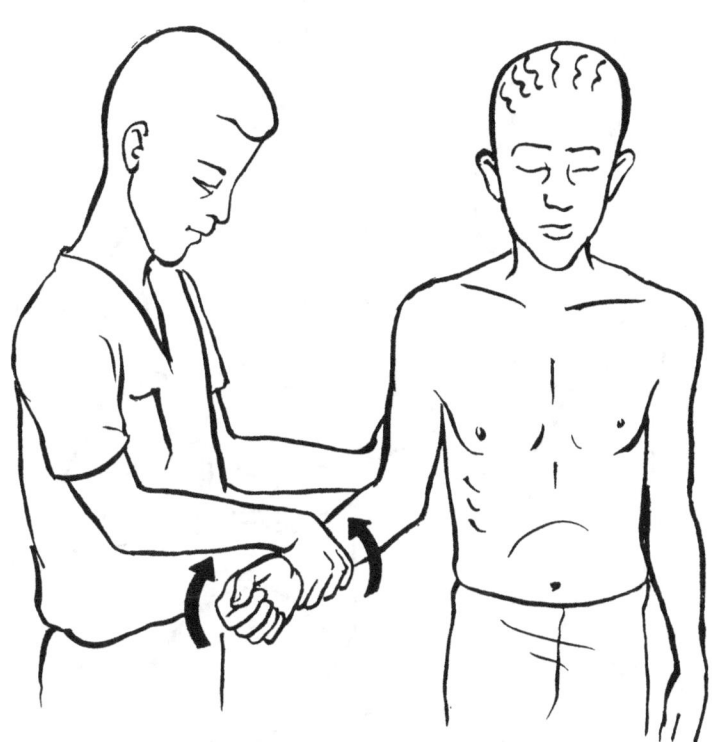

Lippman Test

Description
The patient sits or lies supine. The examiner flexes the patient's elbow to 90° and holds the forearm with one hand. With the other hand the examiner palpates the tendon of the long head of the biceps approximately 3 inches distal to the shoulder joint with the index finger and thumb. The examiner then displaces the tendon from side to side.

Interpretation
A positive test is one in which a sharp pain is produced, indicating bicipital tendonitis.

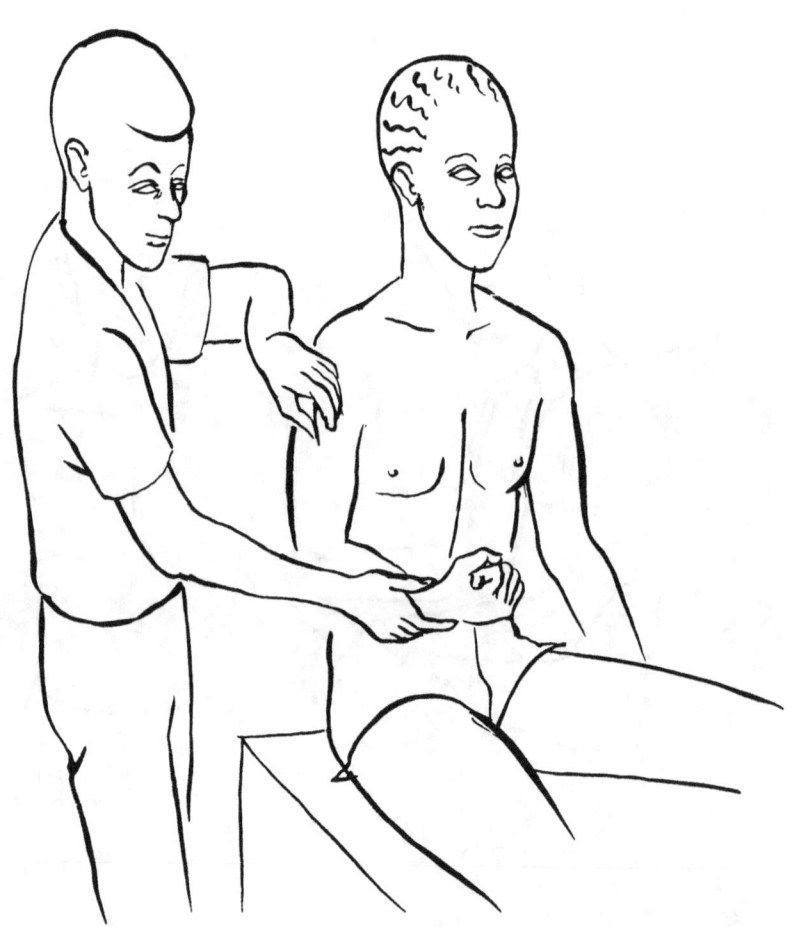

Speed Test

Description

The patient sits or stands. The examiner forward flexes the patient's shoulder to about 90° while extending the elbow and supinating the forearm. The examiner grasps the patient's distal forearm. The patient is then instructed to forward flex the arm while the examiner resists the movement.

Interpretation

A positive test is one which produces increased pain in the bicipital groove, indicating bicipital tendonitis.

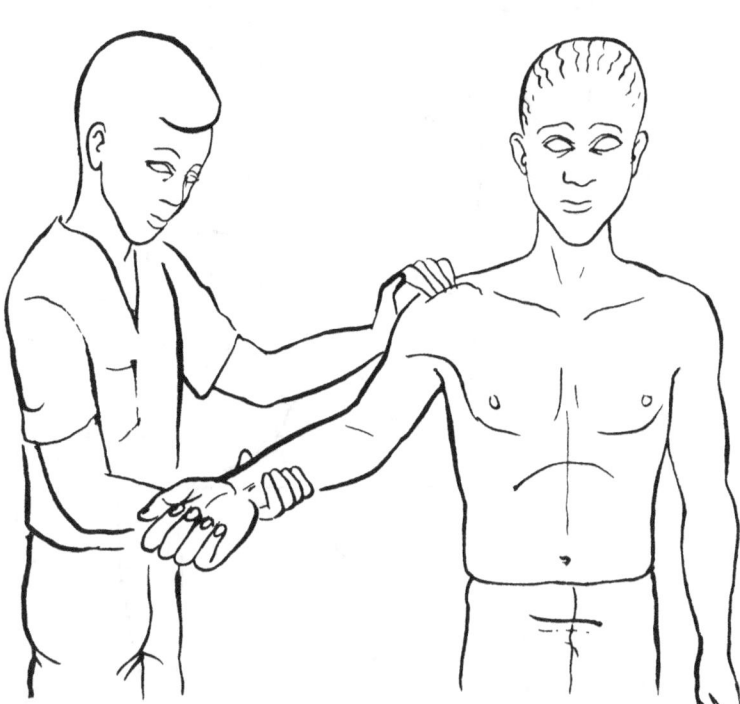

Gilcrest Test

Description

The patient sits or stands. The patient is instructed to lift a 5 lb. weight over the head and then fully externally rotate the arm. The examiner places the fingers of one hand on the long head of the biceps and instructs the patient to lower the arm to the side in the coronal plane.

Interpretation

A positive test is one in which an audible snap is heard and increased discomfort or pain is produced as the arm reaches from 110° to 90°, indicating bicipital tendonitis.

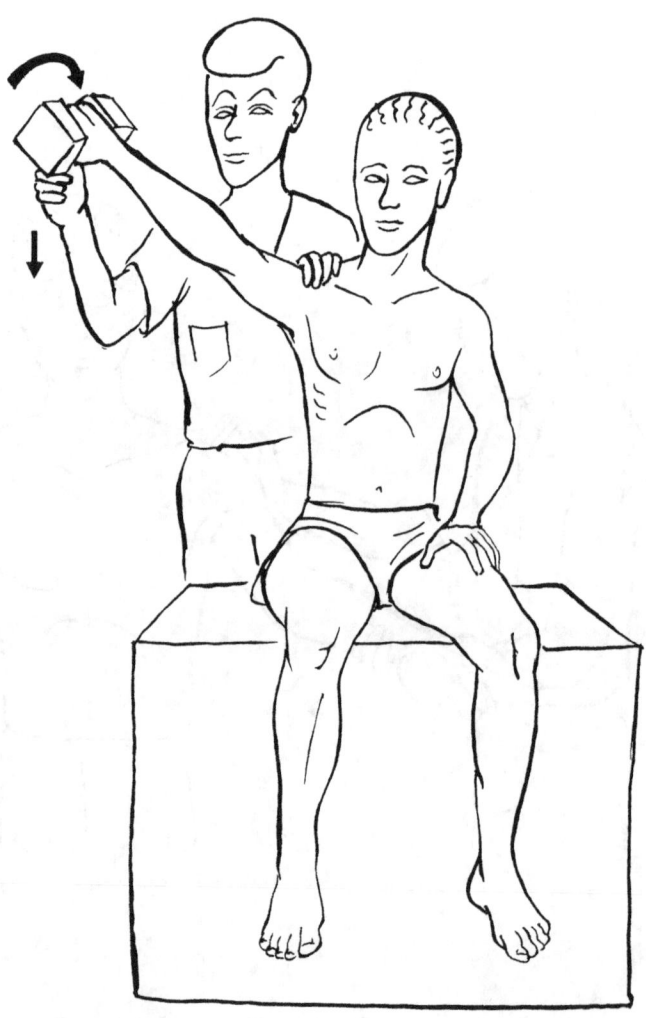

Ludington Test

Description

The patient sits or stands and clasps both hands on top of the head to support the weight of the upper extremities. The patient is then instructed to contract and relax the biceps muscles. While the patient does the contraction and relaxation of the biceps, the examiner palpates the biceps tendon.

Interpretation

A positive test is one in which the biceps tendon is not felt, indicating a rupture of the long head of the biceps tendon.

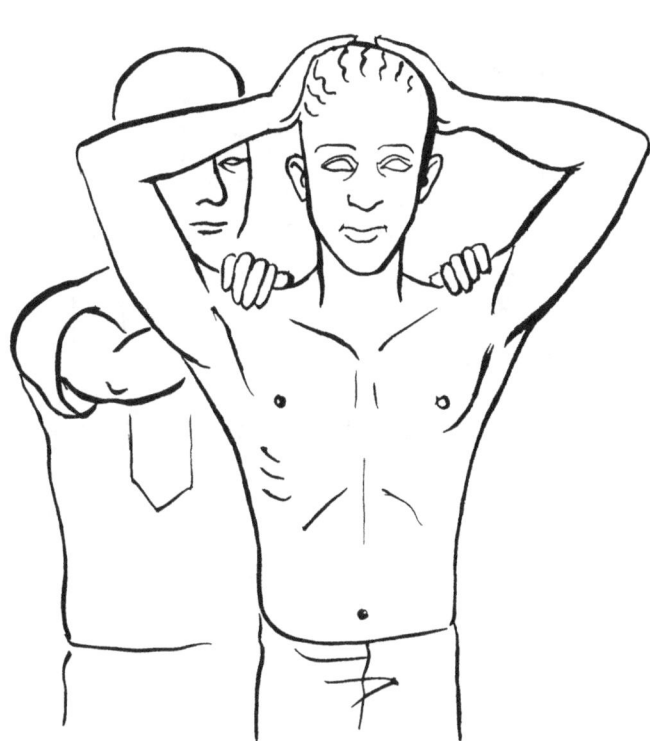

Heuter Test

Description

The patient sits or stands. The patient is instructed to abduct the shoulder to 90° and then flex the elbow to 90°.

Interpretation

A positive test is one in which a distal "bunching up" of muscles occurs, indicating rupture of the long head of the biceps muscles. A proximal "bunching up" of muscles indicates rupture of the distal biceps brachii muscle.

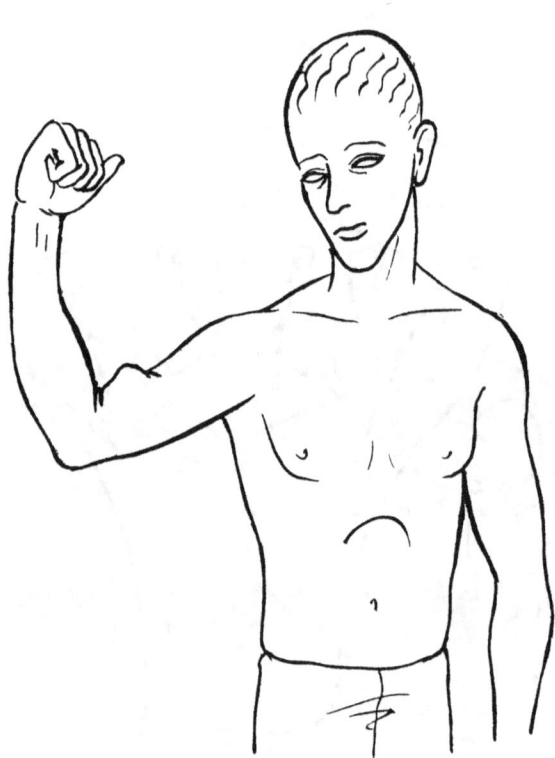

Adson Test

Description

The patient stands or sits. The examiner holds the patient's arm in slight abduction and monitors the radial pulse. The patient is then instructed to take and hold a deep breath, extend the neck, and turn the chin toward the side being tested while the examiner externally rotates and extends the patient's shoulder. The patient is then instructed to turn the head toward the opposite side.

Interpretation

A positive test is one in which the radial pulse disappears, indicating thoracic outlet syndrome.

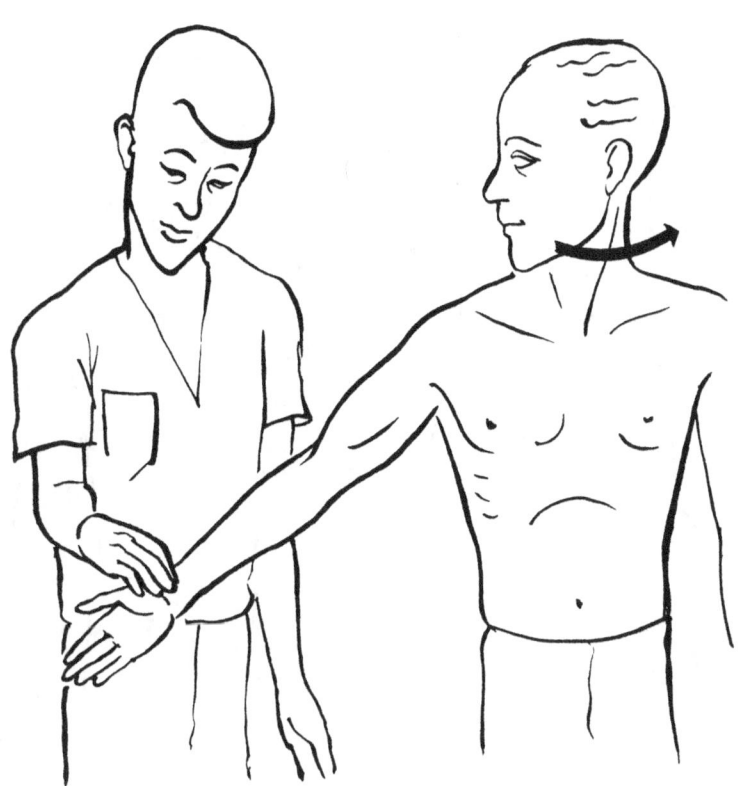

Allen Test

Description
The patient stands or sits. The examiner flexes the patient's elbow to 90° while the patient's shoulder is abducted to 90° and externally rotated. The examiner monitors the radial pulse and instructs the patient to rotate the head away from the test side.

Interpretation
A positive test is one in which the pulse disappears and other symptoms are produced indicating thoracic outlet syndrome.

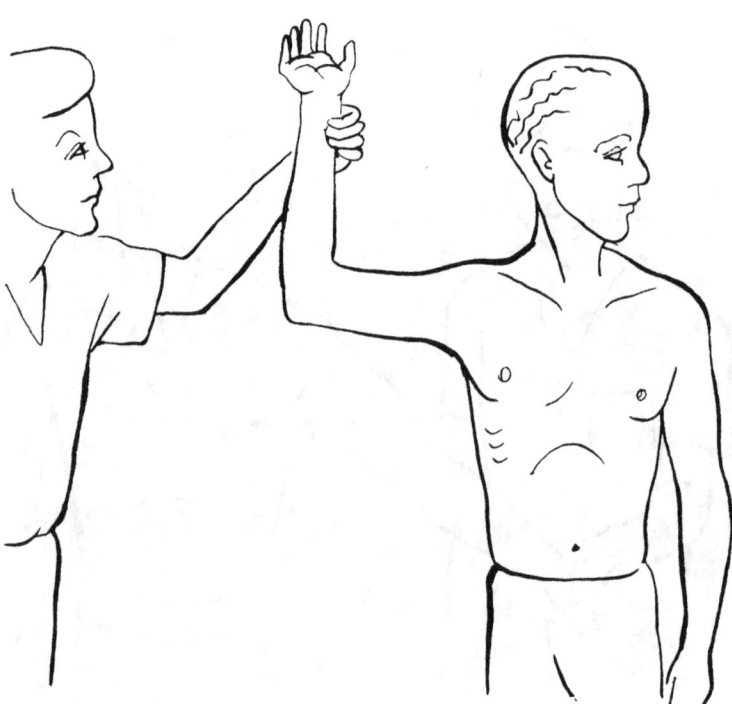

Roos Test

Description

The patient stands. The patient is instructed to abduct the arms to 90°, externally rotate the shoulders, and flex the elbows to 90°. The patient is then instructed to open and close the hands slowly for 3 minutes while maintaining this position.

Interpretation

A positive test is one in which the patient is either unable to maintain the starting position for 3 minutes or experiences pain, heaviness in the arms, or tingling/numbness in the hands, indicating thoracic outlet syndrome.

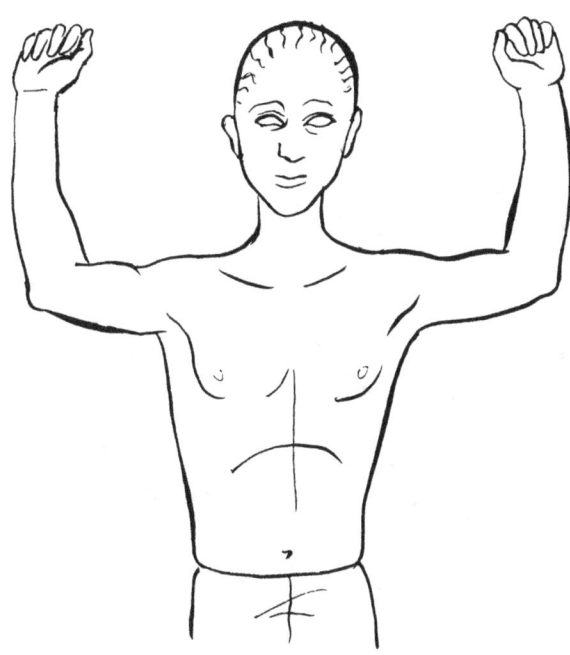

Wright Test

Description
The patient sits. The examiner holds the patient's arm at approximately 45° of shoulder abduction and monitors the radial pulse. While monitoring the radial pulse, the examiner moves the patient's arm in hyperabduction.

Interpretation
A positive test is one in which the radial pulse disappears on hyperabduction of the arm, indicating thoracic outlet syndrome.

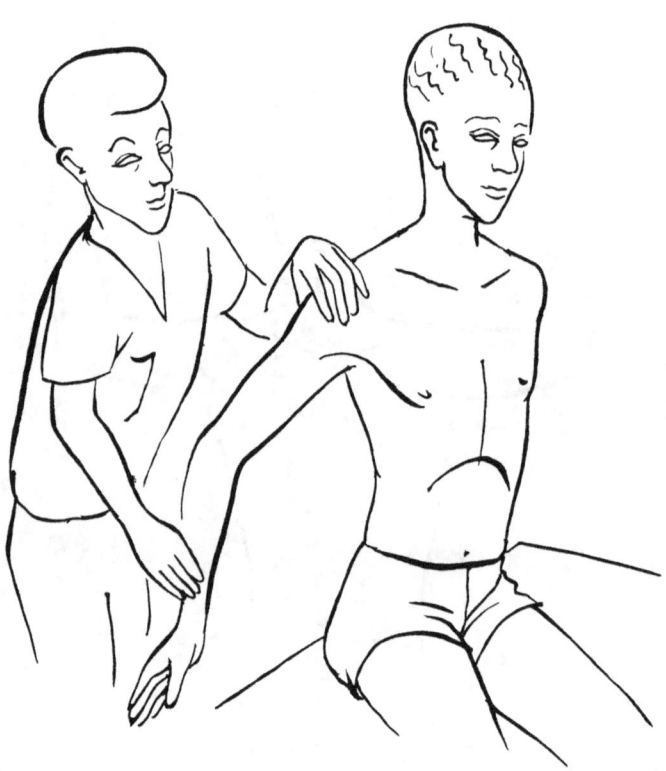

Hyperabduction Test

Description

The patient sits. The examiner holds the patient's arm in hyperabduction and external rotation, and monitors the radial pulse.

Interpretation

A positive test is one in which pain is produced in the arm and the radial pulse disappears, indicating thoracic outlet syndrome.

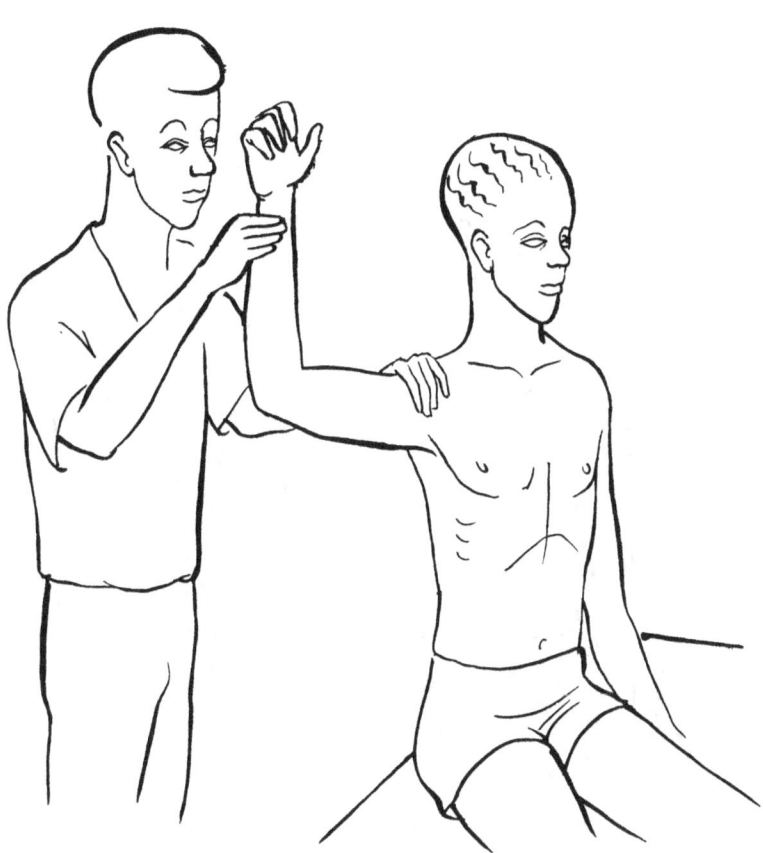

Costoclavicular Test

Description

The patient sits. The examiner moves the patient's shoulder to about 45° abduction. The patient is instructed to adduct the scapula. The examiner monitors the patient's radial pulse and extends the patient's shoulder.

Interpretation

A positive test is one in which the radial pulse decreases and other symptoms are produced indicating thoracic outlet syndrome.

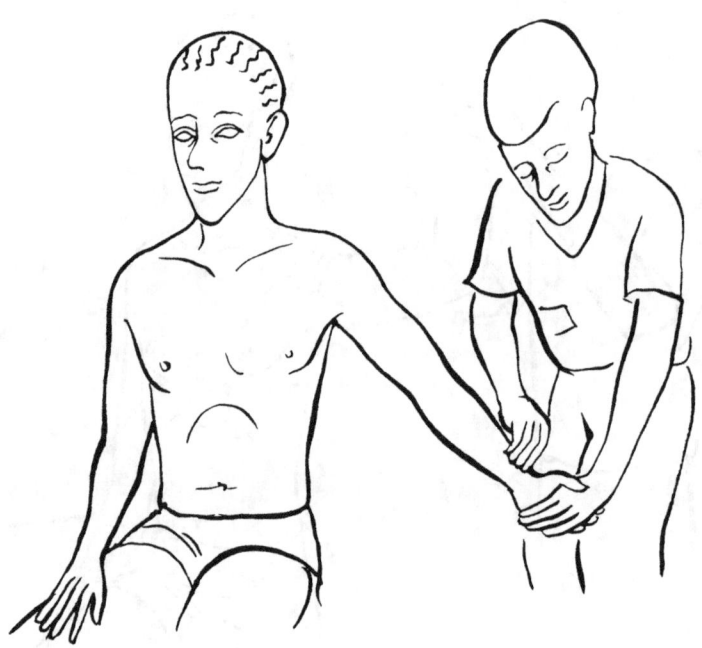

Halstead Test

Description

The patient sits or stands. The examiner monitors the patient's radial pulse and applies a downward force on the arm. The patient is then instructed to extend and rotate the head away from the test side.

Interpretation

A positive test is one in which the radial pulse disappears, indicating thoracic outlet syndrome.

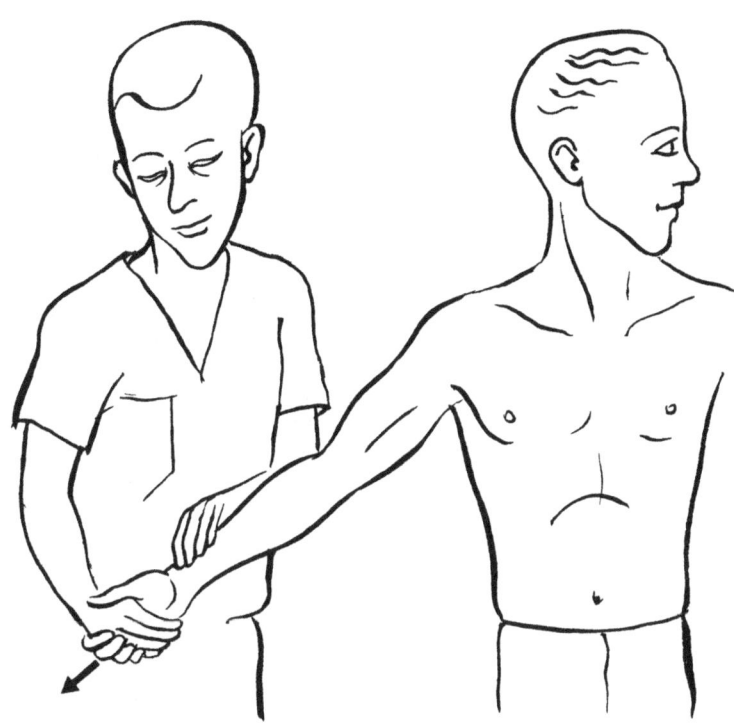

Section 2
Elbow

Section 2

Essays

Ligamentous Stability Test

Description
The patient sits. The examiner holds the patient's elbow with one hand at the posterior aspect of the elbow and holds the wrist with the other hand. The patient is then instructed to flex his/her elbow a few degrees while the examiner forces the patient's forearm laterally, producing a valgus stress on the joint's medial side. The test is then repeated to produce a varus stress on the joint's lateral side.

Interpretation
A positive test is one in which a gap is produced on the medial side during valgus stress, indicating medial collateral ligament instability. If a gap is produced on the lateral side during varus stress, it indicates lateral collateral ligament instability.

Comments
The test is performed on both sides. The involved side is compared with the uninvolved side to check for a positive test.

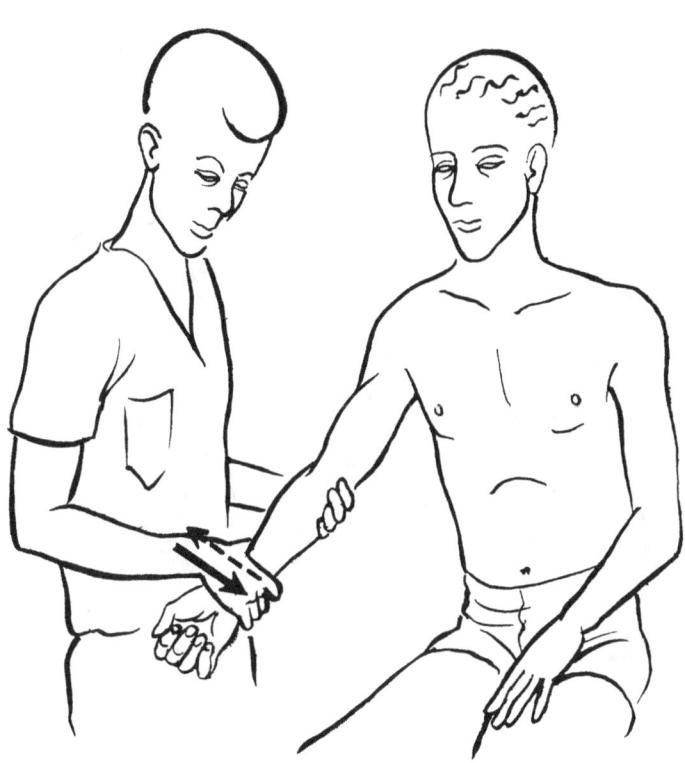

Tennis Elbow Test

Description
The patient sits or stands. The examiner flexes the patient's elbow to approximately 90° and stabilizes the patient's elbow with one hand while placing the thumb of the other hand over the lateral epicondyle. The patient is then instructed to extend the wrist while the examiner resists the movement with the other hand.

Interpretation
A positive test is one in which pain is produced in the common extensor tendon at the lateral epicondyle, indicating lateral epicondylitis (tennis elbow).

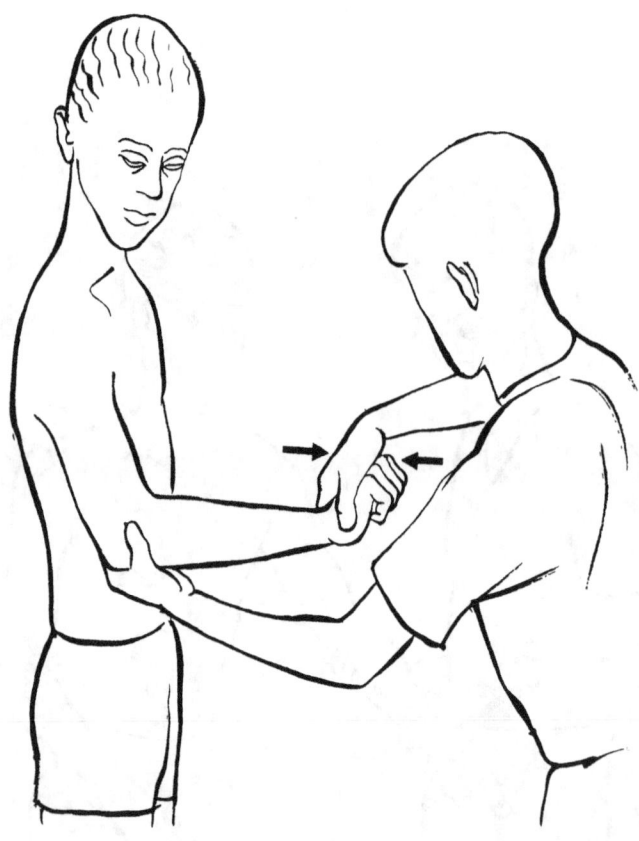

Cozen Test

Description

The patient sits. The examiner flexes the patient's elbow to approximately 90° and stabilizes the patient's elbow with one hand while placing the thumb of the other hand over the lateral epicondyle. The patient is then instructed to make a fist, pronate the forearm, and radially deviate and extend the wrist while the examiner resists the movement.

Interpretation

A positive test is one in which a sudden severe pain is produced in the lateral epicondyle area, indicating lateral epicondylitis (tennis elbow).

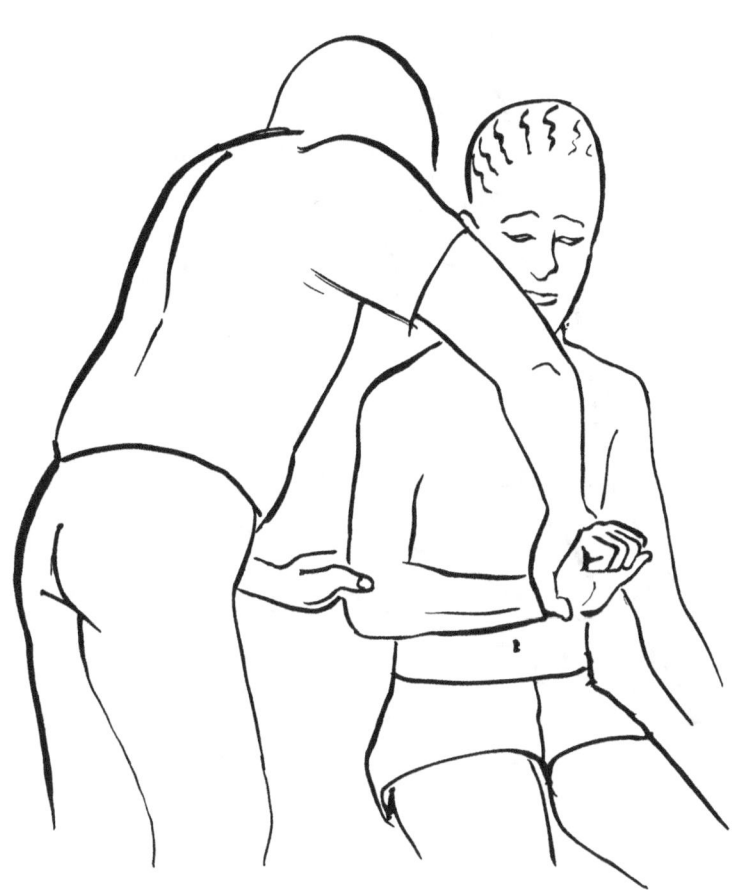

Golfer Elbow Test

Description
The patient sits with elbow held in extension. The examiner holds the patient's arm proximal to the elbow with one hand. The patient is then instructed to flex the wrist while the examiner resists the movement with the other hand.

Interpretation
A positive test is one in which pain is produced in the common flexor tendon at the medial epicondyle, indicating medial epicondylitis (golfer's elbow).

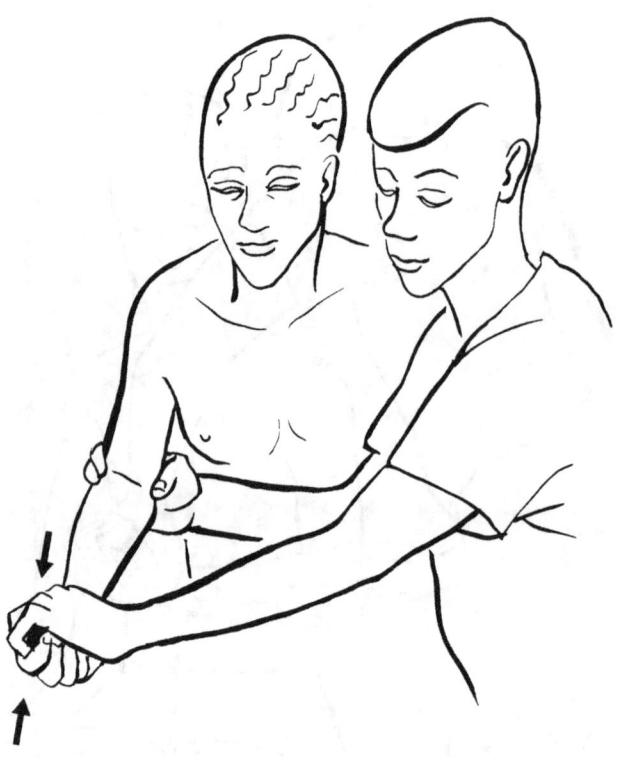

Elbow Flexion Test

Description

The patient sits. The examiner instructs the patient to fully flex the elbow and slightly flex the wrist and to hold this position for 5 minutes.

Interpretation

A positive test is one in which tingling or paresthesia is produced in the last two and a half fingers (ulnar nerve distribution), indicating cubital tunnel syndrome.

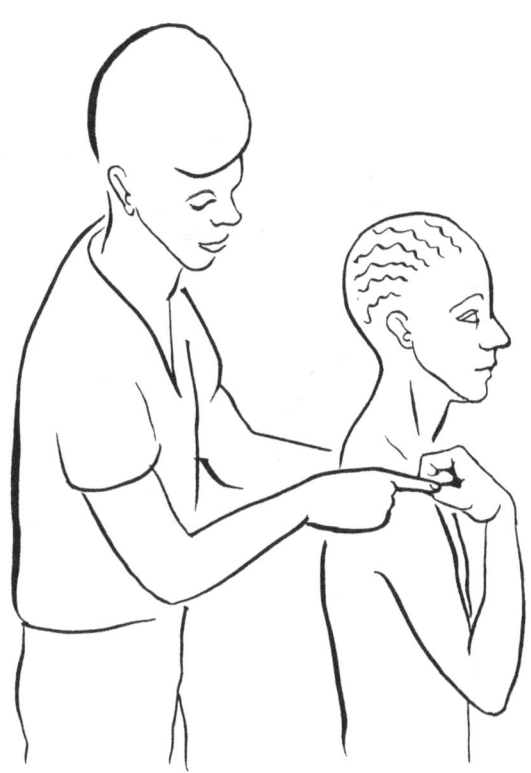

Pinch Grip Test

Description
The patient sits or stands. The patient is instructed to pinch the tips of the index finger and thumb together.

Interpretation
A positive test is one in which the patient has an abnormal pulp-to-pulp pinch of the index finger and thumb instead of tip-to-tip pinch, indicating a pathology of the anterior interosseous nerve, a branch of the median nerve.

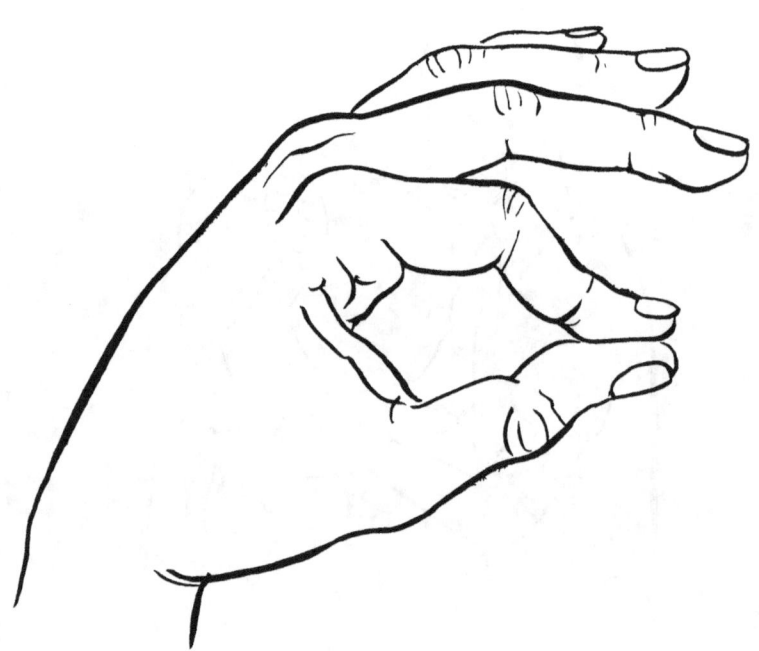

Tinel Test

Description

The patient sits. The examiner holds the patient's arm proximal to the wrist with one hand and with the other hand gently taps the groove between the olecranon process and the medial epicondyle with a reflex hammer.

Interpretation

A positive test is one in which the patient experiences tingling or paresthesia in the last two and a half fingers (ulnar nerve distribution), indicating compression of the ulnar nerve.

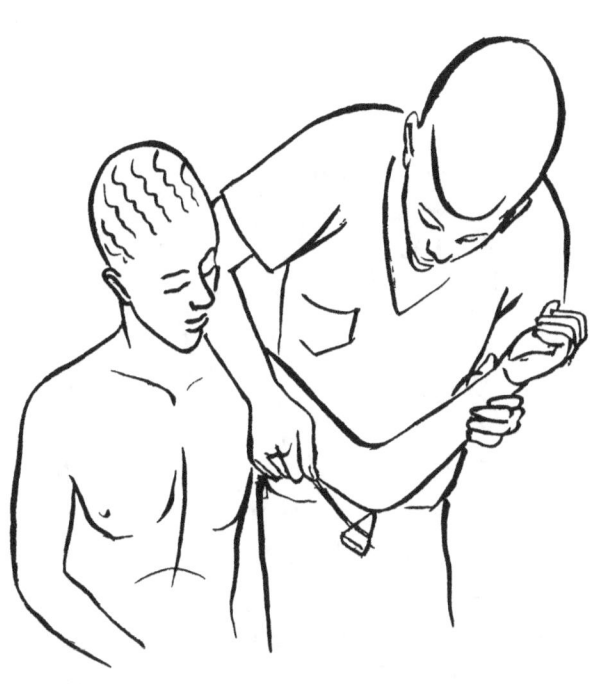

Pronator Teres Syndrome Test

Description
The patient sits. The examiner flexes the patient's elbow to 90° and supinates the forearm. The examiner stabilizes the forearm proximally. The patient is then instructed to pronate the forearm and extend the elbow while the examiner resists the pronation with the other hand.

Interpretation
A positive test is one in which the patient experiences tingling or paresthesia in the median nerve distribution in the forearm and hand, indicating pronator teres syndrome.

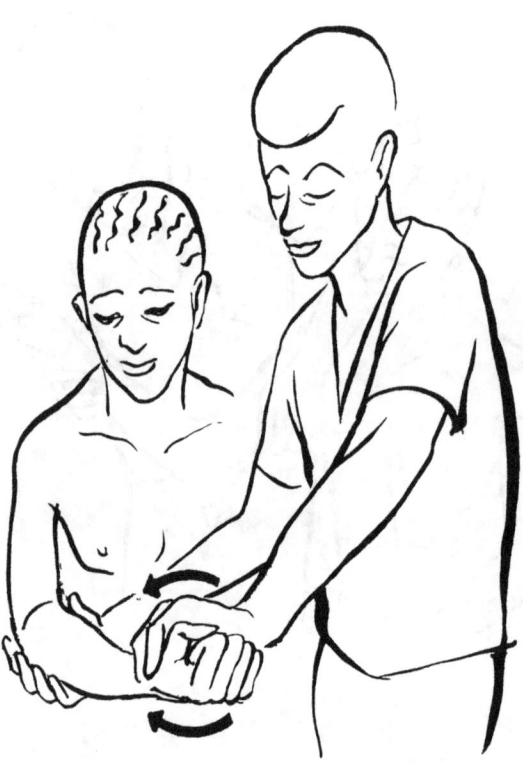

Section 3
Wrist and Hand

Allen Test

Description

The patient sits. The examiner supports the patient's hand with one hand and instructs the patient to open and close the fist quickly several times and then to squeeze the fist tightly. Now the examiner places the thumb of the other hand over the radial artery, and the index and middle fingers over the ulnar artery and presses them over the underlying bones to occlude them. The patient is now instructed to open the hand. The examiner releases one of the arteries at the wrist while maintaining the pressure over the other artery.

Interpretation

A positive test is one in which the blood does not flush immediately or flushes very slowly, indicating a complete or partial occlusion of the tested artery.

Comments

Repeat the test releasing the other artery. Also test the opposite hand for comparison.

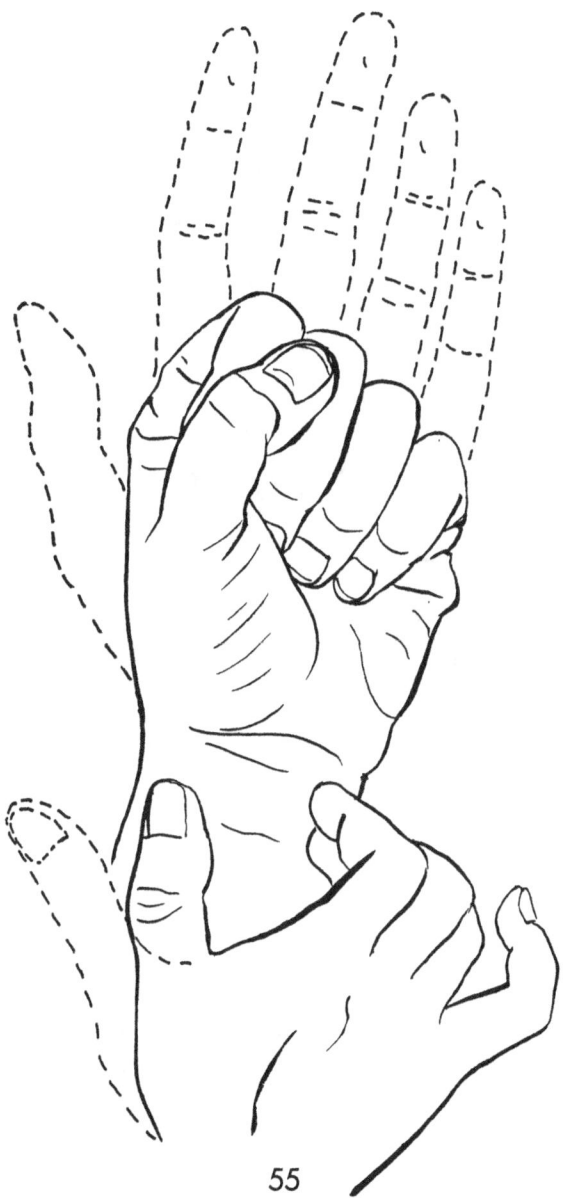

Froment Test

Description

The patient sits. The patient is instructed to secure a piece of paper placed between the thumb and the radial side of the index finger. The examiner then pulls on the paper.

Interpretation

A positive test is one in which the patient flexes the interphalangeal joint of the thumb due to paralysis of the adductor pollicis muscle and fails to hold the paper, indicating ulnar nerve lesion.

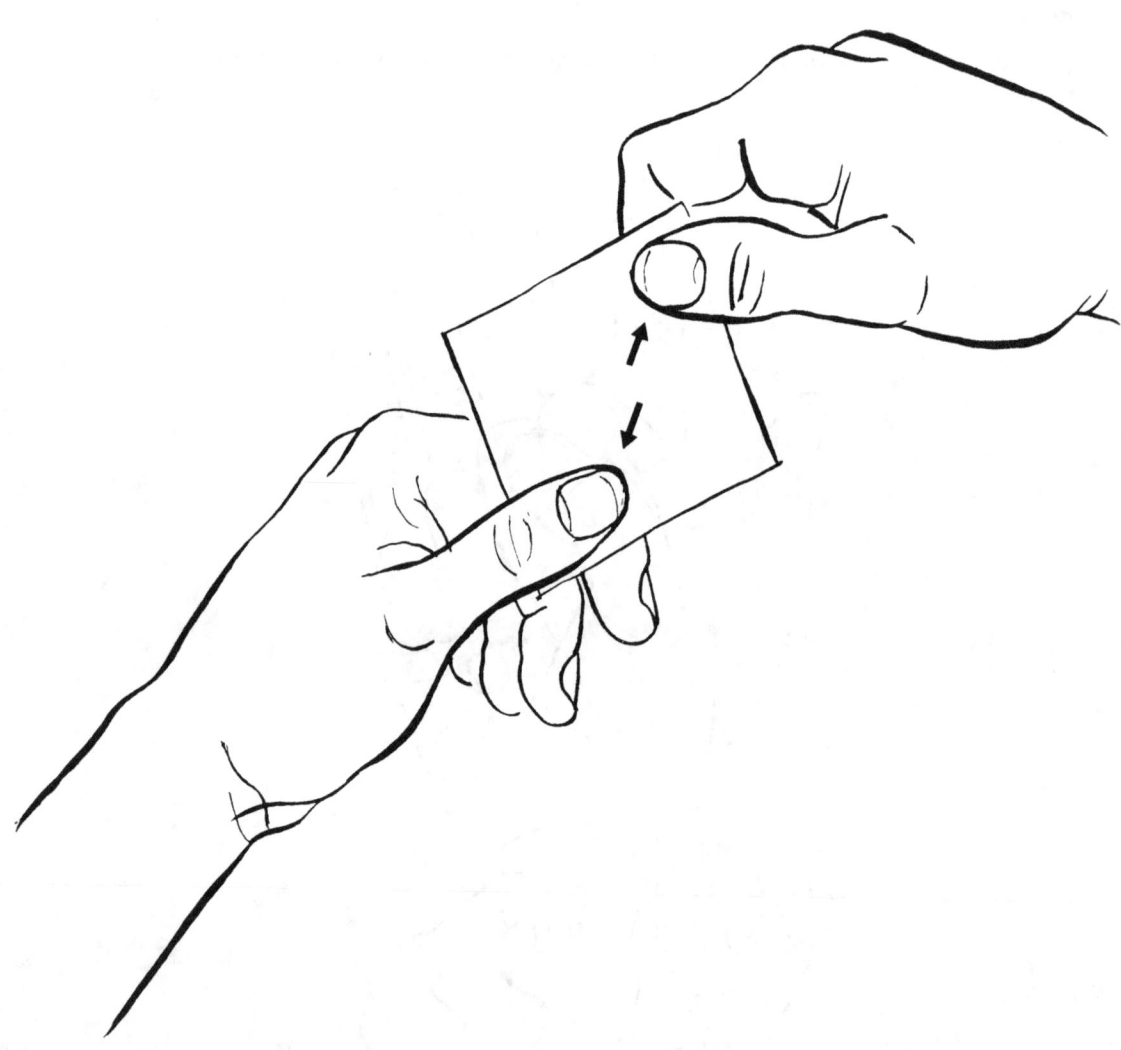

Egawa Test

Description
The patient sits. The patient is instructed to slightly flex the third digit and then alternatively deviate the finger radially and ulnarly.

Interpretation
A positive test is one in which the patient is unable to perform this movement, indicating ulnar nerve paralysis.

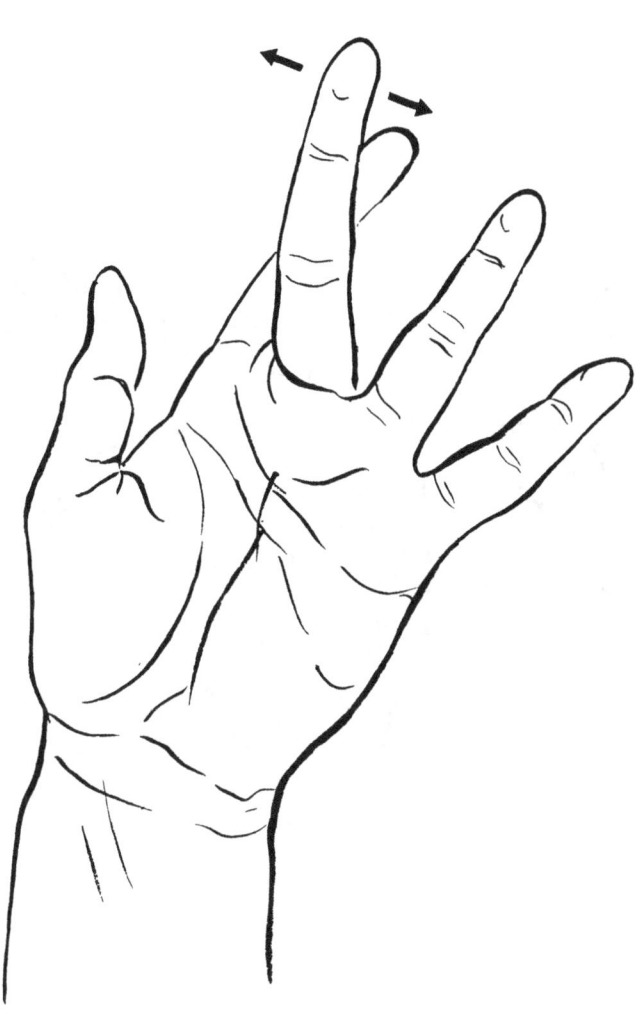

Phalen Test

Description

The patient sits. The examiner holds both the patient's forearms distally. The patient is then instructed to flex both the wrists as much as possible, and to maintain the flexed position for at least a minute.

Interpretation

A positive test is one which produces pain and/or tingling in the first three and a half fingers (median nerve distribution), indicating carpal tunnel syndrome.

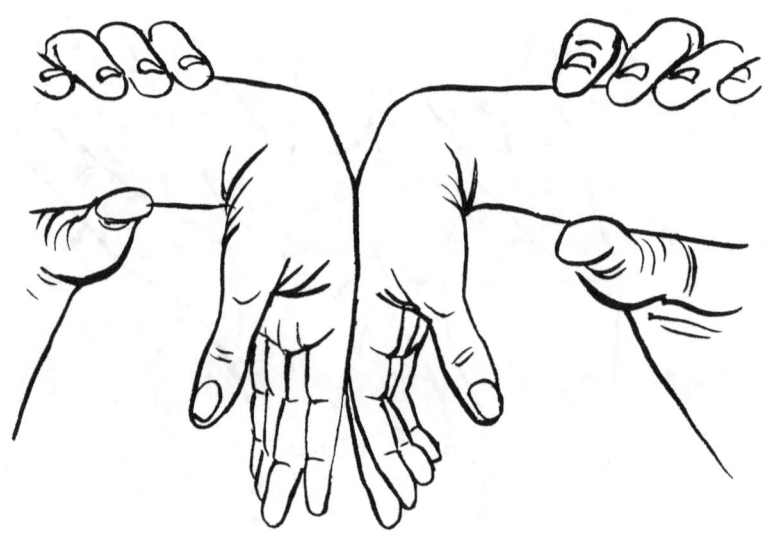

Tinel Test

Description

The patient sits. The examiner stabilizes the patient's forearm with one hand with the patient's wrist held in neutral position. The examiner then taps over the volar carpal ligament with the index finger of the other hand.

Interpretation

A positive test is one which produces pain and/or tingling in the first three and a half fingers (median nerve distribution), indicating carpal tunnel syndrome.

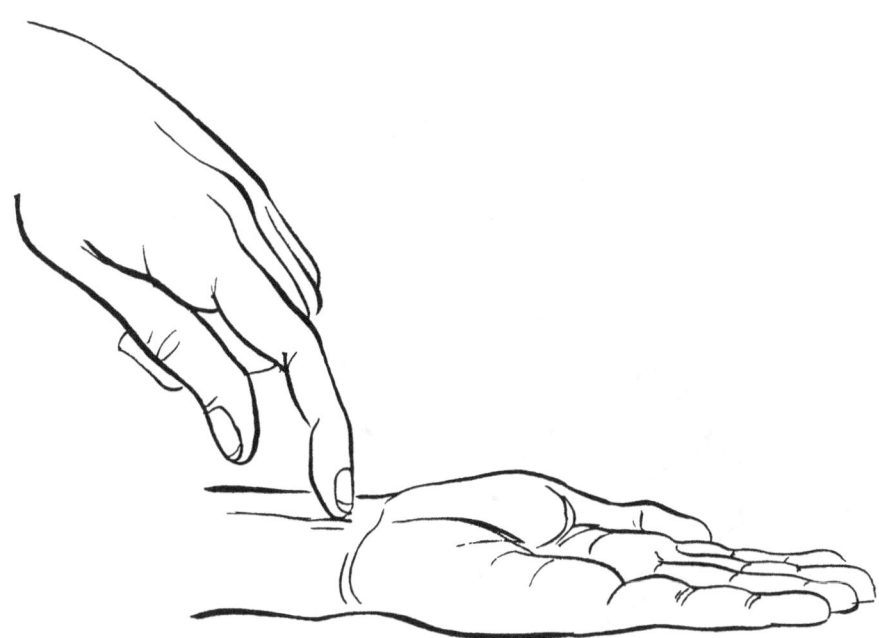

Watson Test

Description
The patient sits. The examiner stabilizes the patient's distal radius and ulna with one hand. The examiner grasps the patient's scaphoid with the thumb and index finger of the other hand and moves it anteriorly and posteriorly. The test is then repeated on the uninvolved side.

Interpretation
A positive test is one in which the scaphoid moves excessively compared to the uninvolved side, indicating instability or subluxation of the scaphoid.

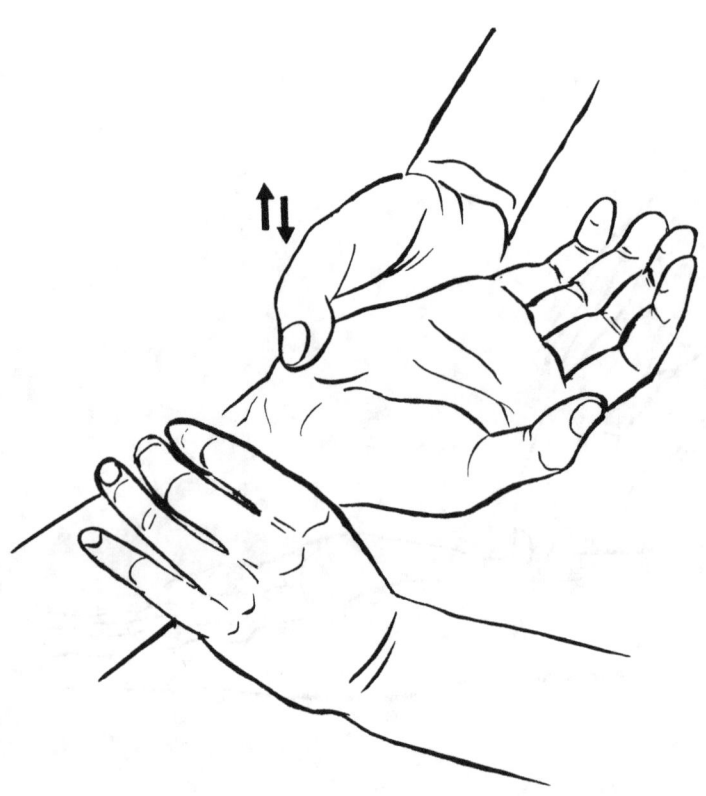

Lunatotriquetral Ballottement Test

Description

The patient sits. The examiner grasps the patient's triquetrum between the thumb and index finger of one hand and the lunate similarly with the other hand. The examiner then attempts to displace the triquetrum anteriorly and posteriorly on lunate.

Interpretation

A positive test is one which produces laxity, crepitus, and pain, indicating a partial or complete tear of the lunatotriquetral interosseous membrane.

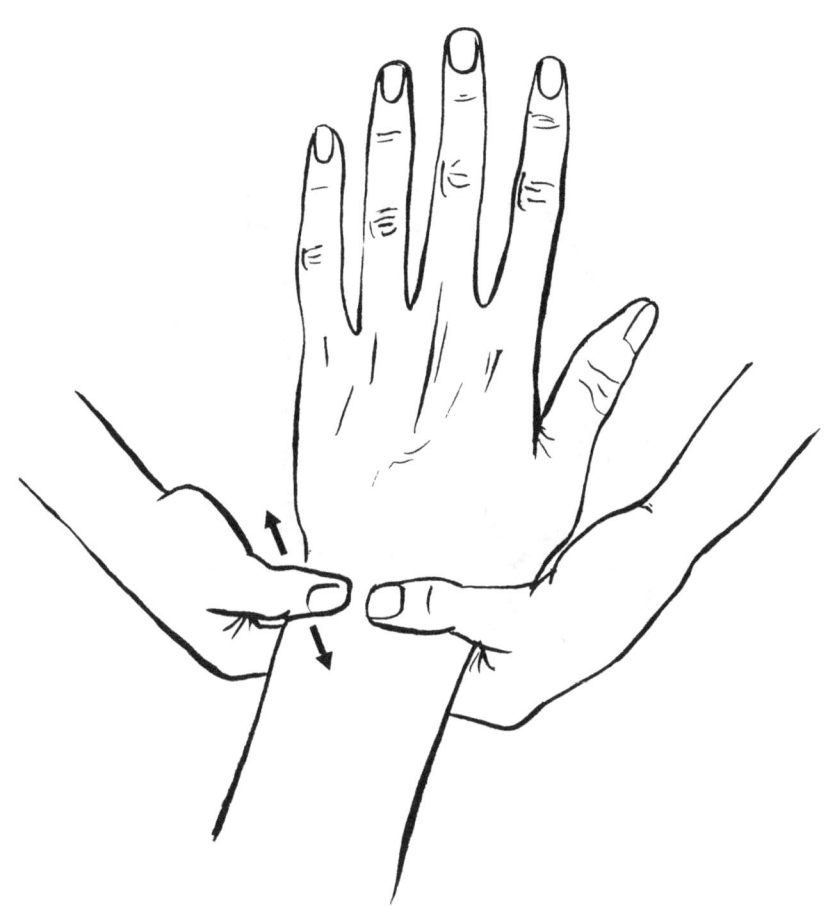

Murphy Test

Description
The patient sits. The patient is then instructed to make a fist.

Interpretation
A positive test is one in which the head of the third metacarpal is level with the second and fourth metacarpals, indicating lunate dislocation.

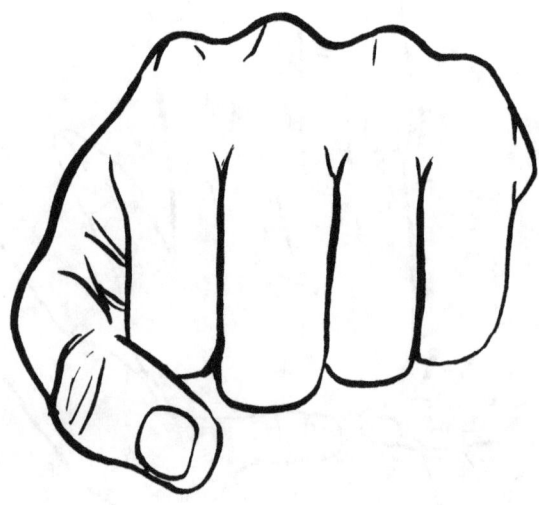

Grind Test

Description

The patient sits. The examiner stabilizes the patient's hand with one hand. The examiner grasps the patient's thumb distal to the metacarpophalangeal joint with the other hand and then applies axial compression and rotation to the metacarpophalangeal joint.

Interpretation

A positive test is one which produces pain, indicating degenerative joint disease in the metacarpophalangeal or metacarpotrapezial joint.

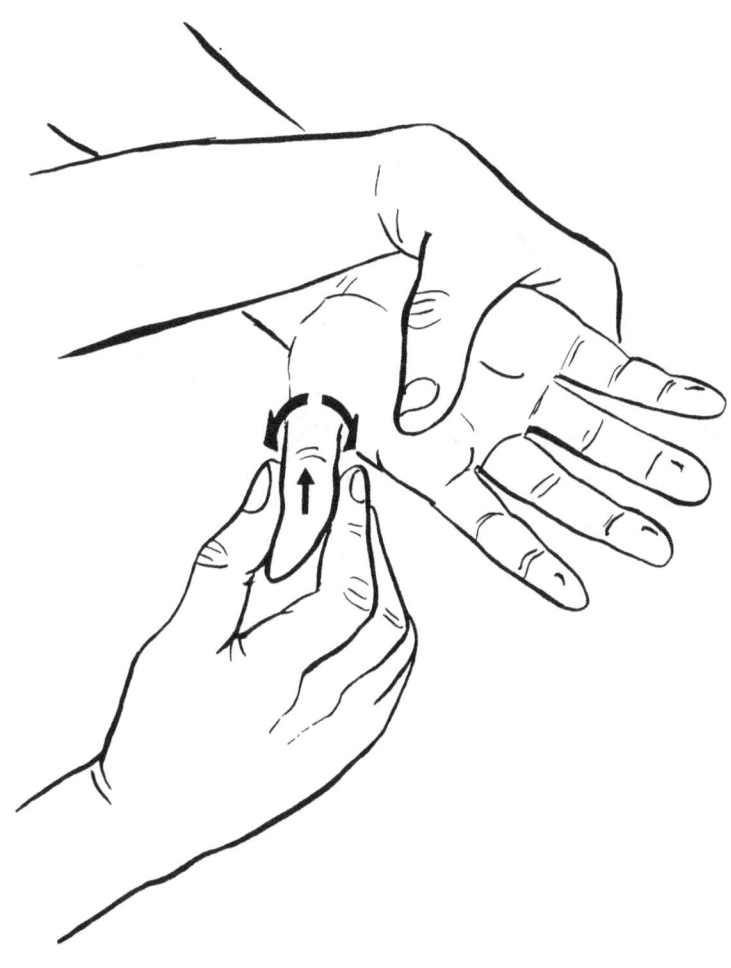

Finkelstein Test

Description

The patient sits. The examiner stabilizes the patient's forearm. The patient is then instructed to clench the thumb under the grasping fingers. The examiner then moves the patient's wrist in ulnar deviation.

Interpretation

A positive test is one in which a sharp pain is produced at the radial styloid, indicating deQuervain's disease (tenosynovitis of the first dorsal compartment).

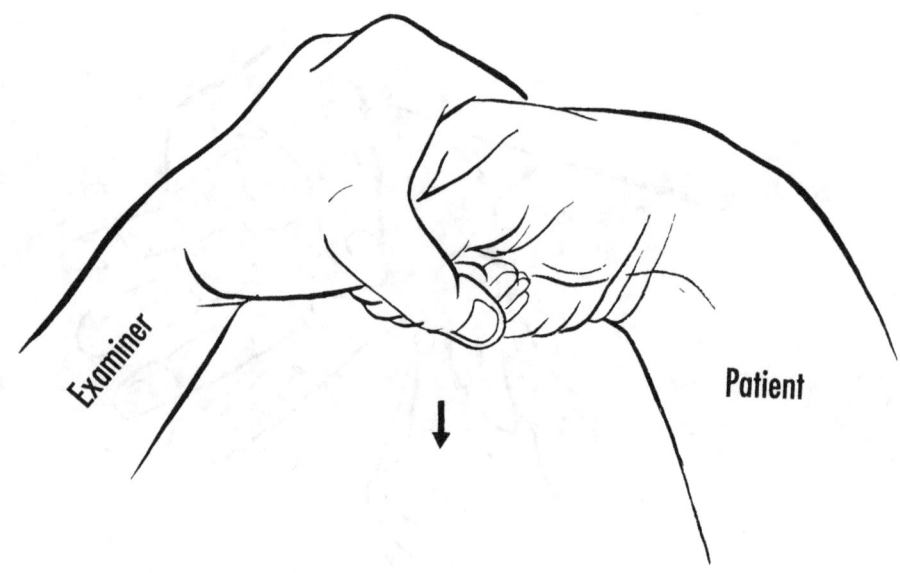

Retinacular/Capsular Test

Description

The patient sits. The examiner stabilizes the patient's proximal interphalangeal joint in neutral position and then moves the distal interphalangeal joint into flexion.

Interpretation

A positive test is one in which the distal interphalangeal joint does not flex, indicating either joint capsule contracture or retinacular tightness.

Comments

Perform Capsular Test to differentiate between the two structures.

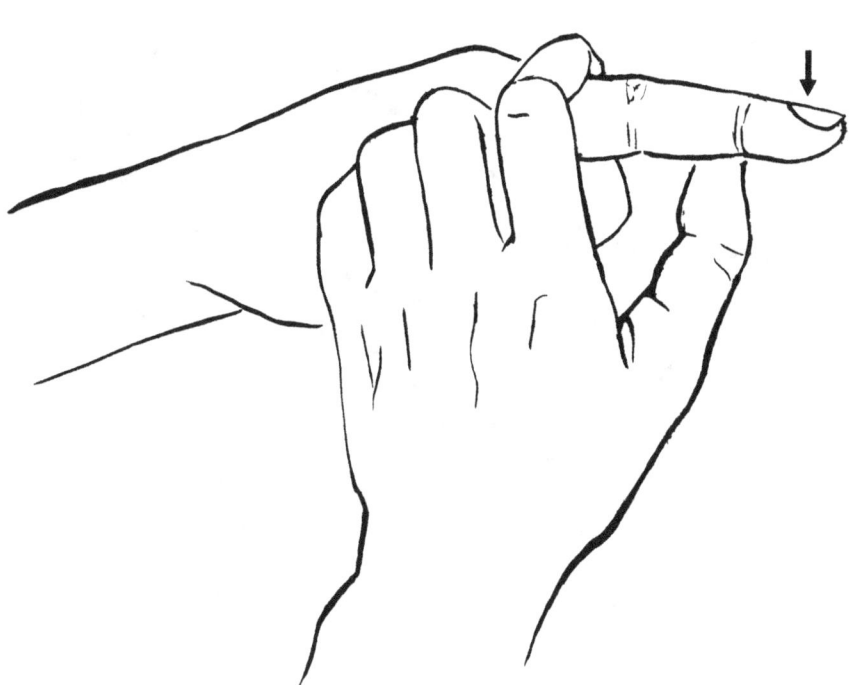

Capsular Test

Description
The patient sits. With one hand the examiner stabilizes the patient's metacarpophalangeal joint in neutral position and slightly flexes the proximal interphalangeal joint to relax the retinaculum. With the other hand the examiner then moves distal interphalangeal joint into flexion.

Interpretation
A positive test is one in which the distal interphalangeal joint does not flex, indicating joint capsule contracture.

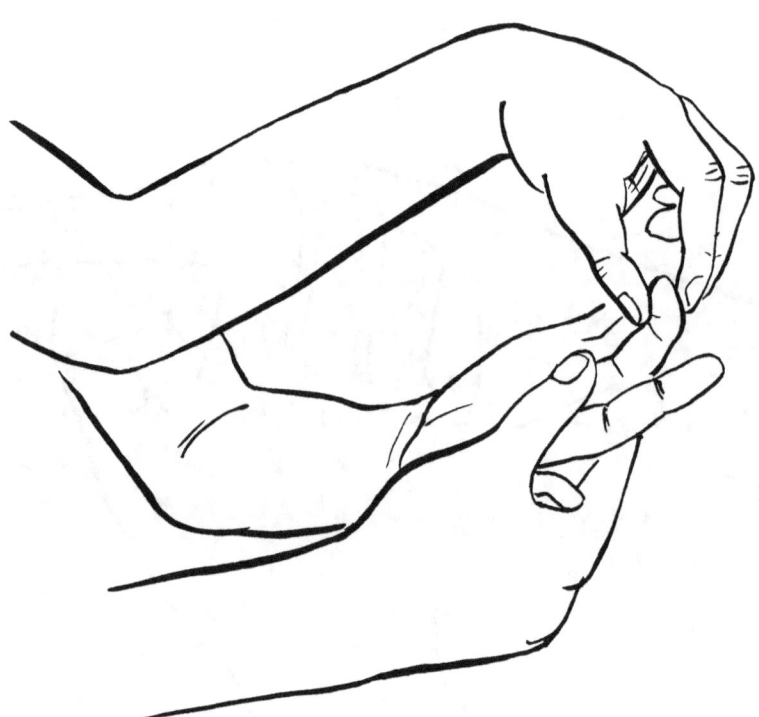

Flexor Digitorum Superficialis Test

Description
The patient sits. The examiner holds the patient's fingers in extension. The patient is then instructed to flex the involved finger at the proximal interphalangeal joint.

Interpretation
A positive test is one in which the finger cannot be flexed at the proximal interphalangeal joint, indicating either a cut or absent flexor digitorum superficialis tendon.

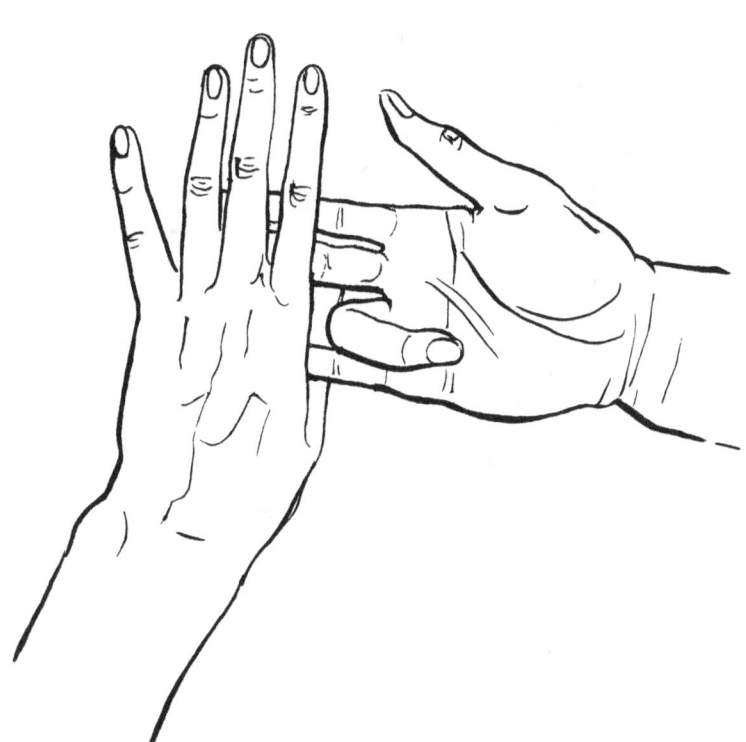

Flexor Digitorum Profundus Test

Description
The patient sits. The examiner holds the patient's finger in extension at the proximal interphalangeal joint. The patient is then instructed to flex the finger at the distal interphalangeal joint.

Interpretation
A positive test is one in which the finger cannot be flexed at the distal interphalangeal joint, indicating either a cut or absent flexor digitorum profundus tendon.

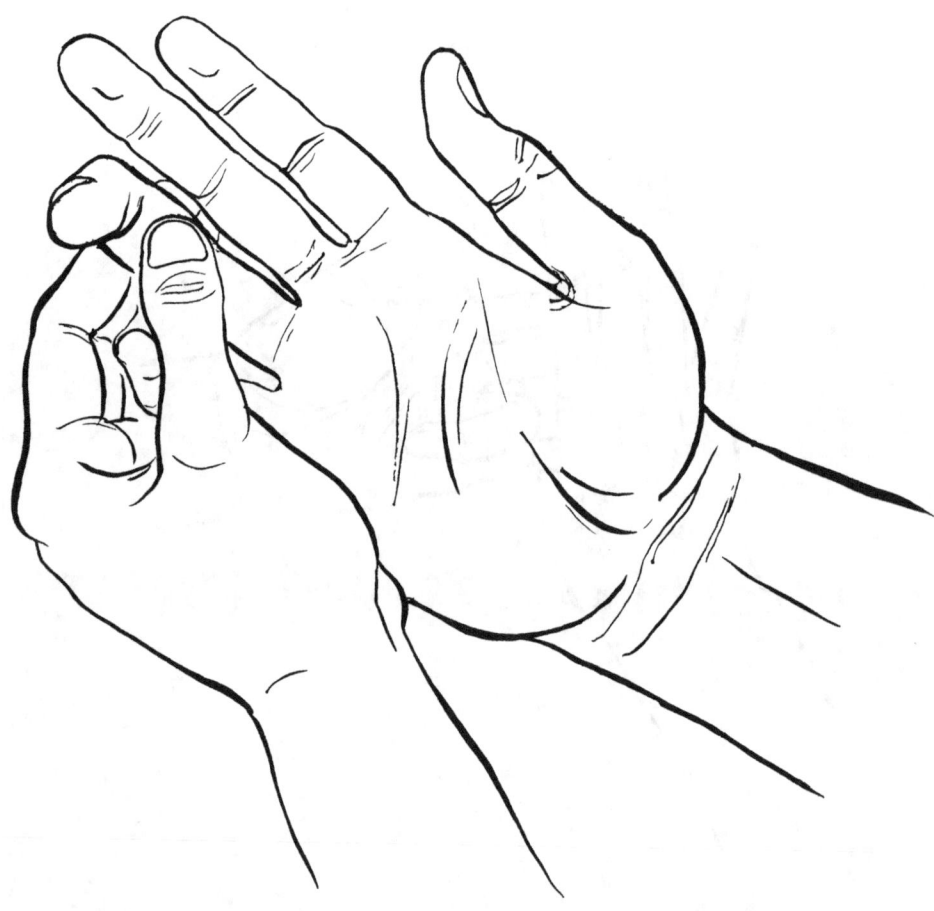

Bunnel-Littler Test

Description

The patient sits. The examiner holds the patient's hand with the metacarpophalangeal joint in slight extension position with one hand. With the other hand the examiner then moves the proximal interphalangeal joint into flexion.

Interpretation

A positive test is one in which the proximal interphalangeal joint cannot be flexed, indicating either a tightness of the intrinsics or joint capsule contracture.

Comments

To differentiate between the two structures, perform the Intrinsic Tightness Test.

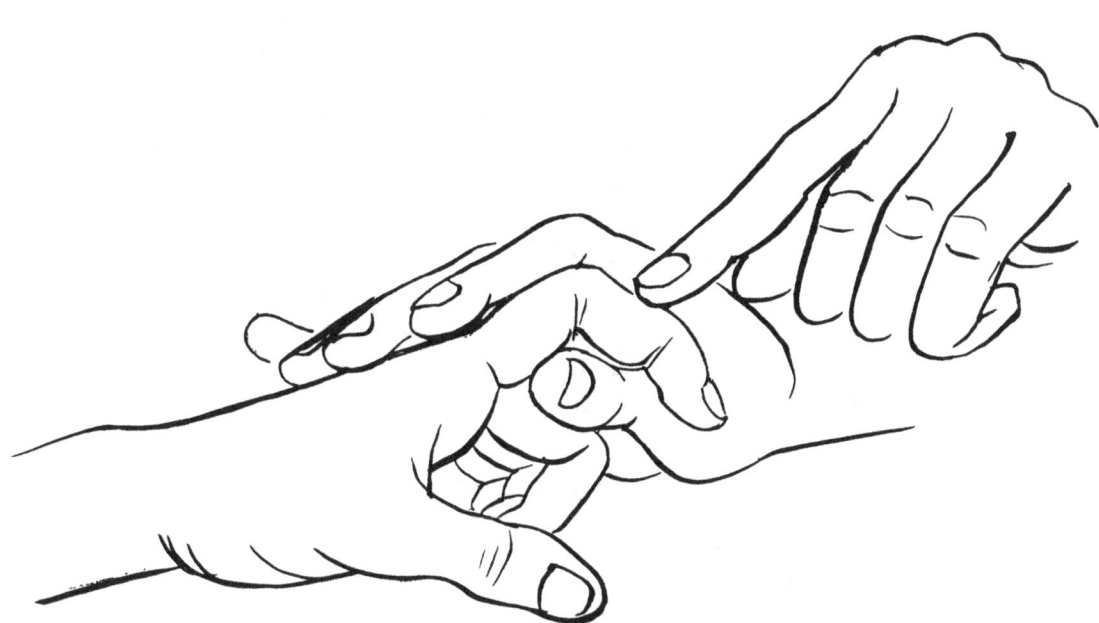

Intrinsic Tightness Test

Description

The patient sits. The examiner holds the patient's hand with the metacarpophalangeal joint in slightly flexed position with one hand. With the other hand the examiner then moves the proximal interphalangeal joint into flexion.

Interpretation

A positive test is one in which the proximal interphalangeal joint can be fully flexed, indicating tightness of the intrinsics.

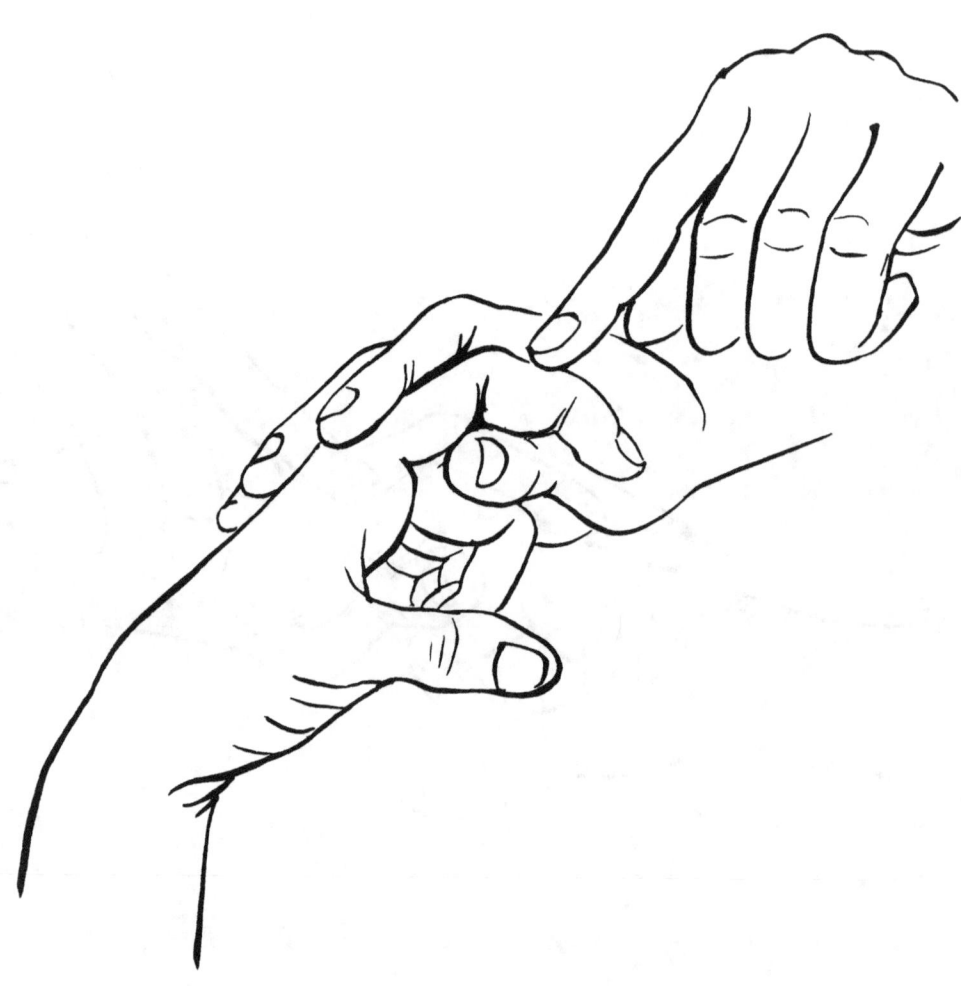

Linburg Test

Description

The patient sits. The patient is instructed to flex the thumb as much as possible onto the hypothenar eminence and to actively stretch the index finger into extension.

Interpretation

A positive test is one which elicits limitation of extension and pain, indicating Linburg's syndrome which is an anomalous tendinous condition, an interconnection between the flexor pollicis longus and the index digitorum profundus.

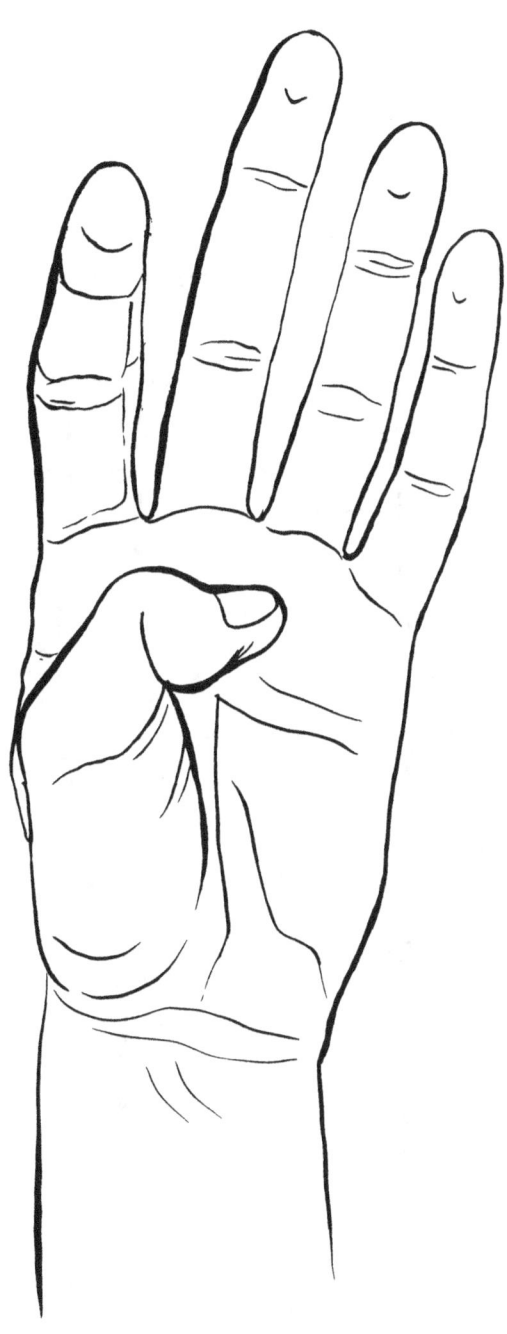

Wrinkle Test

Description
The patient sits and places the fingers in water at comfortable temperature for approximately 5 minutes and then removes them from the water.

Interpretation
A positive test is one in which the skin over the pulp does not wrinkle, indicating denervation.

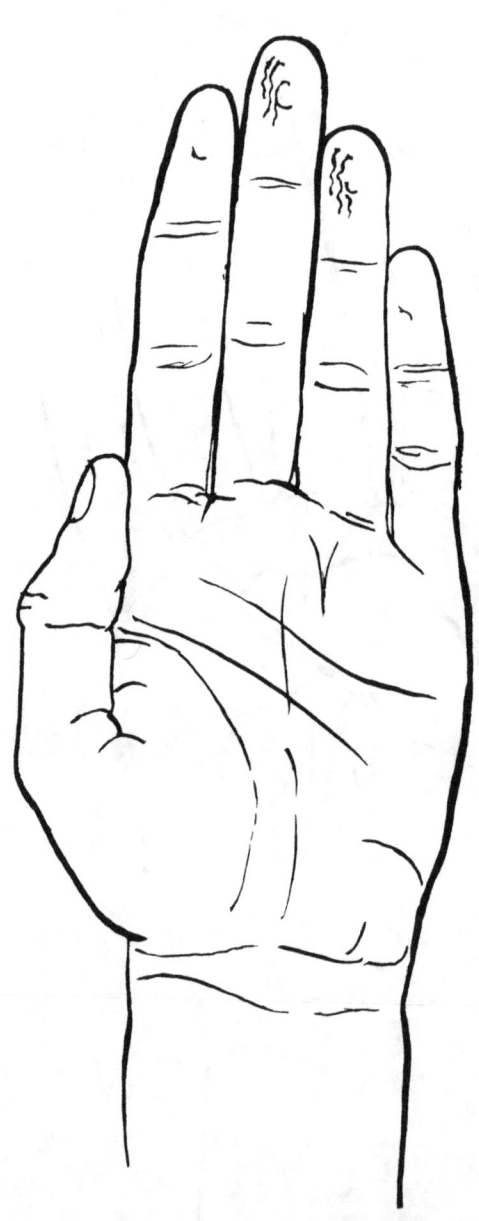

Weber Test

Description

The patient sits. The examiner touches the patient's skin with two blunt points simultaneously placed along a longitudinal line of the fingers. The patient, with eyes closed, is asked to specify whether he/she feels one or two points.

Interpretation

A positive test is one in which the patient does not recognize one or two points correctly, two out of three times, indicating a proprioceptive impairment.

Comments

The two-point discrimination instrument can be made by spreading a paper clip.

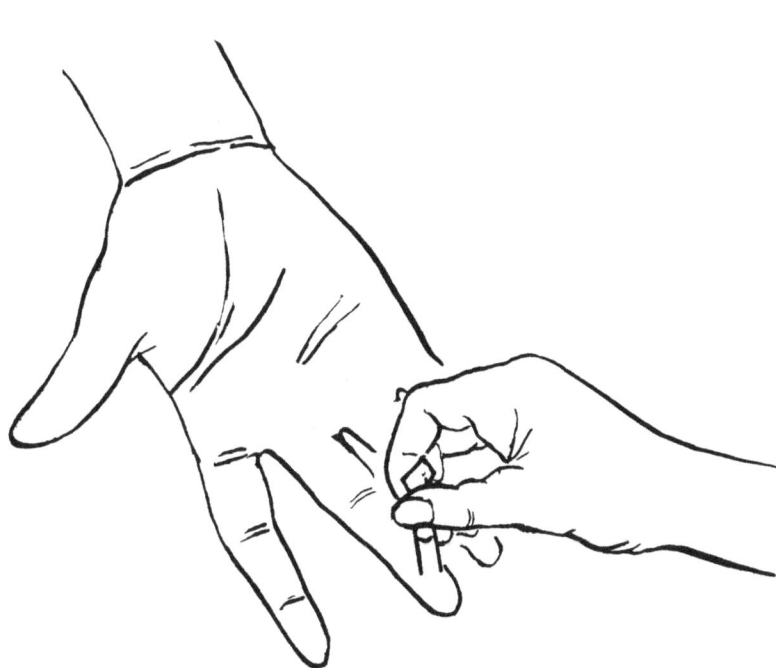

Section 4
Hip

Fabere/Patrick Test

Description

The patient lies supine. The examiner stabilizes the patient's pelvis with one hand. With the other hand the examiner places the foot of the patient's involved side on the opposite knee. In this way, the hip joint is flexed, abducted, and externally rotated. The examiner then slowly lowers the involved leg toward the table.

Interpretation

A positive test is one in which pain is produced in the anterior hip, indicating hip dysfunction. Pain in the posterior and lateral sides of the hip indicates sacroiliac joint and low lumbar dysfunction.

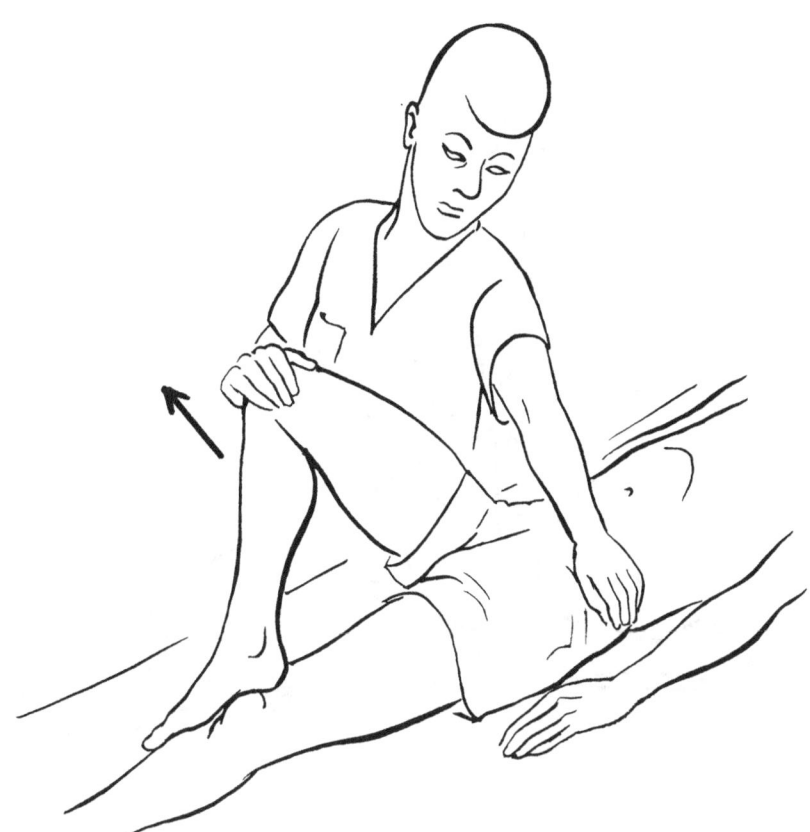

Hibb Test

Description
The patient lies prone. The examiner holds the patient's distal tibiofibula and passively flexes the patient's knee beyond 90°, then internally rotates the hip.

Interpretation
A positive test is one in which pain is elicited in the hip joint, indicating hip joint dysfunction. Pain in the sacroiliac joint indicates a sacroiliac joint dysfunction.

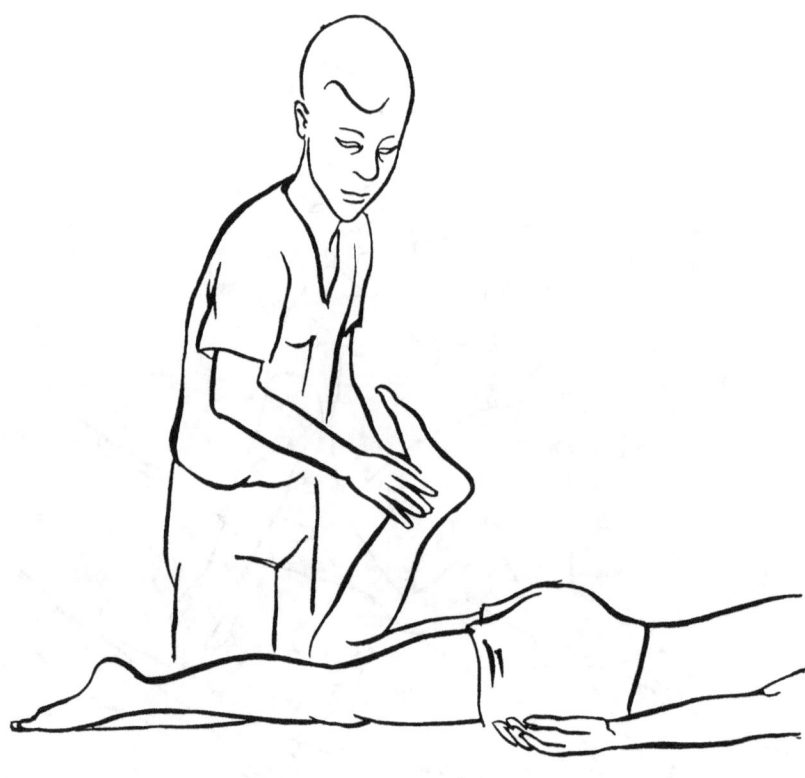

Buttock Test

Description

The patient lies supine. The examiner performs a straight leg raising test (refer to page 245). If the straight leg raising test is positive, the examiner then flexes the patient's knee a few degrees and further flexes the hip.

Interpretation

A positive test is one in which hip flexion does not increase with knee flexion, indicating a lesion in the buttock such as bursitis, tumor or abscess, *not* a dysfunction in the lumbar spine.

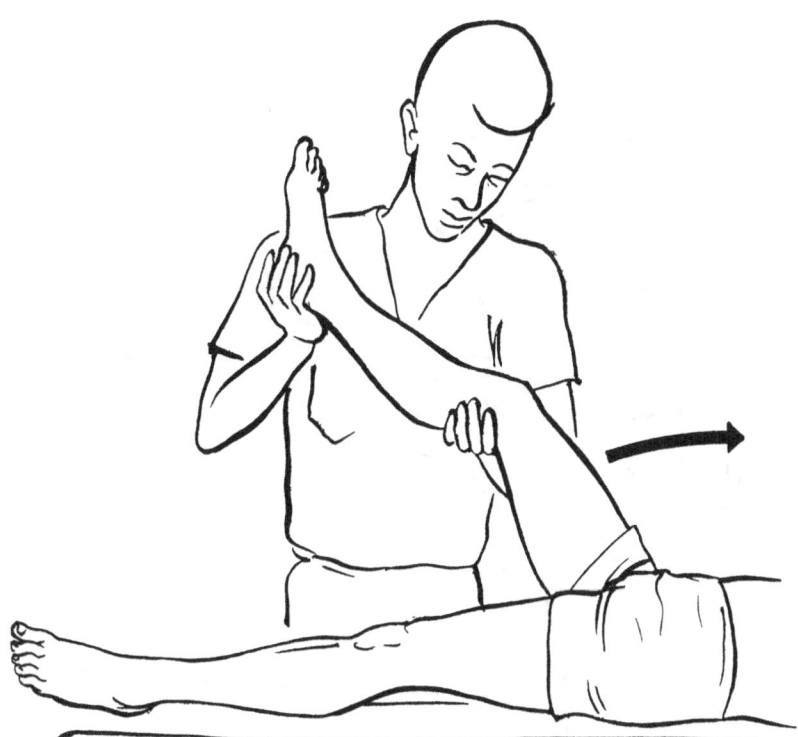

Torque Test

Description
The patient lies supine close to the edge of the table. The examiner extends the patient's hip over the edge of the table until the pelvis begins to move. The examiner grasps the patient's lower leg distally with one hand and places the other hand over the proximal femur anteriorly. The examiner then internally rotates the hip to the end of range with the distal hand and applies a slow posterolateral pressure with the proximal hand for 20 seconds to stress the capsular ligament.

Interpretation
A positive test is one in which excessive movement is observed in the hip joint, indicating instability of the hip joint.

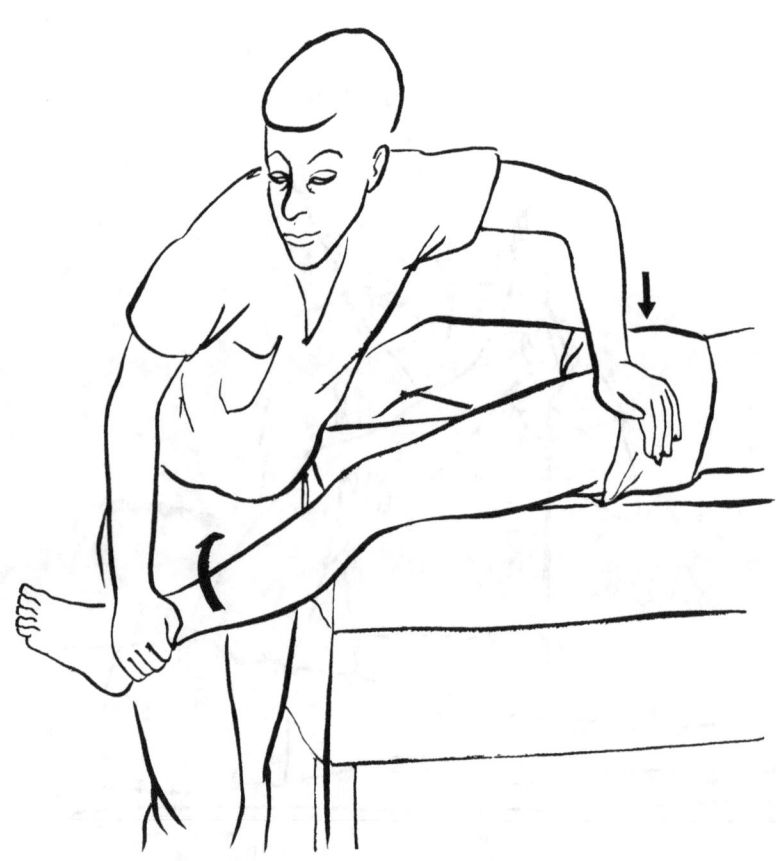

Thomas Test

Description
The patient lies supine with both knees and hips extended. The patient is instructed to flex the uninvolved hip toward the chest as far as possible and to hold the leg in this position.

Interpretation
A positive test is one in which the extended contralateral hip becomes flexed, indicating a fixed flexion contracture of that hip.

Comments
Perform Rectus Femoris Test to confirm the hip flexor contracture.

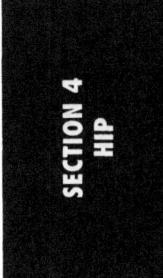

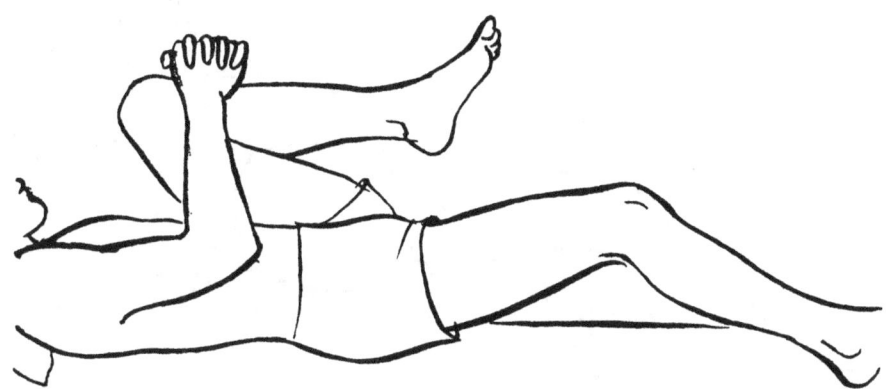

Rectus Femoris Test

Description
This test is performed only if the Thomas Test is positive. The patient lies supine with hips extended and knees hanging off the end of the table. The patient is then instructed to flex the uninvolved hip toward the chest as far as possible and to hold the leg in this position. The examiner observes the knee angle maintained by the involved hanging leg.

Interpretation
A positive test is one in which the knee of the involved leg slightly extends, indicating tightness of the rectus femoris muscle.

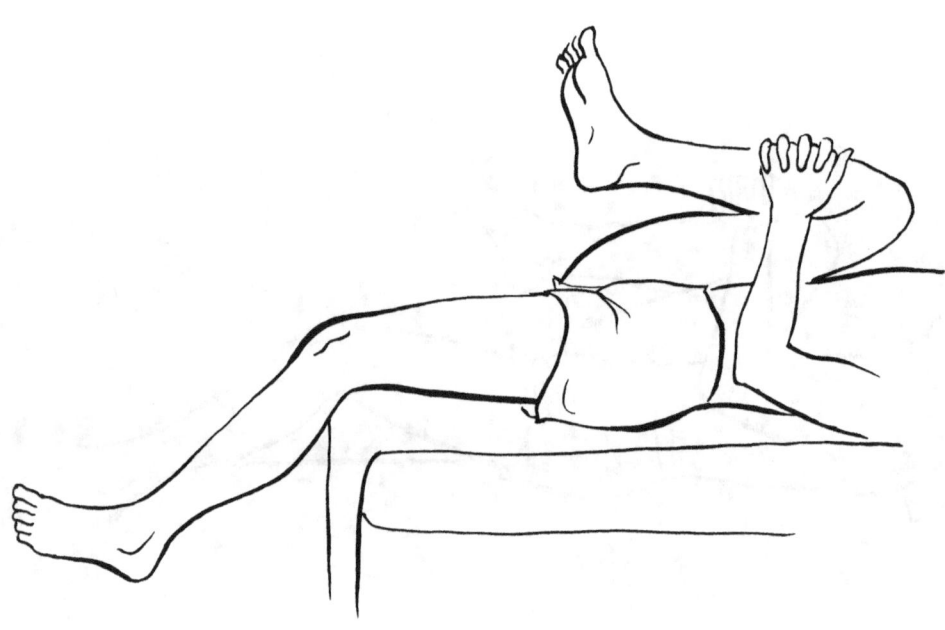

Ely Test

Description

The patient lies prone. The examiner passively flexes the patient's knee.

Interpretation

A positive test is one in which the hip flexes simultaneously on the side the knee is flexed, indicating tight rectus femoris muscle on the tested side.

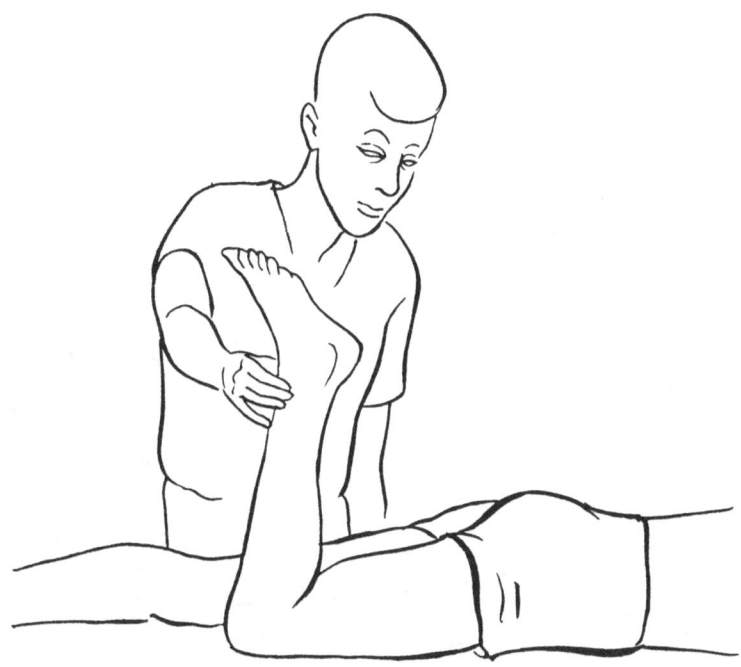

Tripod Test

Description
The patient sits over the edge of the treatment table with both knees flexed to 90°. The examiner holds the patient's distal tibiofibula and passively extends the knee.

Interpretation
A positive test is one in which the patient extends his/her trunk as the examiner extends the patient's knee, indicating hamstring muscles contracture.

Comments
The test may also be positive when there is a problem with the sciatic nerve.

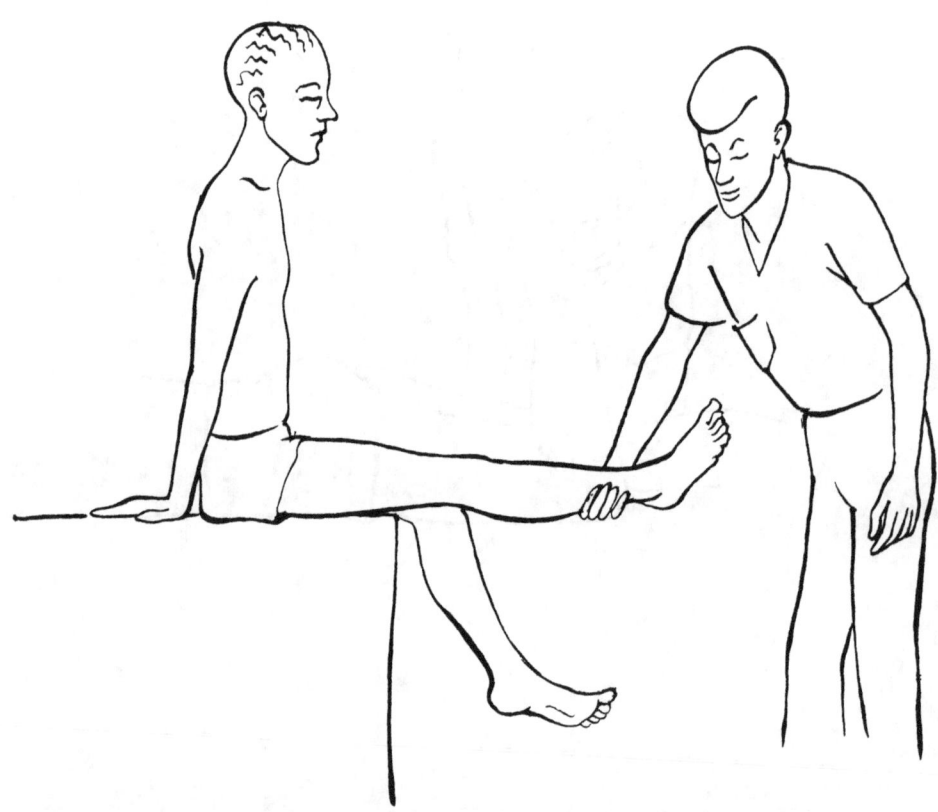

90-90 Straight Leg Test

Description

The patient lies supine. The patient is instructed to flex the hip to 90° while the knee is kept at 90° of flexion, and grasp behind the distal thigh with both hands. The patient is then instructed to extend the knee through available range.

Interpretation

A positive test is one in which the knee remains more than 20° from full extension, indicating a hamstring tightness.

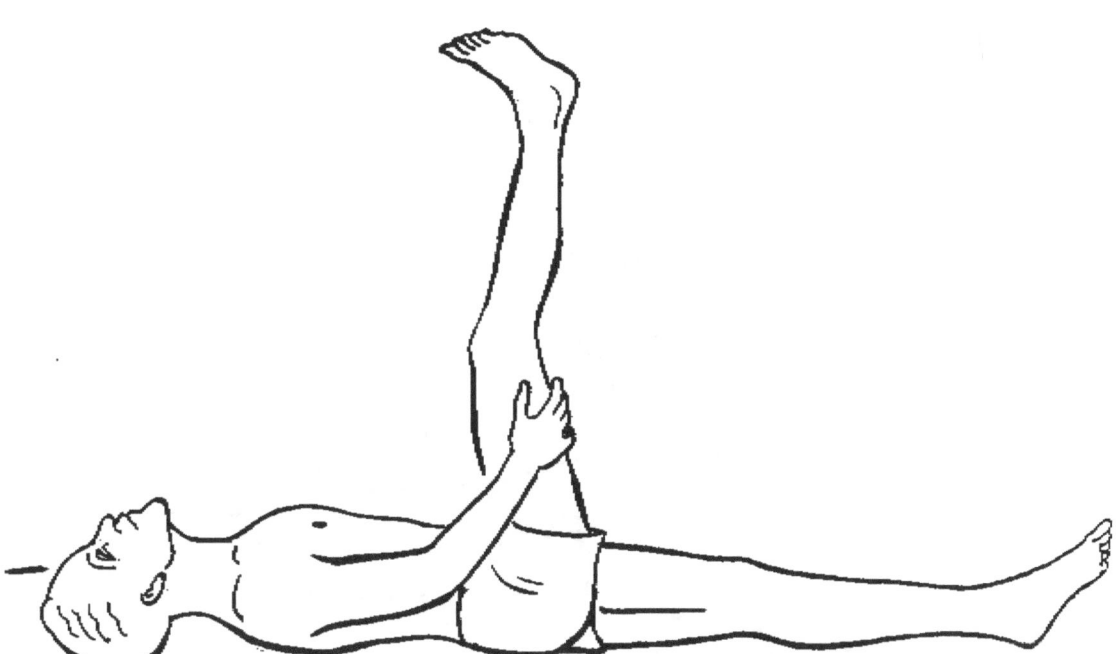

Ober Test

Description

The patient lies on the uninvolved side. The examiner flexes the patient's uninvolved knee enough so as to obliterate any lumbar lordosis. The examiner grasps the patient's involved leg with one hand while with the other hand stabilizes the patient's pelvis. The examiner then extends and abducts the involved hip passively so that the thigh is in line with the body and then adducts the hip.

Interpretation

A positive test is one in which the thigh does not adduct, indicating shortening of the iliotibial band.

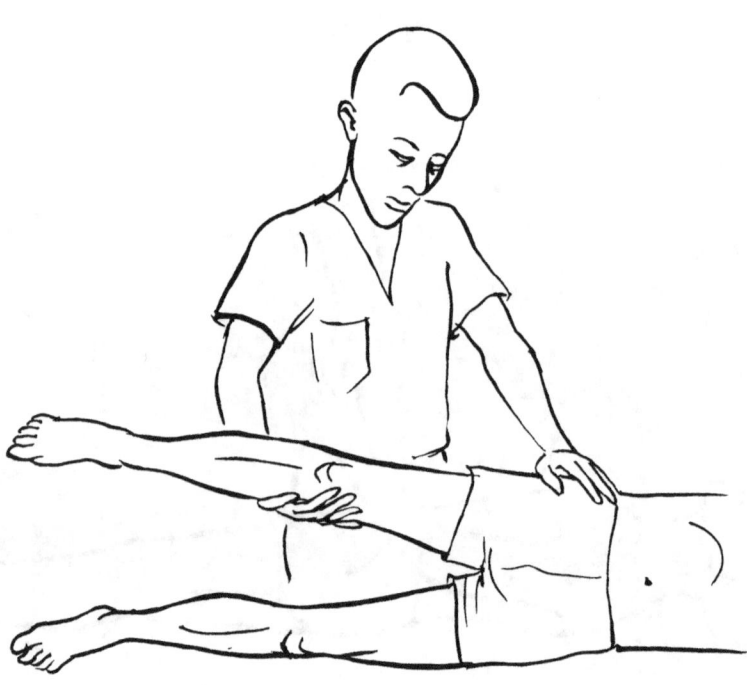

Noble Compression Test

Description

The patient lies supine. The examiner flexes the patient's involved knee to 45°-90° and then applies pressure with the thumb to the lateral femoral epicondyle or 1 to 2 cm proximal to it. While maintaining the pressure, the examiner extends the patient's knee.

Interpretation

A positive test is one in which a severe pain is produced over the lateral femoral epicondyle at about 30° of knee flexion, indicating the iliotibial band friction syndrome near the knee.

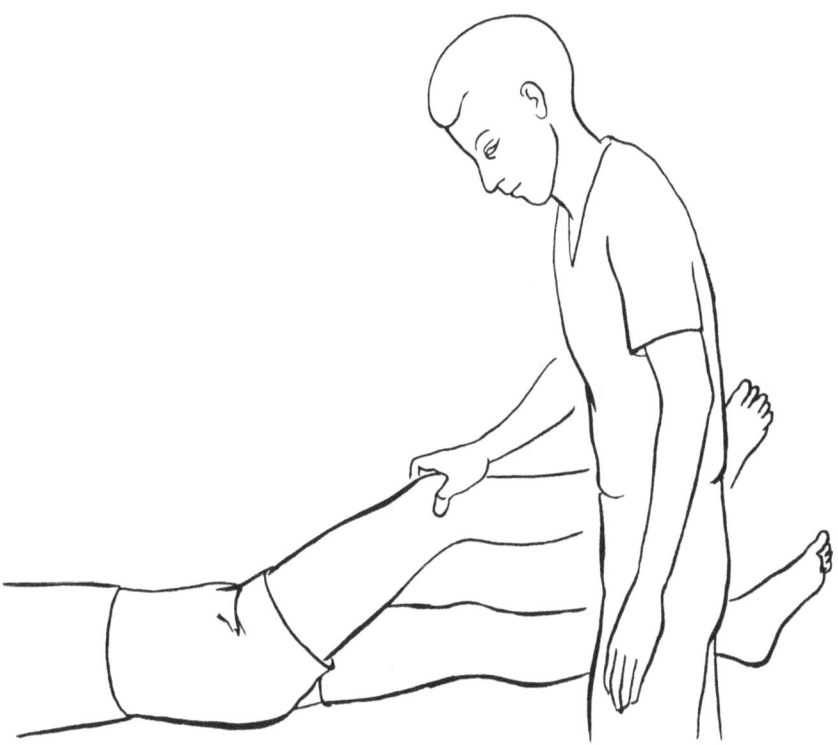

Trendelenburg Test

Description

The patient stands. The examiner squats behind the patient and observes the dimples overlying the posterior superior iliac spines. The patient is then instructed to stand on one leg. The test is then repeated on the opposite side by asking the patient to stand on the other leg.

Interpretation

A positive test is one in which the pelvis on the unsupported side remains in position or actually descends, indicating weakness of the gluteus medius muscle on the supported side.

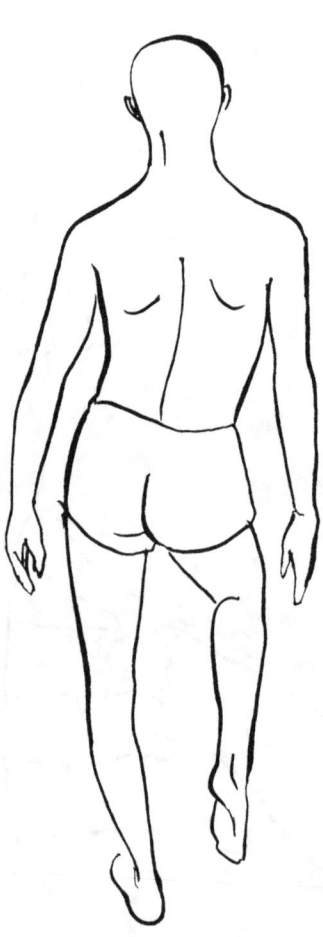

Scour Test

Description

The patient lies supine with the involved knee fully flexed. The examiner grasps the patient's knee of the involved side and applies axial compression to the patient's hip, then scours the femoral head around the acetabular rim from the point of maximal flexion, adduction, and internal rotation.

Interpretation

A positive test is one in which crepitation and "bumps" are felt in the smoothness of the range of motion of the hip, indicating degenerative joint disease.

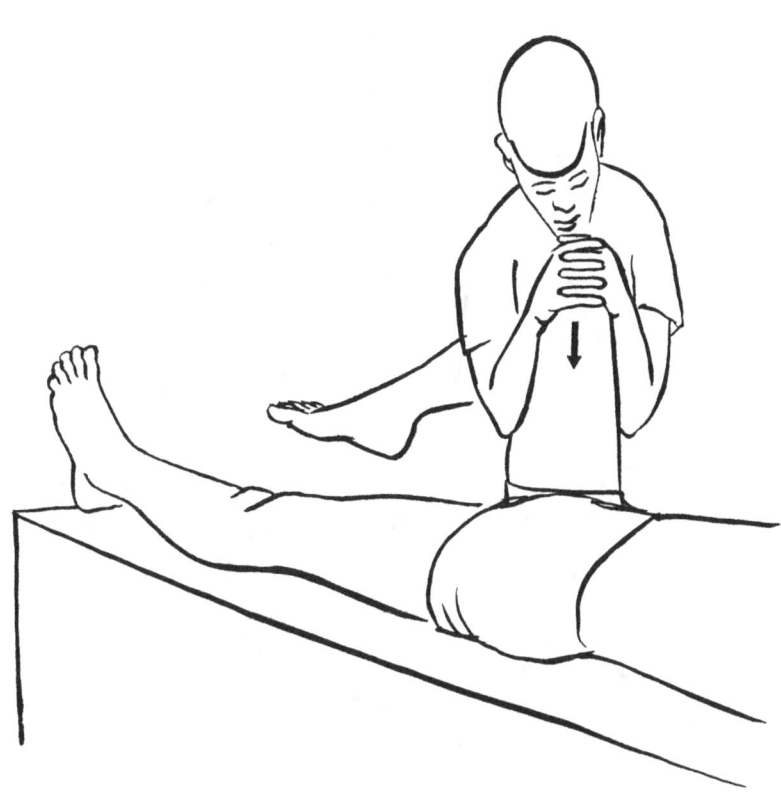

Craig Test

Description

The patient lies prone. The examiner holds the patient's distal tibiofibula with one hand and flexes the knee to 90°. With the other hand the examiner stabilizes the patient's pelvis, palpates the posterior aspect of the greater trochanter of the femur, and then passively rotates the hip internally and externally until the greater trochanter is parallel with the examination table or until it reaches its most lateral position. The degree of anteversion, the angle between the femoral neck and the femoral condyles, is then estimated.

Interpretation

A positive test is one in which the degree of anteversion is higher than the normal (adult normal range 8° to 15°), indicating excessive medial rotation of the hip and decreased lateral rotation of the hip. Increased anteversion leads to squinting patellae and toeing-in.

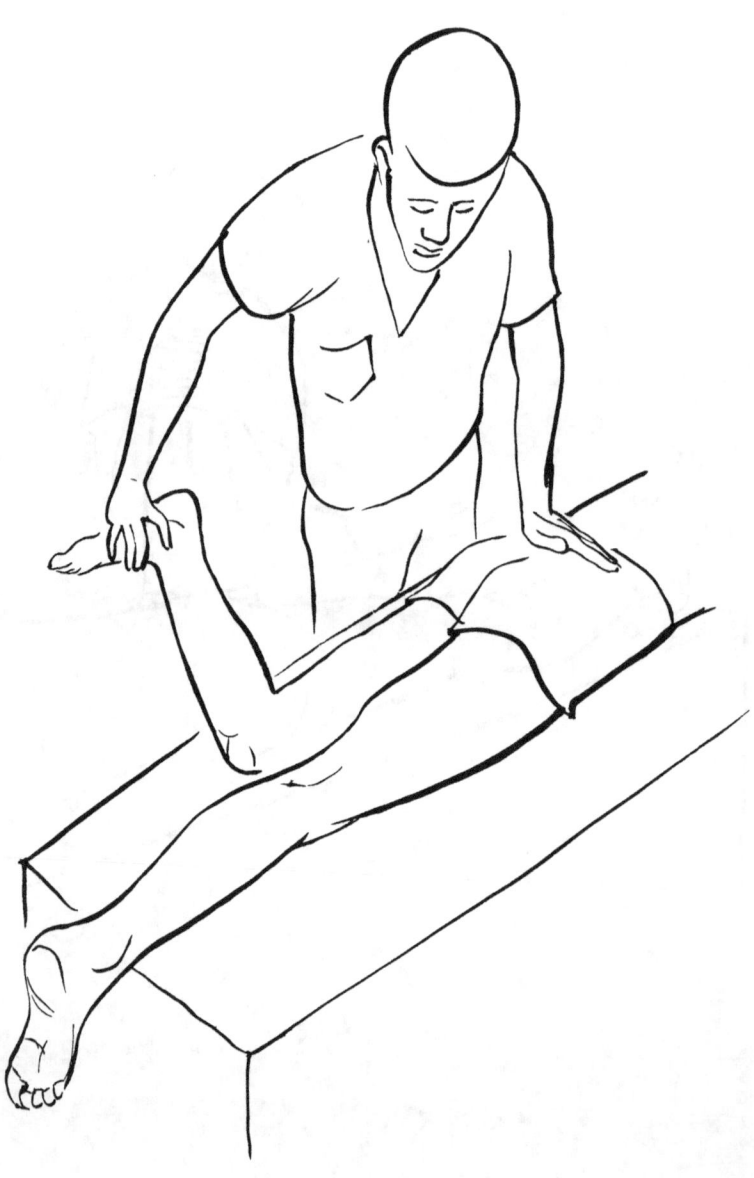

Leg Length Discrepancy Test

Description

The patient lies supine. The patient's legs are placed in precisely comparable positions. The examiner measures the distance from the anterior superior iliac spine to the medial malleoli of the ankle and compares the left and right leg length.

Interpretation

A positive test is one which reveals unequal distances in the left and right between these fixed points, indicating one leg shorter than the other.

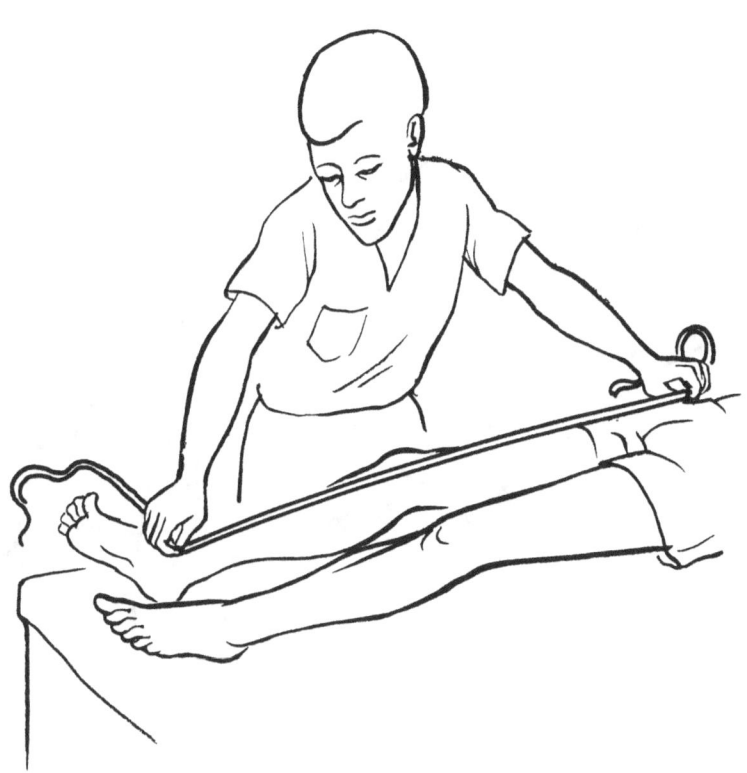

Ischial Bursitis Test

Description

The patient lies on the uninvolved side with both the hips flexed to about 45°. The examiner holds the patient's pelvis with one hand and palpates the patient's ischial tuberosity with the other hand.

Interpretation

A positive test is one in which pain is elicited on palpation of the ischial tuberosity, indicating ischial bursitis.

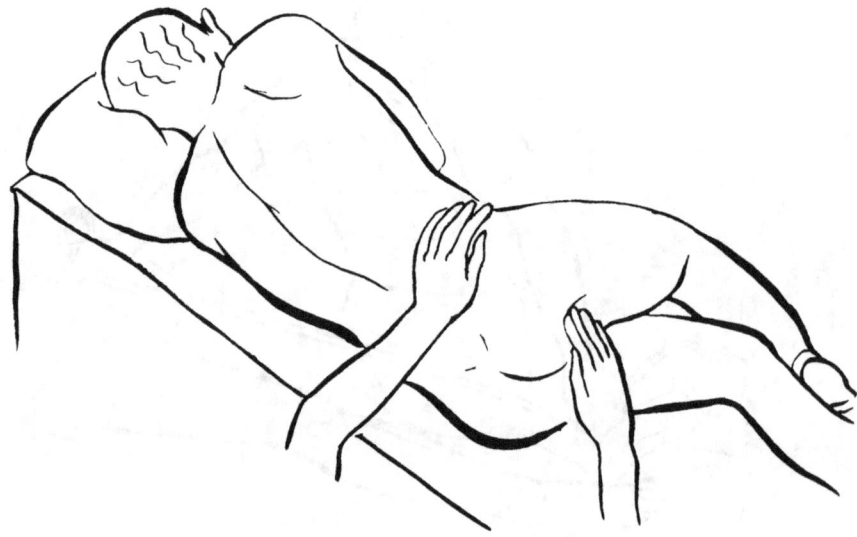

Trochanteric Bursitis Test

Description

The patient lies on the uninvolved side with both hips and knees flexed. The examiner holds the patient's pelvis with one hand and palpates the patient's greater trochanter with the other hand.

Interpretation

A positive test is one in which pain is elicited on palpation of the greater trochanter, indicating trochanteric bursitis.

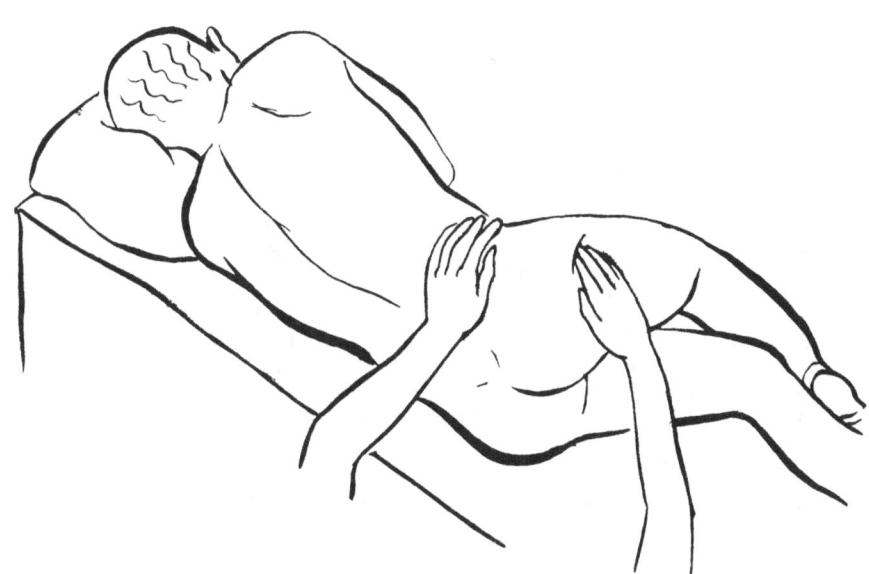

Piriformis Test

Description

The patient lies on the uninvolved side. The examiner flexes the patient's hip to 90° and fully flexes the knee. The examiner stabilizes the patient's pelvis with one hand and with the other hand pushes the knee downward.

Interpretation

A positive test is one which produces pain in the buttock, indicating piriformis syndrome.

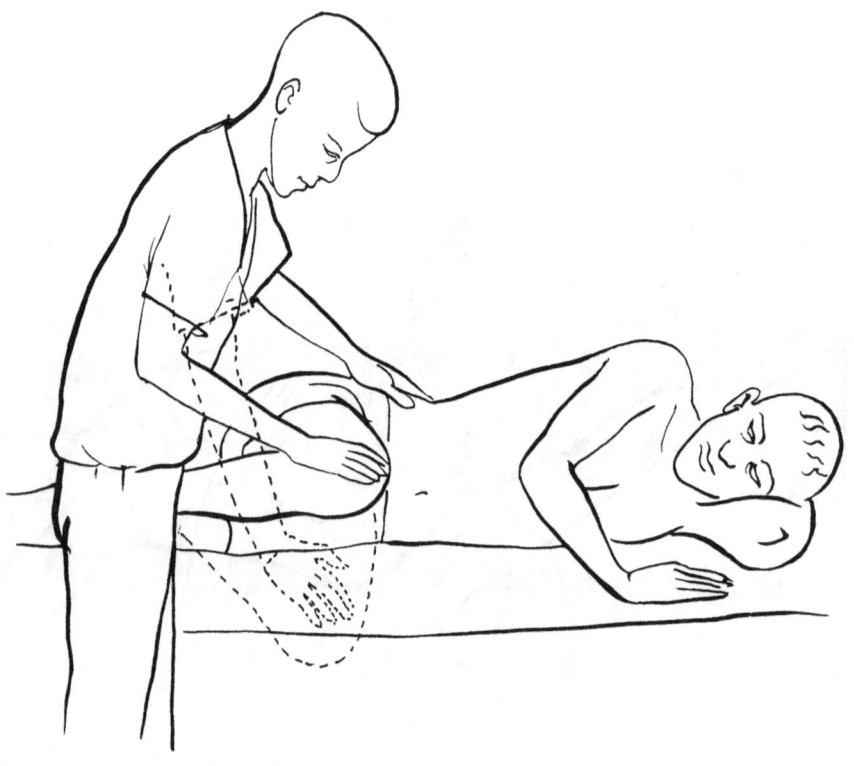

Sciatic Nerve Test

Description

The patient lies on the uninvolved side with the involved hip and knee flexed to about 90°. The examiner holds the patient's pelvis with one hand. With the other hand the examiner palpates the patient's greater trochanter and ischial tuberosity and then presses firmly with the thumb into the soft tissue at the midpoint between the greater trochanter and the ischial tuberosity.

Interpretation

A positive test is one in which tenderness is produced in the sciatic nerve, indicating a herniated disc in the lumbar spine, a piriformis muscle spasm, or a direct trauma to the nerve itself.

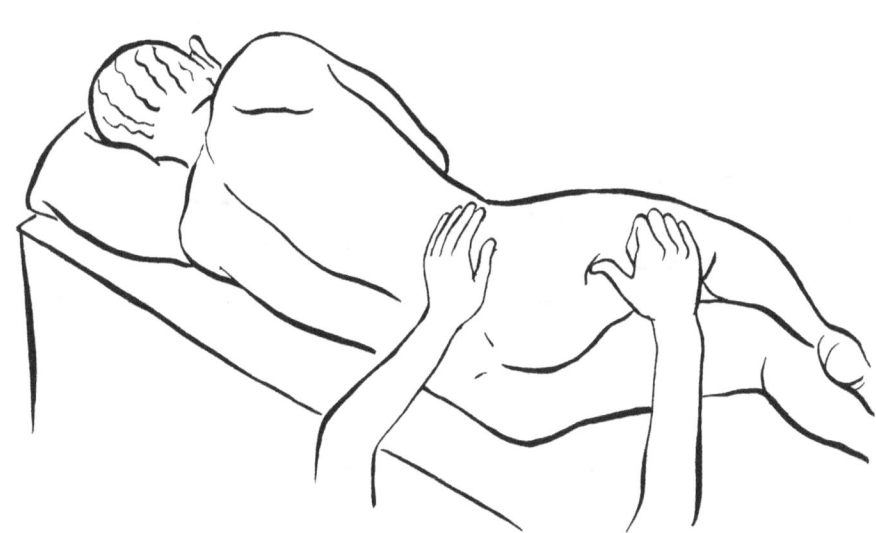

Femoral Nerve Stretch Test

Description
The patient lies prone. The examiner grasps the patient's distal tibiofibula and passively flexes the patient's knee and hyperextends the hip.

Interpretation
A positive test is one in which pain is produced in the lateral hip or anterior thigh, indicating an impingement of the femoral nerve.

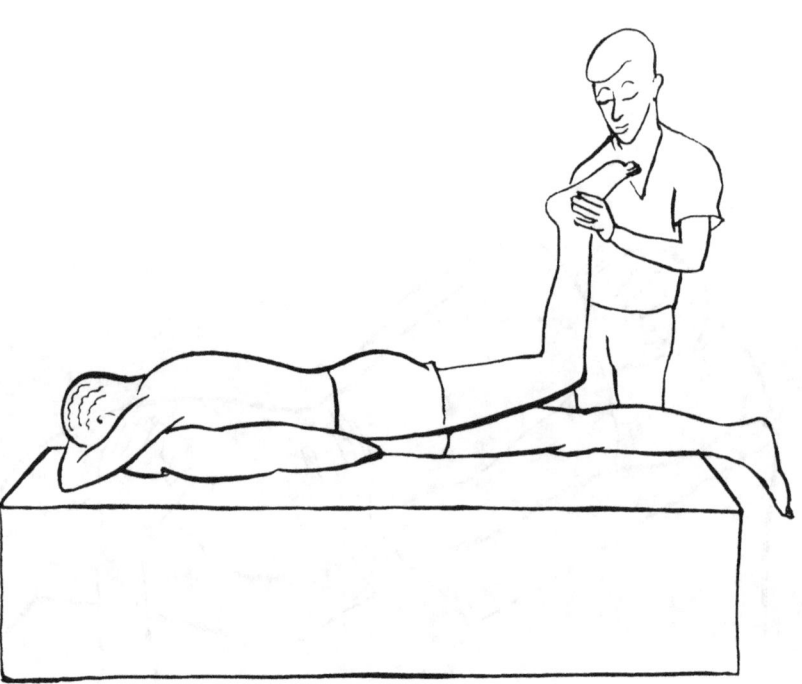

Ortolani Click Test
(Pediatrics Only)

Description

The patient lies supine. The examiner holds the patient's legs at the knees and flexes the hips. The examiner then abducts and externally rotates the patient's hips.

Interpretation

A positive test is one in which a "click" is produced, indicating a congenital hip dislocation.

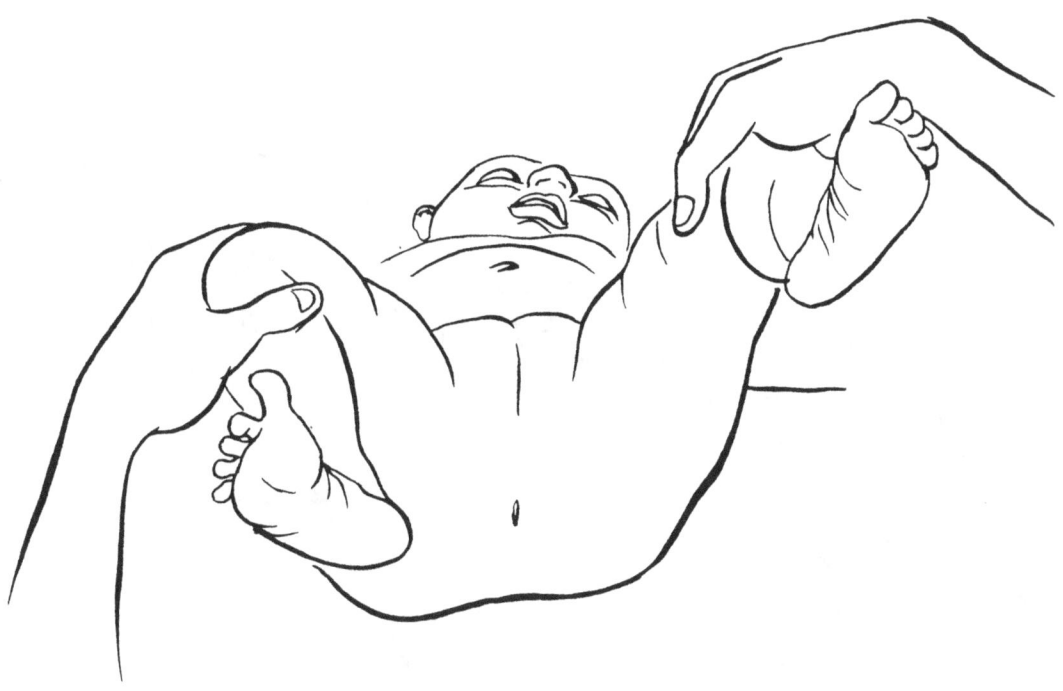

Barlow Test
(Pediatrics Only)

Description
This is a modified Ortolani Click Test. The patient lies supine. The examiner flexes the patient's hips to 90° and fully flexes the knees. The examiner places the middle finger of each hand over the patient's greater trochanter while the thumb is placed adjacent to the medial side of the thigh just proximal to the knee. The examiner stabilizes the patient's one leg with one hand and with the other hand moves the hip into abduction while simultaneously applying pressure over the greater trochanter. The examiner then applies posterior and lateral pressure on the medial thigh with the thumb.

Interpretation
A positive test is one in which the femoral head slips out over the posterior lip of the acetabulum and then reduces again when the pressure is removed, indicating an unstable hip.

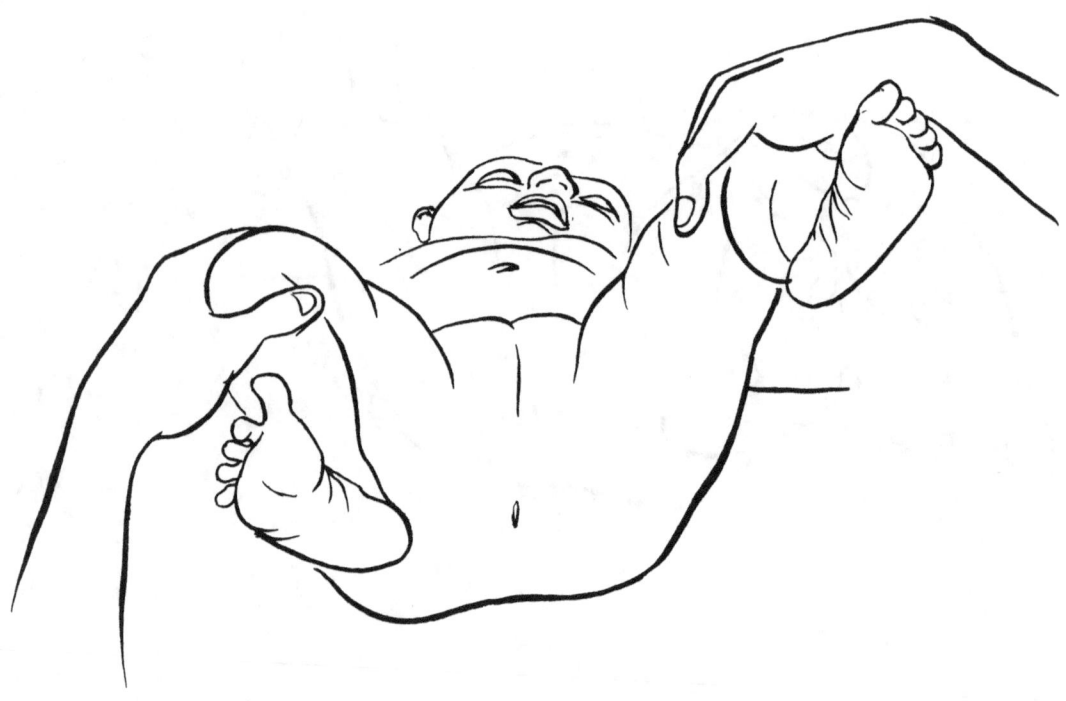

Allis Test
(Pediatrics Only)

Description

The patient lies supine. The examiner flexes the patient's knees and hips with feet flat on the table. The examiner observes the height of the knees.

Interpretation

A positive test is one in which one knee is higher than the other, indicating congenital dislocation of the hip.

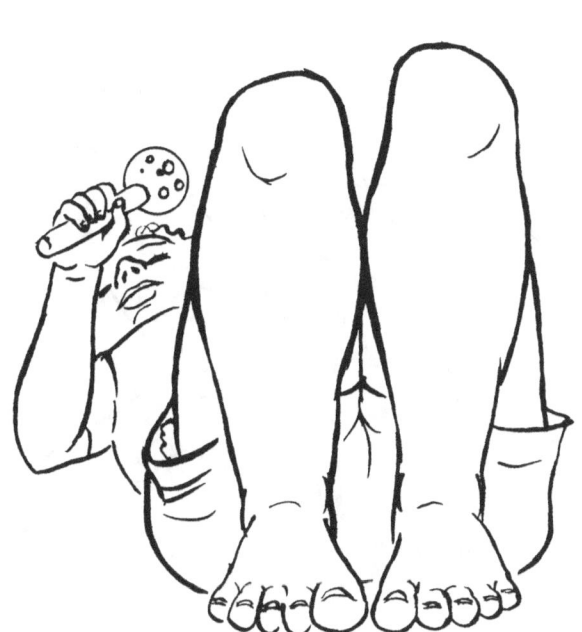

Telescoping Test
(Pediatrics Only)

Description

The patient lies supine. The examiner holds the patient's proximal tibiofibula, flexes the patient's knee and hip to 90°, and pushes the femur toward the table. The examiner then lifts the patient's femur and leg up and away from the table. The test is repeated on the other leg.

Interpretation

A positive test is one in which there is a lot of relative movement in one hip, indicating dislocated hip.

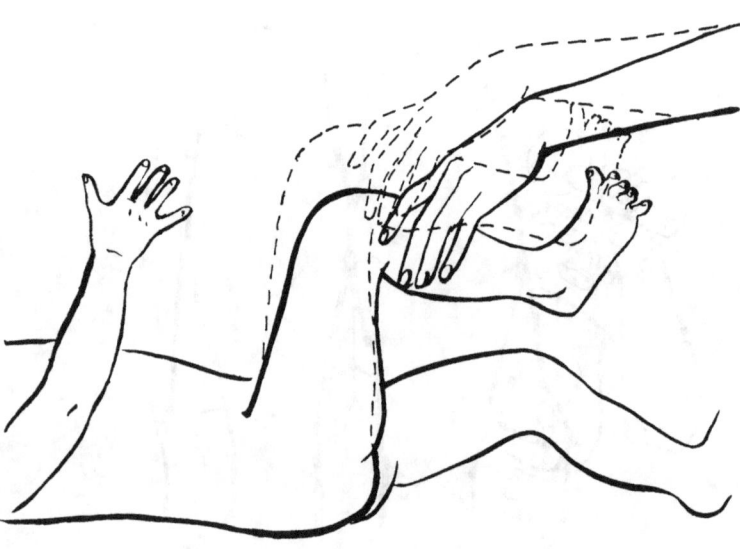

Section 5
Knee

Stroke Test

Description

The patient lies supine. The examiner commences just below the joint line on the medial side of the patella stroking proximally toward the patient's hip as far as the suprapatellar pouch with one hand, and repeats two or three times with the palm and fingers. With the other hand the examiner strokes down the lateral side of the patella.

Interpretation

A positive test is one in which a wave of fluid passes to the medial side of the joint and bulges below the medial distal border of the patella, indicating minimal effusion in the knee.

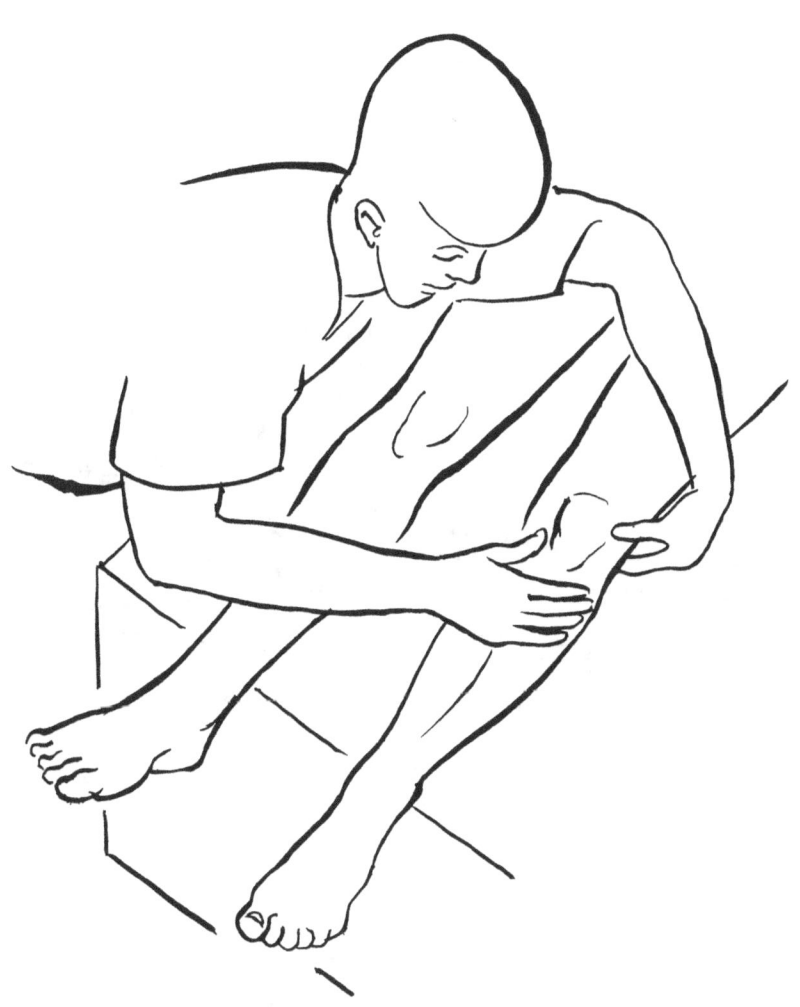

Effusion Test

Description

The patient lies supine with knees extended and quadricep muscles relaxed. The examiner then pushes the patella into the trochlear groove with both thumbs and quickly releases it.

Interpretation

A positive test is one in which the fluid under the patella first moves to the sides of the joint and then flows back to its former position forcing the patella to rebound, indicating joint effusion.

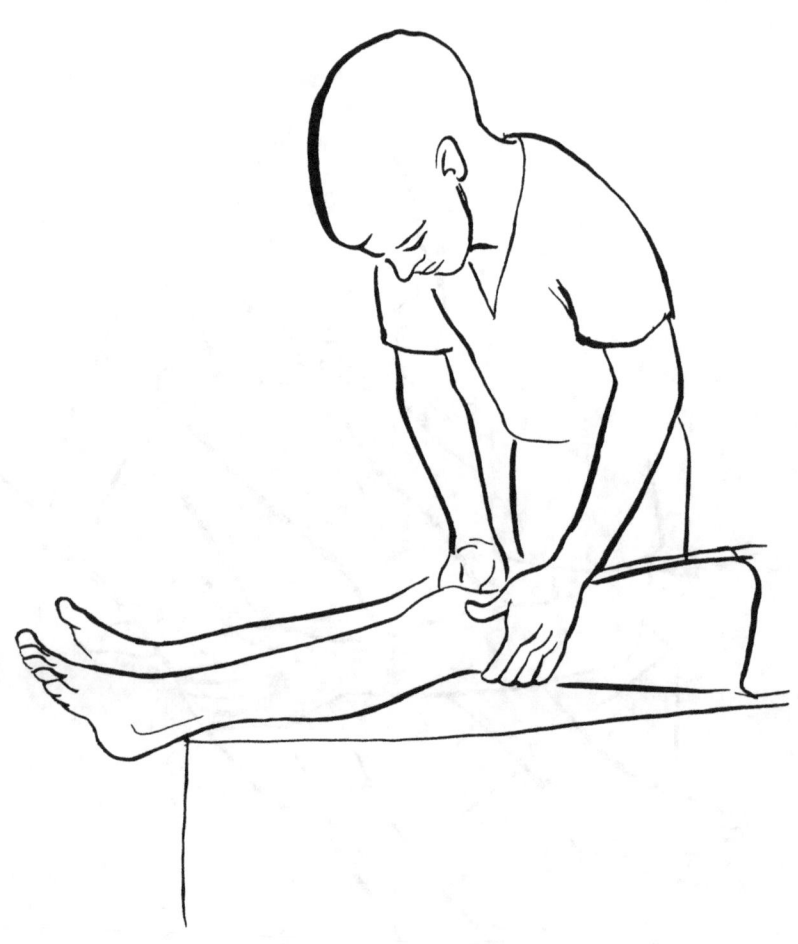

Fluctuation Test

Description

The patient lies supine with knees extended. The examiner places the palm of one hand over the suprapatellar pouch and the palm of the other hand anterior to the joint with the thumb and index finger just beyond the margins of the patella. The examiner first presses down with one hand and then up with the other hand.

Interpretation

A positive test is one in which the synovial fluid fluctuates under the hands, moving from one hand to the other hand, indicating significant effusion in the knee joint.

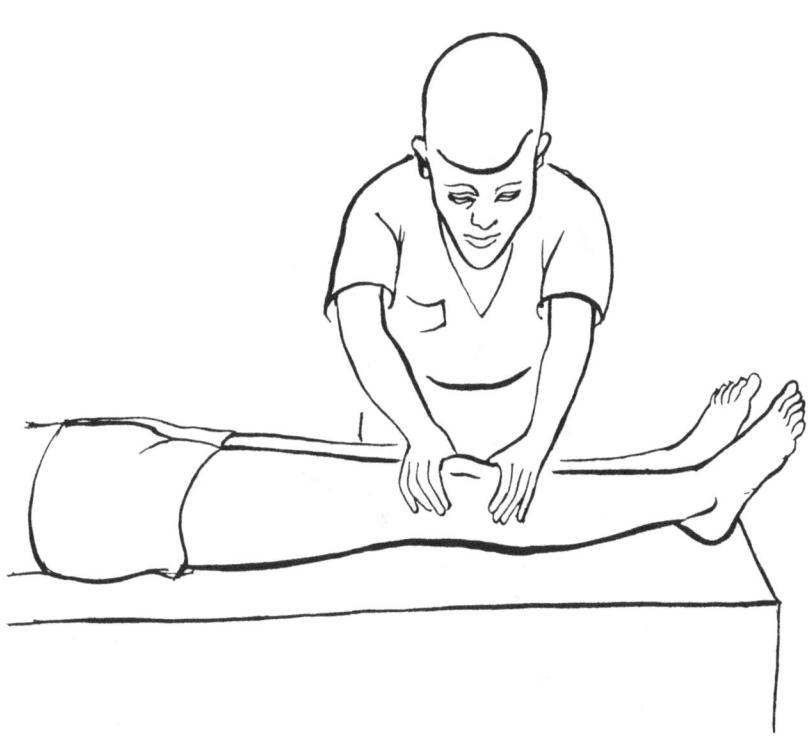

Patellar Tap Test

Description

The patient lies supine with knees extended. The examiner applies a slight pressure over the proximal patella to force fluid down into the knee joint. The examiner then taps the patella toward the condyle with a reflex hammer.

Interpretation

A positive test is one in which a floating of the patella is felt, indicating a large amount of swelling in the knee.

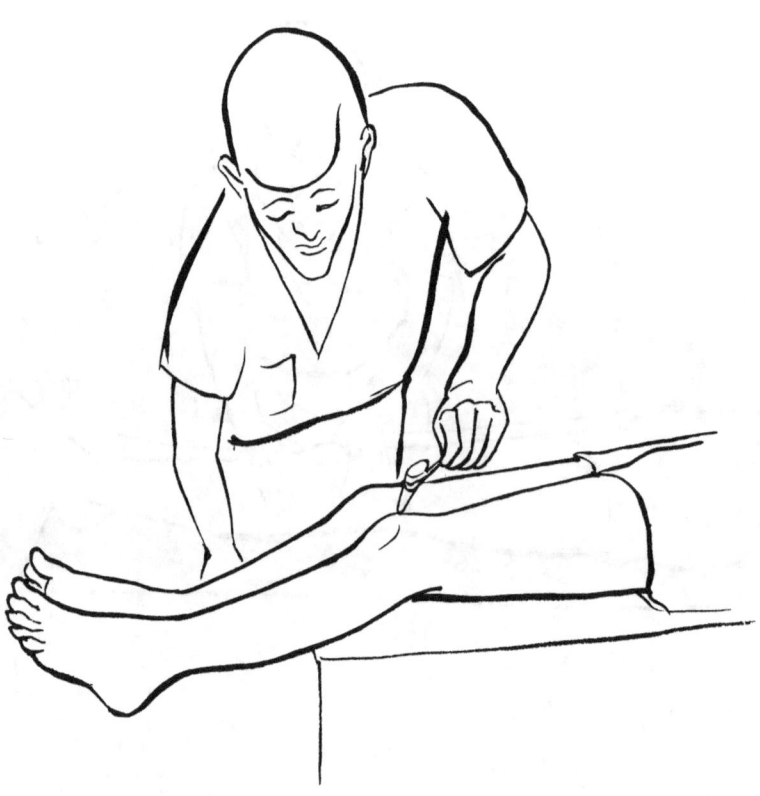

Tinel Test

Description

The patient lies supine with knees extended and quadricep muscles relaxed. The examiner taps around the medial side of the tibial tubercle where the infrapatellar branch of the saphenous nerve runs.

Interpretation

A positive test is one which either elicits or provokes pain at the medial side of the tibial tubercle, indicating a neuroma in the peripheral nerve secondary to a knee surgery.

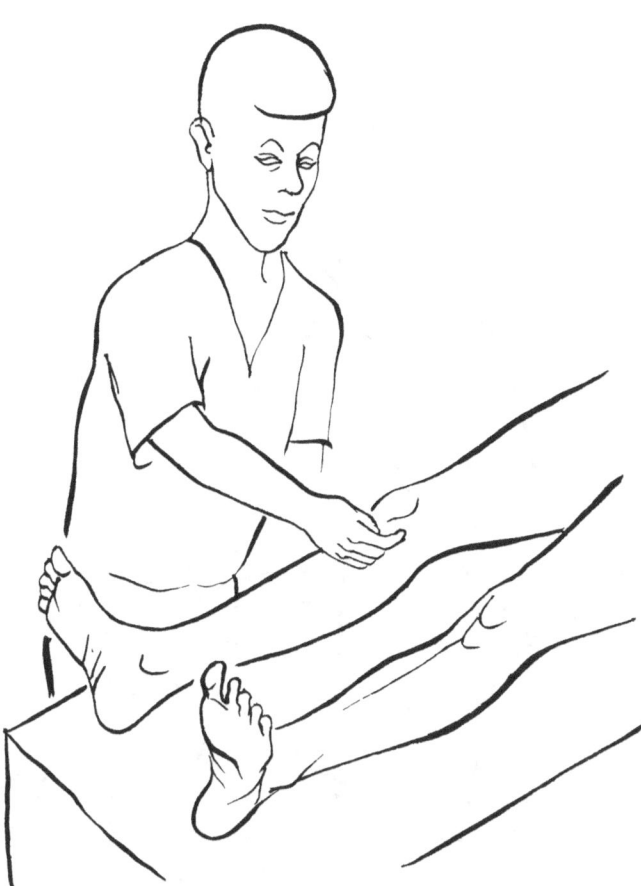

McConnel Test

Description
The patient sits on the examination table. The examiner sits in a chair. The examiner flexes the patient's knee to approximately 20° while the patient's lower leg rests on the examiner's thigh. The patient is then instructed to contract the quadricep muscles isometrically.

Interpretation
A positive test is one in which pain is produced and the patella sits laterally, indicating patello-femoral dysfunction. Pain is eased by a medial glide of the patella.

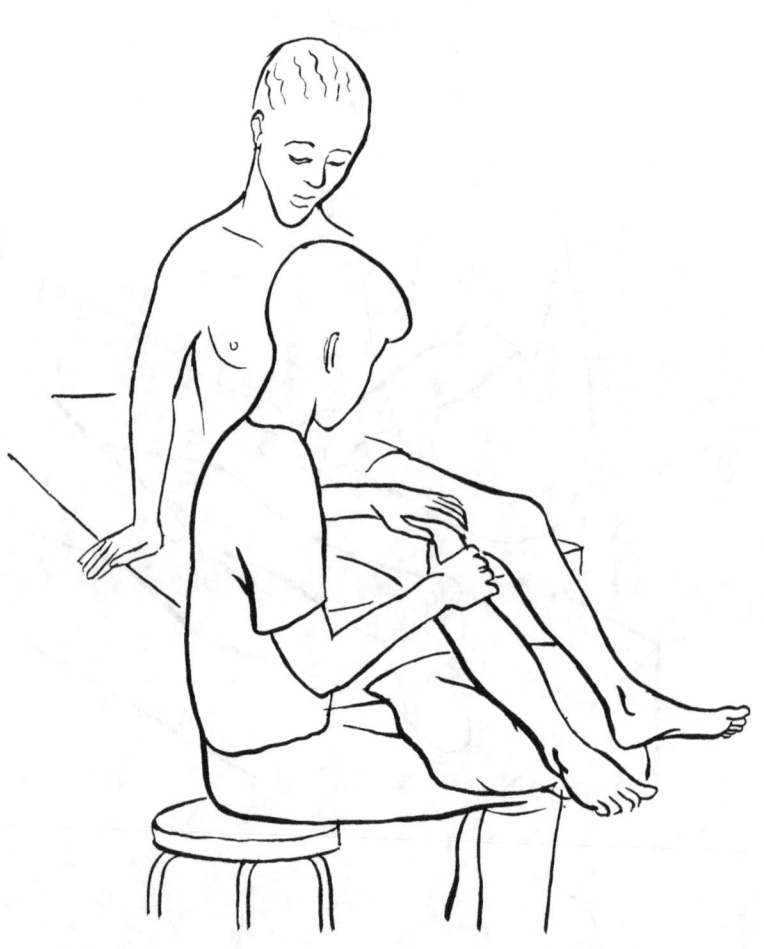

Patella Femoral Grinding Test

Description

The patient lies supine with knees and hips extended and quadricep muscles relaxed. The examiner first pushes the patella distally in the trochlear groove and then instructs the patient to tighten the quadricep muscles. Further, the examiner applies resistance to the patella as it moves under the examiner's fingers.

Interpretation

A positive test is one in which the articulating surfaces cause a palpable crepitation when the patella moves and the patient complains of pain/discomfort, indicating osteochondral defects or degenerative changes within the trochlear groove.

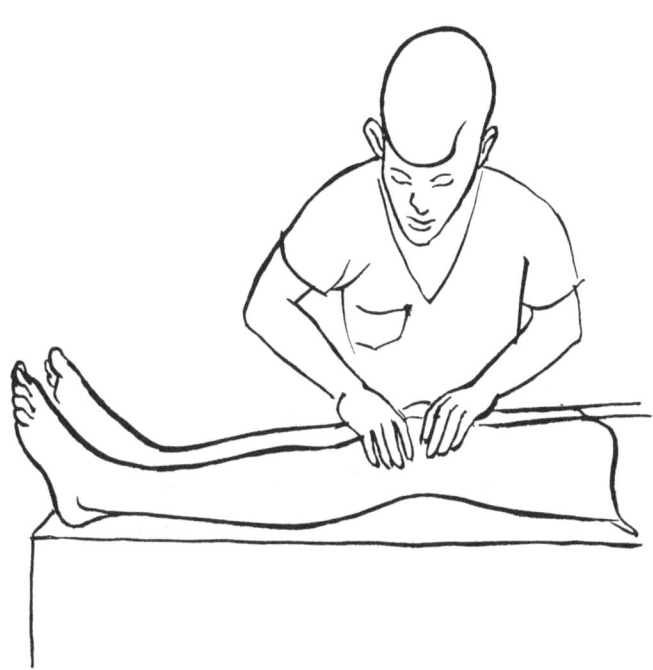

Clarke Test

Description

The patient lies supine with knees and hips extended and quadricep muscles relaxed. The examiner presses down slightly proximal to the upper pole or base of the patella with the web space of the hand. The patient is then instructed to contract the quadricep muscles while the examiner pushes down.

Interpretation

A positive test is one in which the patient experiences retropatellar pain and cannot hold the contraction, indicating chondromalacia patella.

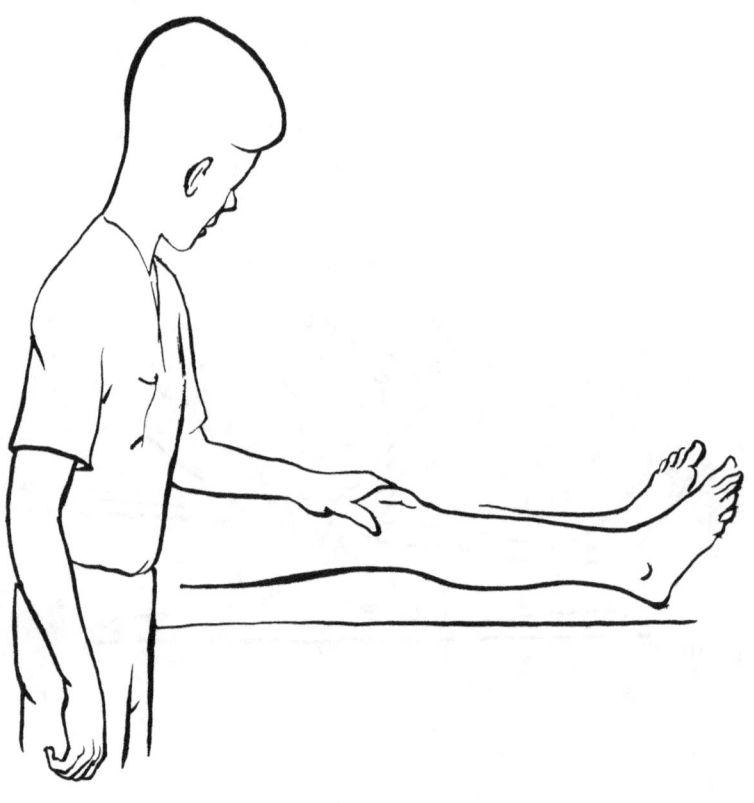

Waldron Test

Description

The patient stands. The examiner palpates the patient's patella and instructs the patient to perform several slow deep knee bends.

Interpretation

A positive test is one in which a crepitus is produced along with pain as the patient goes through the range of motion, indicating chondromalacia patella.

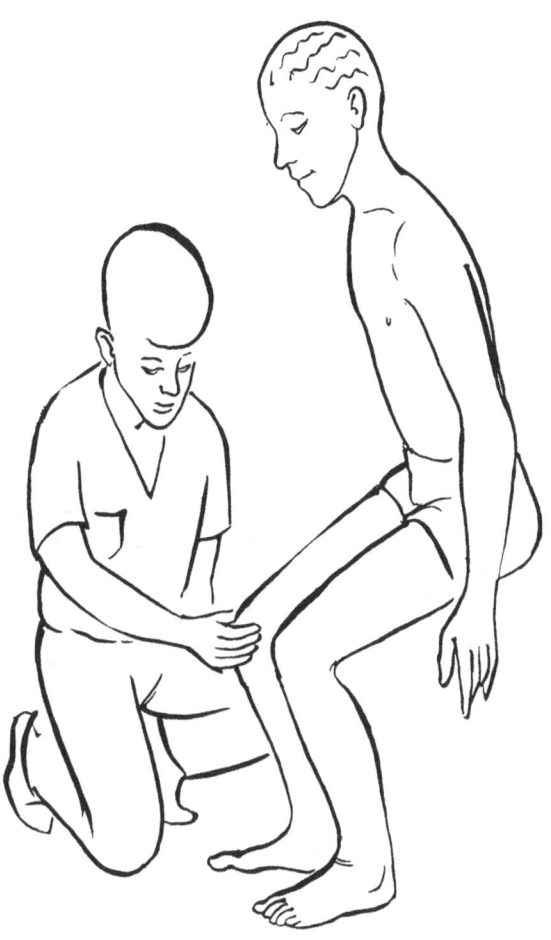

Zohler Test

Description

The patient lies supine with knees and hips extended. The examiner pulls the patient's patella distally with both hands and holds it in this position. The patient is then instructed to contract the quadricep muscles.

Interpretation

A positive test is one in which pain is produced, indicating chondromalacia patella.

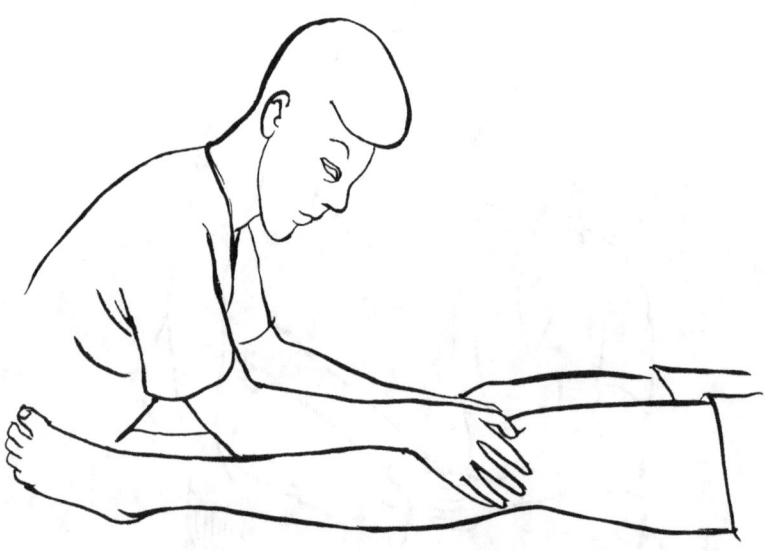

Apprehension Test

Description

The patient lies supine with knees extended and quadricep muscles relaxed. The examiner presses against the medial border of the patella with both thumbs.

Interpretation

A positive test is one in which the patient becomes apprehensive and distressed, indicating patellar dislocation or subluxation.

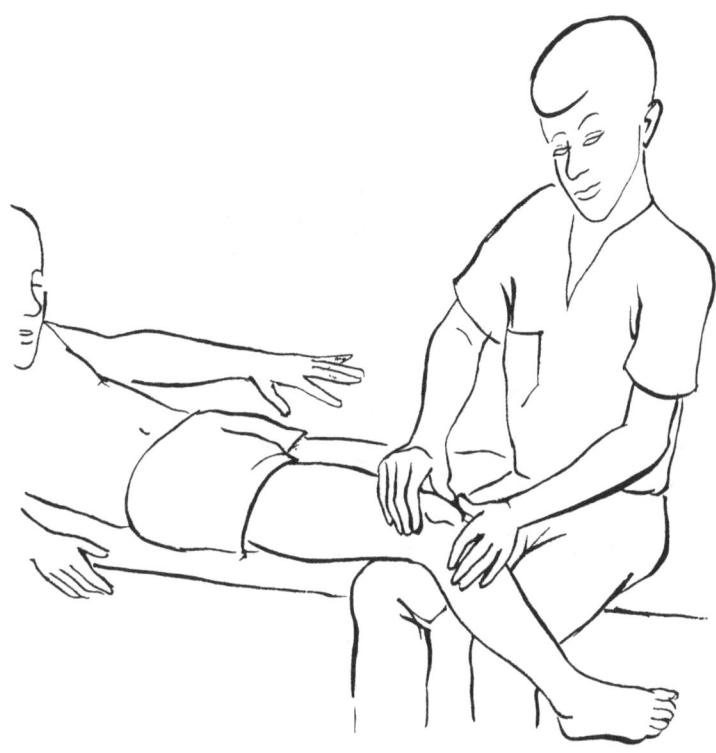

Fairbank Apprehension Test

Description
The patient lies supine. The examiner grasps the patient's distal tibiofibula with one hand and flexes the patient's knee to about 30°. The quadricep muscles are relaxed. With the other hand the examiner pushes the patella laterally.

Interpretation
A positive test is one in which the patient becomes apprehensive and distressed, indicating patellar dislocation or subluxation.

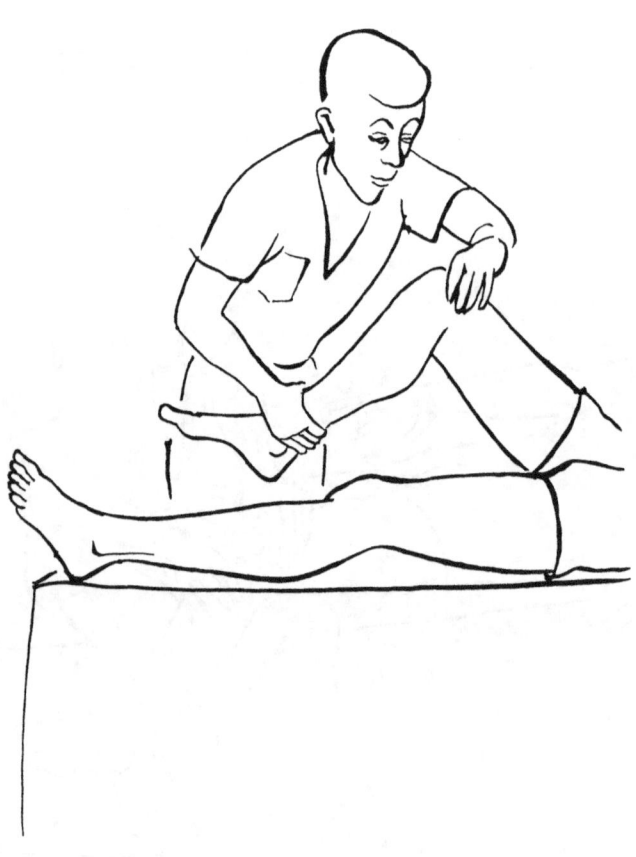

Dreyer Test

Description

The patient lies supine. The patient is instructed to flex the hip actively while maintaining the knee in extension. If the patient is unable to flex the hip, the examiner stabilizes the quadriceps tendon with both hands just above the knee level and then instructs the patient to flex the hip.

Interpretation

A positive test is one in which the patient is able to flex the hip only when the quadriceps tendon is stabilized, indicating a possible fracture of the patella.

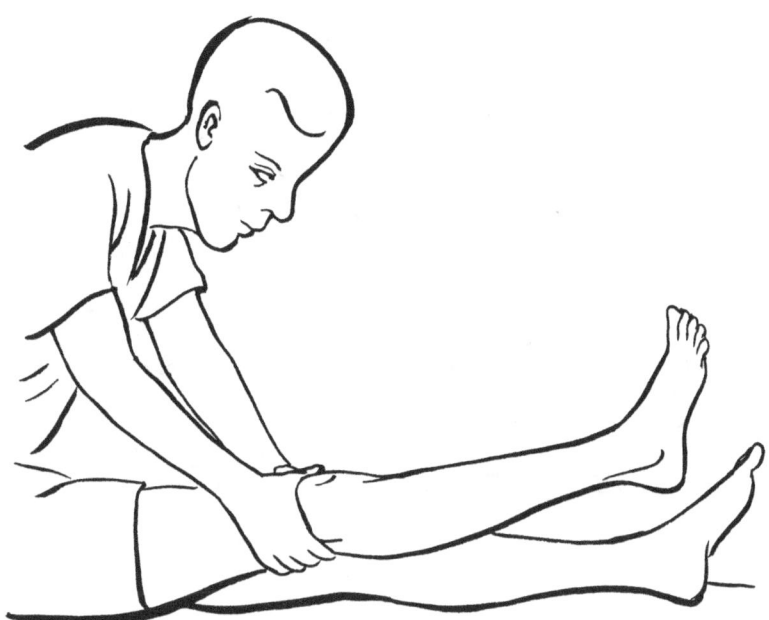

Mediopatellar Plica Test

Description

The patient lies supine. The examiner grasps the patient's distal tibiofibula with one hand and flexes the patient's knee to 30°. With the other hand the examiner then moves the patient's patella medially.

Interpretation

A positive test is one in which the patient experiences pain, indicating mediopatellar plica.

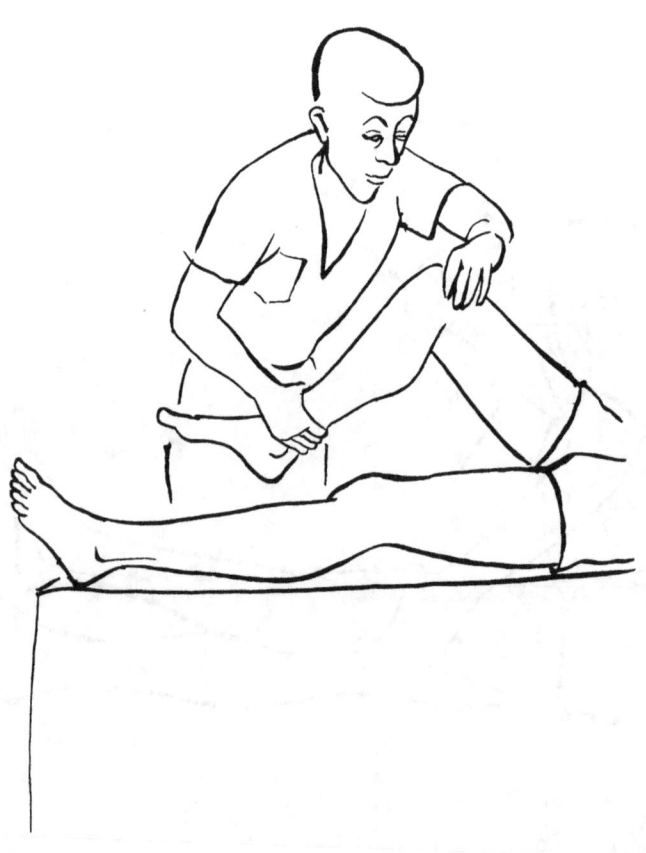

Plica "Stutter" Test

Description

The patient sits on the edge of the table with knees flexed to 90°. The examiner places the fingers over the patella. The patient is then instructed to slowly extend the knee while the examiner palpates the patella with the fingers.

Interpretation

A positive test is one in which the patella stutters or jumps at 60° to 45° of flexion, indicating patellar plica.

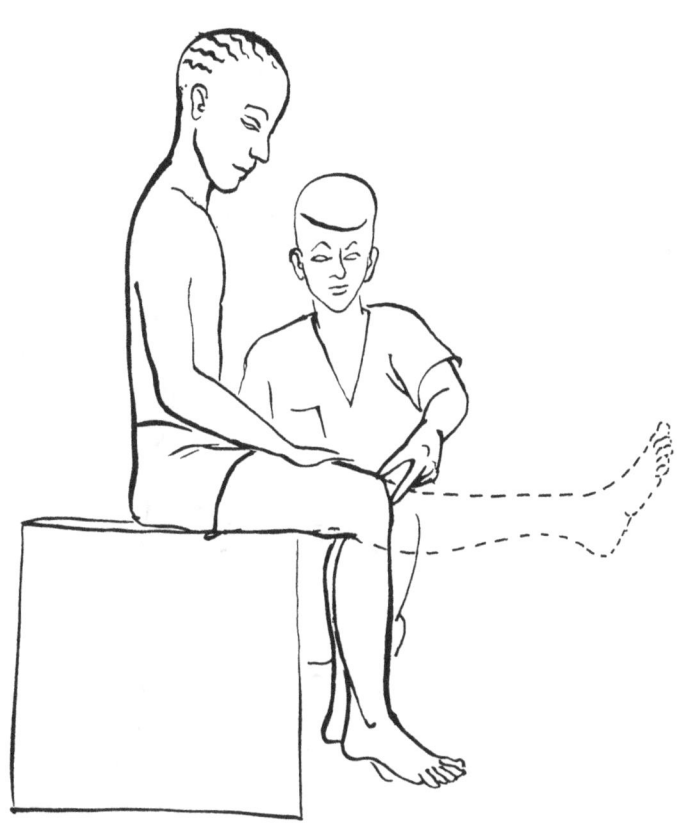

Noble Compression Test

Description
The patient lies supine. The examiner flexes the patient's involved knee to 45°-90° and then applies pressure with the thumb to the lateral femoral epicondyle or 1 to 2 cm proximal to it. While maintaining the pressure, the examiner extends the patient's knee.

Interpretation
A positive test is one in which the patient experiences severe pain over the lateral femoral condyle at about 30° of flexion as the knee is extended from the 90° flexed position, indicating iliotibial band syndrome.

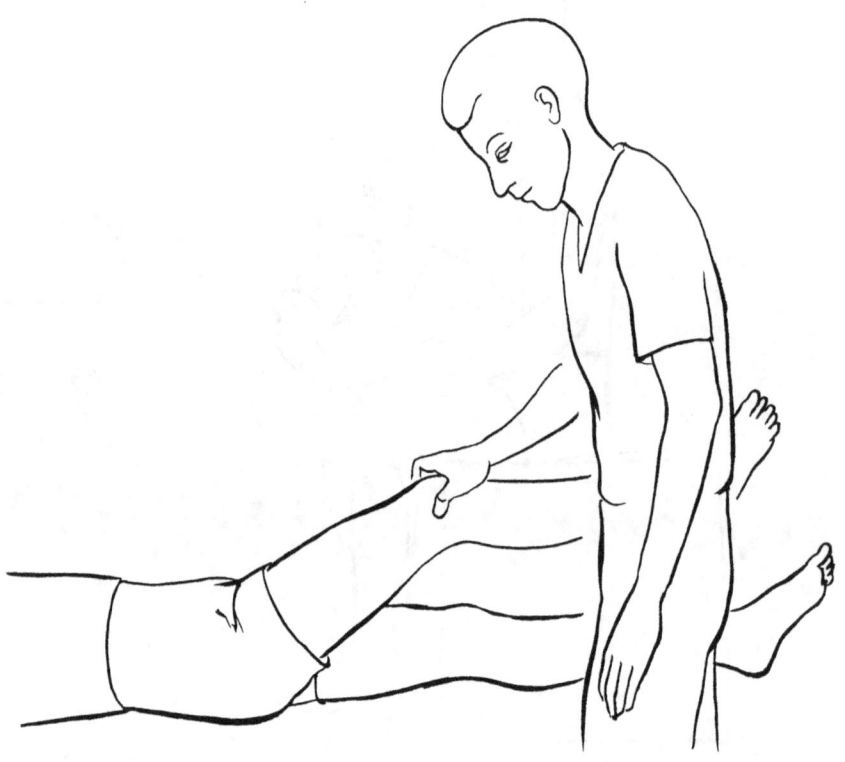

Bounce Home Test

Description

The patient lies supine. The examiner holds the patient's heel with one hand and places the other hand posteriorly distal to the knee. The examiner fully flexes the patient's knee and then allows it to extend.

Interpretation

A positive test is one in which the knee is unable to fully extend, but rather offers a leathery resistance to full extension, indicating a possible torn meniscus or loose body within the knee joint.

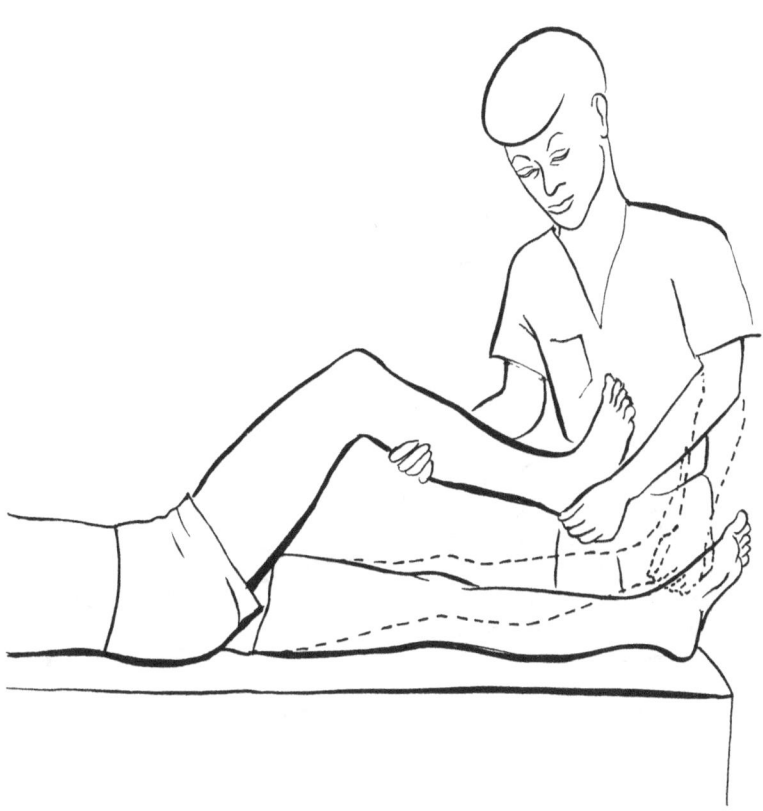

Apley Compression Test

Description

The patient lies prone. The examiner flexes the patient's knee to 90°. The examiner then grasps the patient's foot with both hands and performs forceful compression through the foot to the knee joint. Simultaneously, the examiner performs internal and external rotation of the tibia.

Interpretation

A positive test is one in which pain is elicited with "clicking" or "snapping," indicating meniscal tear.

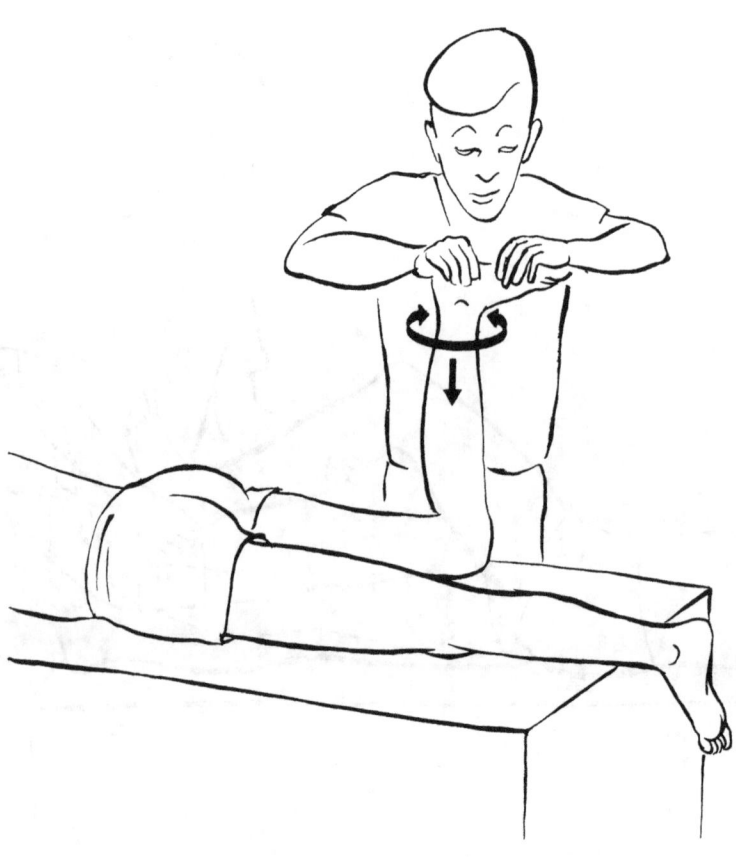

Steinmann Test

Description

The patient sits on the edge of the treatment table with knee flexed to 90°. The examiner holds the patient's distal tibiofibula with one hand and the proximal tibiofibula with the other hand. The examiner first rotates the tibia externally and then internally.

Interpretation

A positive test is one in which pain is elicited on internal and external rotation of the tibia, indicating meniscal tear.

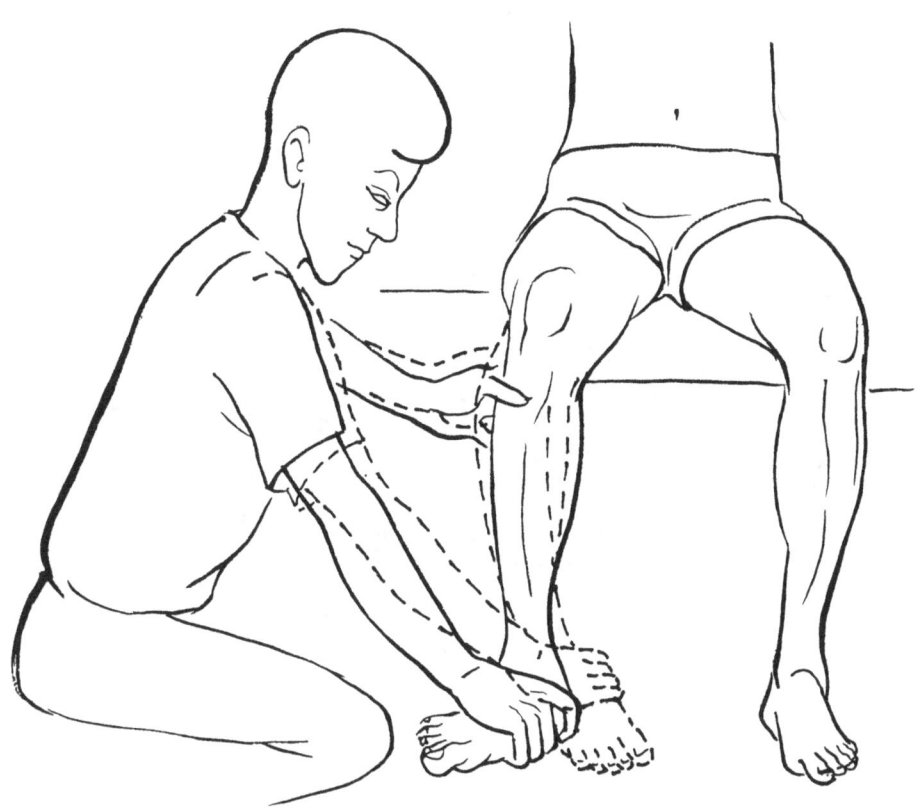

Spring Test

Description

The patient lies supine with knees extended. The examiner stabilizes the patient's distal femur with one hand and with the other hand grasps the distal tibiofibula and attempts to extend the patient's knee forcefully.

Interpretation

A positive test is one in which the forceful extension is inhibited, indicating a displaced meniscus.

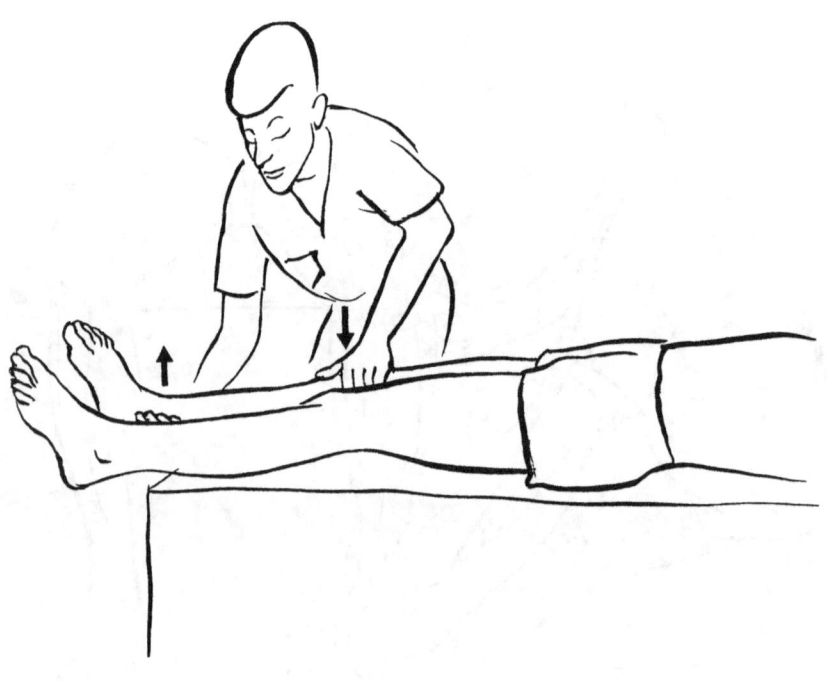

Steinmann Tenderness Displacement Test

Description

The patient sits on the edge of the treatment table with knee flexed to 90°. The patient is instructed to first fully extend the knee and then to flex the knee past 90°.

Interpretation

A positive test is one in which the tenderness moves anteriorly as the knee is extended and posteriorly as the knee is flexed, indicating meniscal tear.

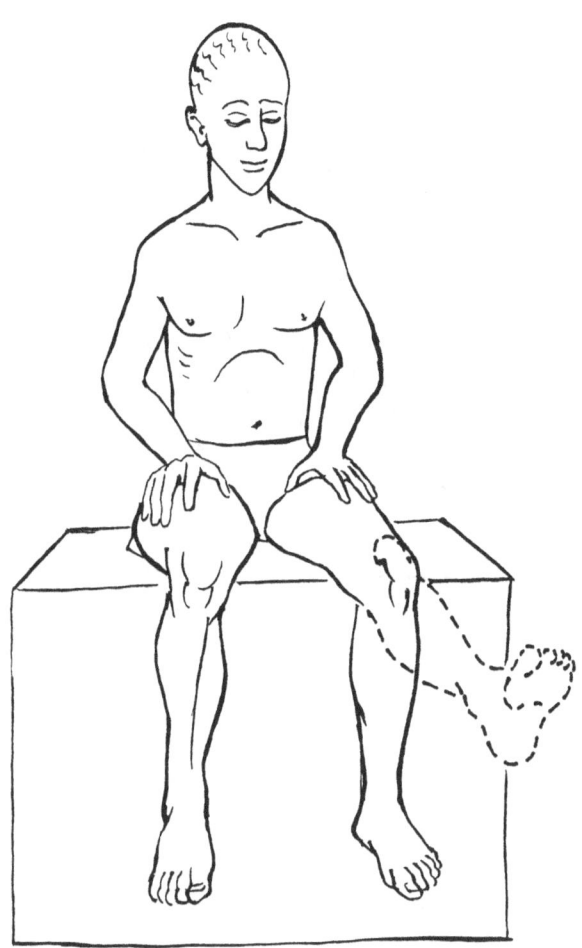

Hyperflexion Meniscus Test

Description
The patient lies prone. The examiner holds the patient's distal tibiofibula and hyperflexes the knee with tibiofibula either externally or internally rotated.

Interpretation
A positive test is one which causes a painful click, indicating meniscal lesion.

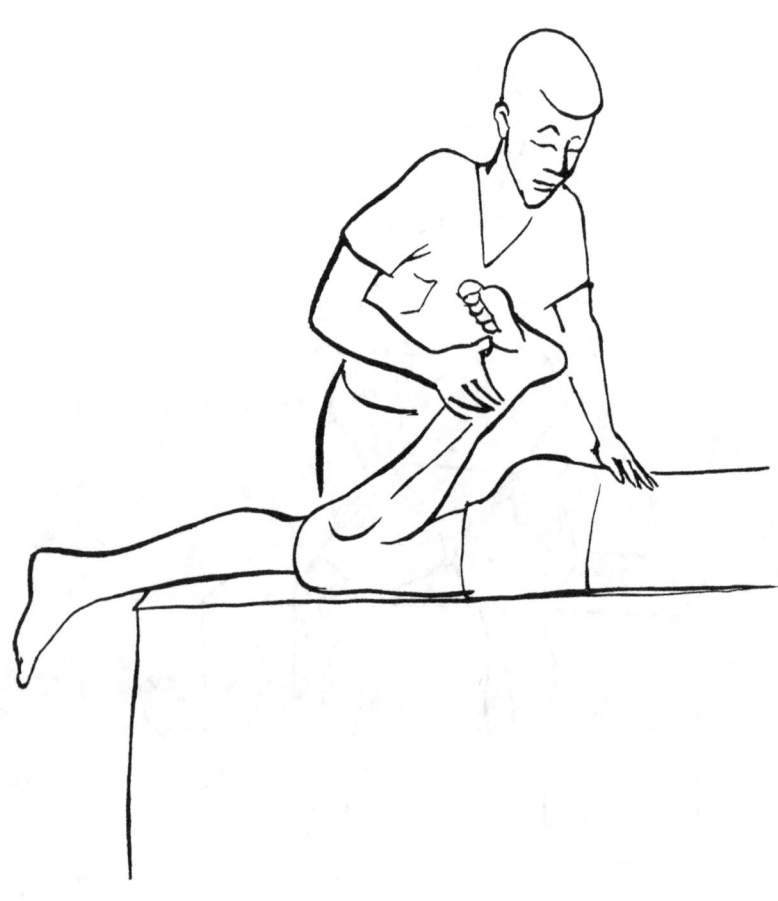

Cabot Popliteal Test

Description

The patient lies supine. The examiner positions the patient's leg in the figure four position. The examiner holds the patient's lower leg proximal to the ankle with one hand and palpates the joint line with the thumb and index finger of the other hand. The patient is then instructed to extend the knee while the examiner resists the movement.

Interpretation

A positive test is one in which pain is produced at the knee joint line, indicating lesion in the meniscus.

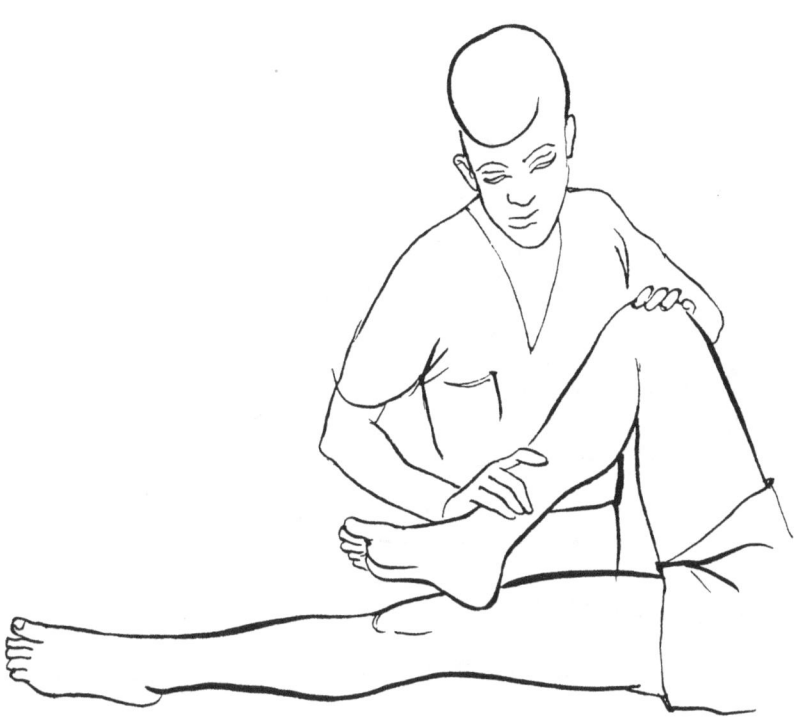

Payr Test

Description

The patient lies supine. The examiner holds the patient's lower leg distal to the ankle and flexes the patient's knee, then abducts and externally rotates the hip. With the other hand the examiner then applies a gentle over pressure at the knee forcing it toward the table.

Interpretation

A positive test is one in which pain is produced in the medial aspect of the knee, indicating torn medial meniscus.

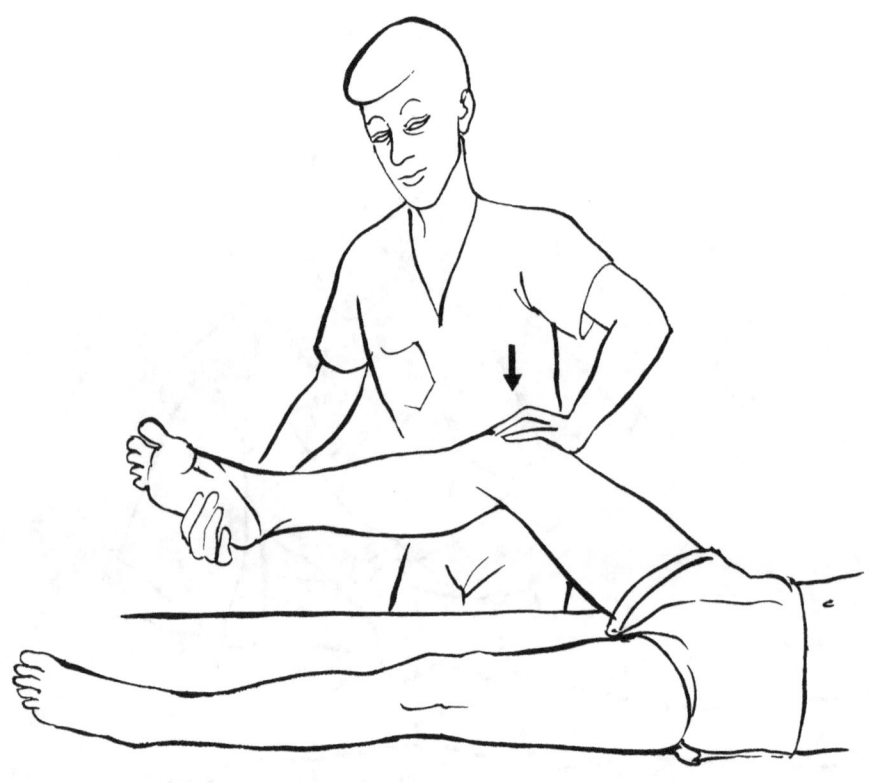

McMurray Test

Description

The patient lies supine. The examiner grasps the bottom of the patient's foot with one hand and palpates the knee joint lines with the other hand. The examiner then fully flexes the patient's knee and externally rotates the tibia while applying a valgus force. While maintaining the valgus force and external rotation the examiner extends the patient's knee.

Interpretation

A positive test is one in which a palpable or audible "popping" is elicited in the joint, indicating a posterior tear of the medial meniscus.

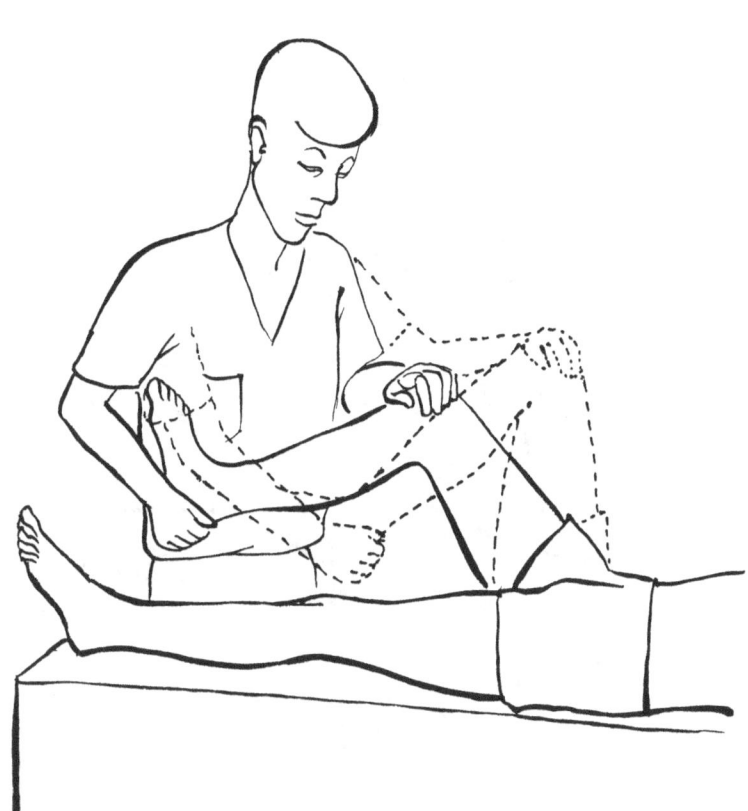

Bohler Test

Description

The patient lies supine. The examiner stabilizes the patient's knee with one hand and holds the distal tibiofibula with the other hand. The examiner then applies varus and valgus stresses to the patient's knee.

Interpretation

A positive test is one in which pain is produced laterally on valgus stress, indicating lesion in the lateral meniscus, and medially on varus stress, indicating lesion in the medial meniscus.

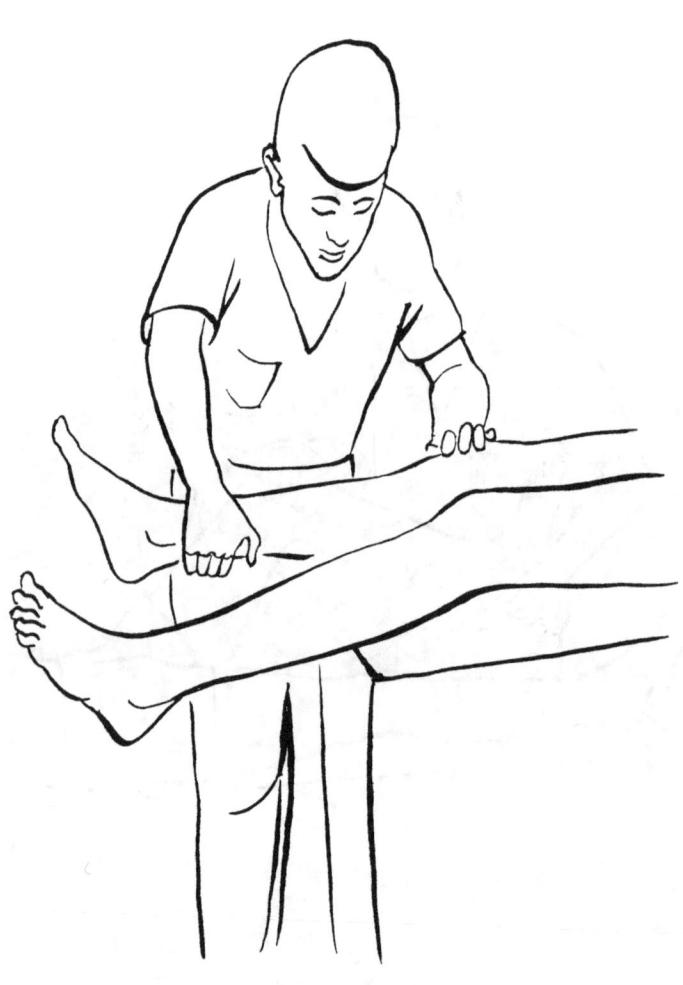

Bragard Test

Description

The patient lies supine. The examiner grasps the bottom of the patient's foot with one hand and holds the distal femur with the other hand. The examiner flexes the patient's knee and externally rotates the tibia. The examiner then extends the patient's knee.

Interpretation

A positive test is one in which pain and tenderness are produced on the medial joint line which decreases on medial rotation of the tibia and flexion of the knee, indicating lesion in the medial meniscus.

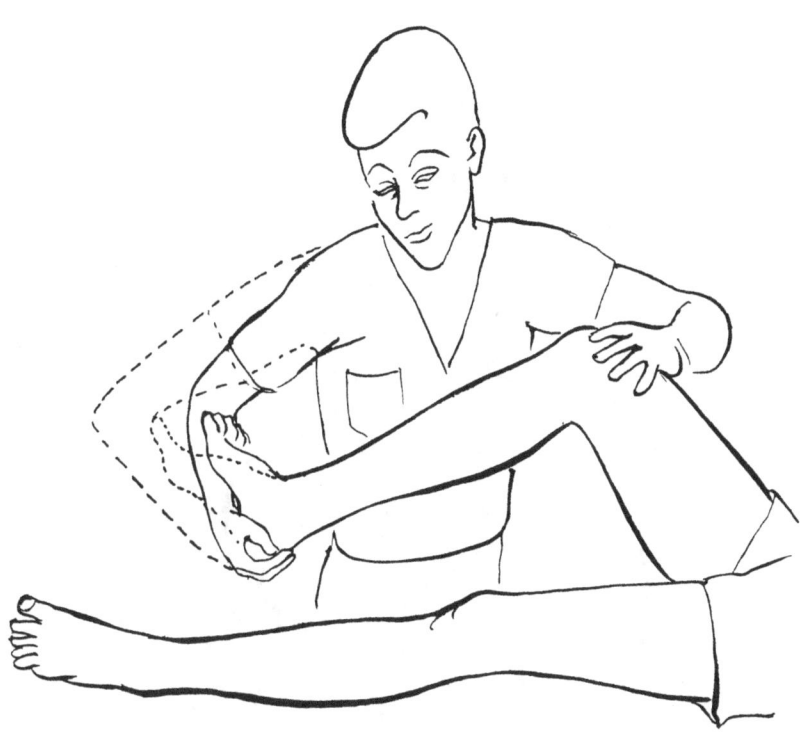

Retracting Meniscal Test

Description

The patient lies supine with knee and hip flexed to 90°. The examiner places one finger over the patient's knee joint line anterior to the medial collateral ligament. The examiner holds the patient's distal lower leg and then passively rotates the patient's tibia internally and externally several times.

Interpretation

A positive test is one in which the meniscus does not disappear under the examiner's finger, indicating a torn medial meniscus.

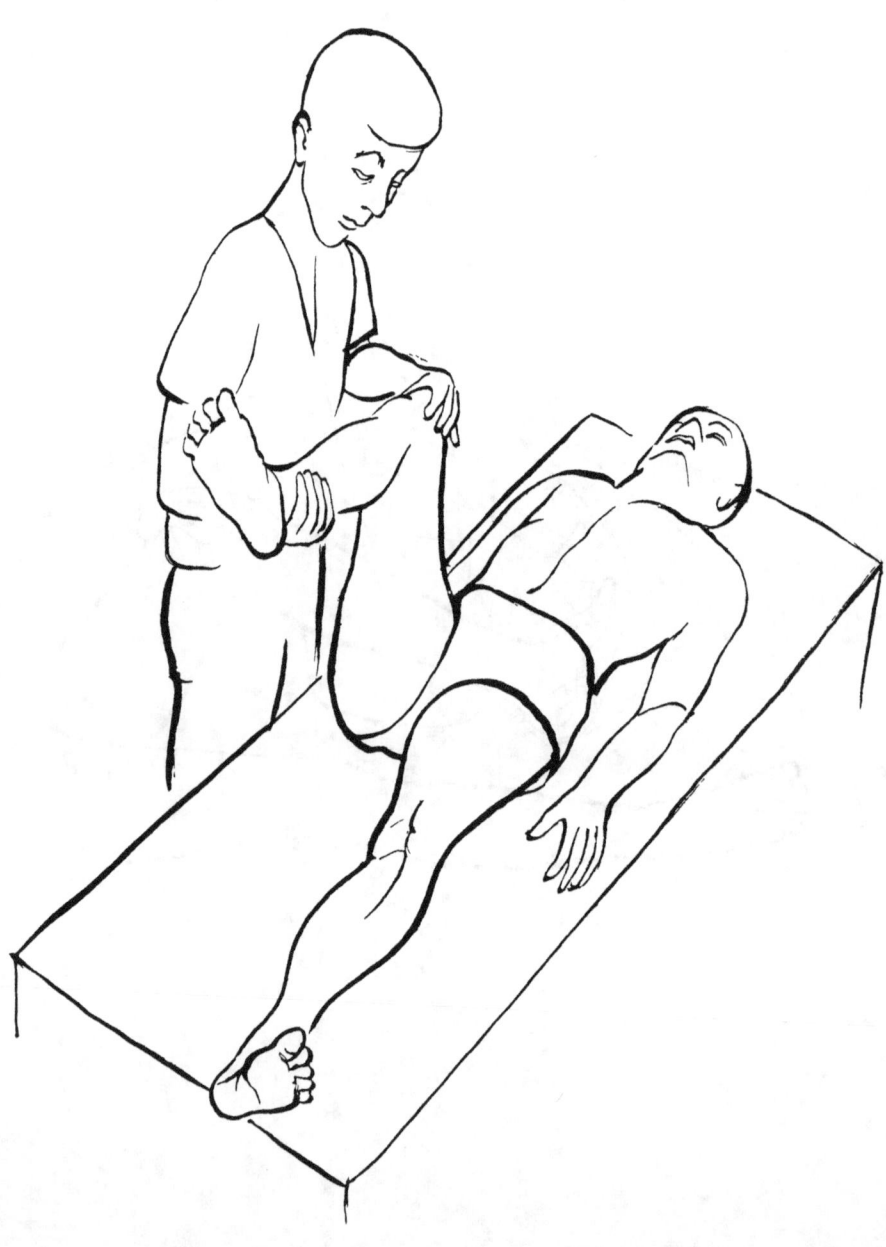

O'Donoghue Test

Description

The patient lies supine. The examiner grasps the bottom of the patient's foot with one hand and with the other hand holds the proximal tibiofibula. The examiner flexes the patient's knee to 90° and rotates the tibia internally and externally twice. The examiner then fully flexes the knee and rotates it both ways again.

Interpretation

A positive test is one in which pain is increased on rotation in either or both positions, indicating either a capsule irritation or a meniscus tear.

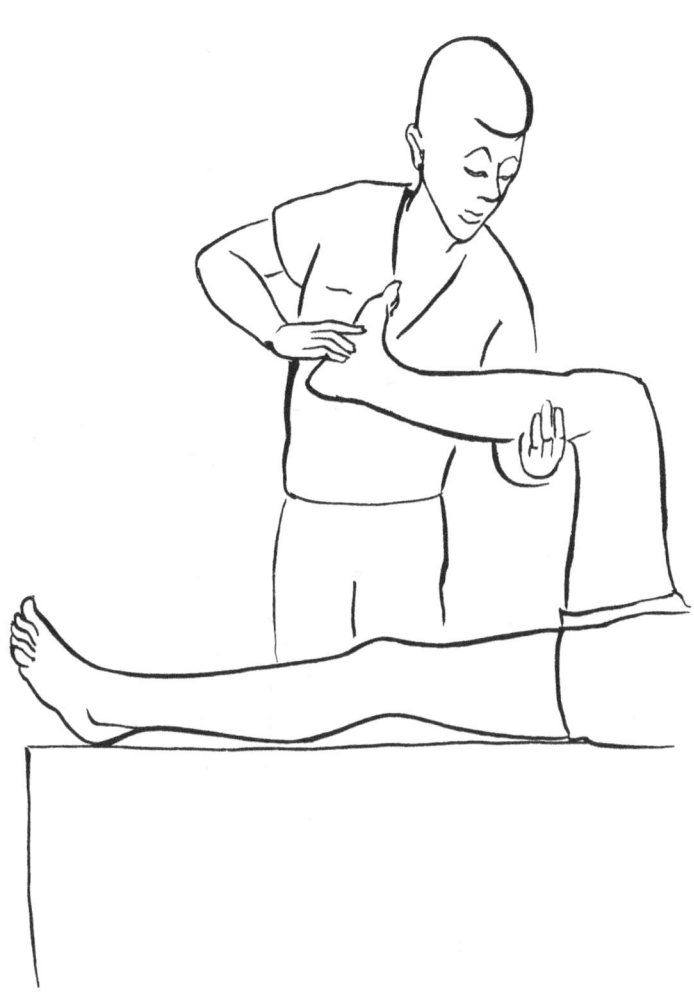

Helfet Test

Description

The patient sits with the involved leg hanging over the edge of the table. The examiner notices the position of the tibial tuberosity relative to the anterior ridge of the lateral femoral condyle. The patient is then instructed to repeatedly flex and fully extend the knee through 45°. The examiner again notices the position of the tibial tuberosity relative to the anterior ridge of the lateral femoral condyle.

Interpretation

A positive test is one in which the tibia does not externally rotate as the knee is extended, indicating a blocked rotation due to injury to the meniscus or the cruciate ligament.

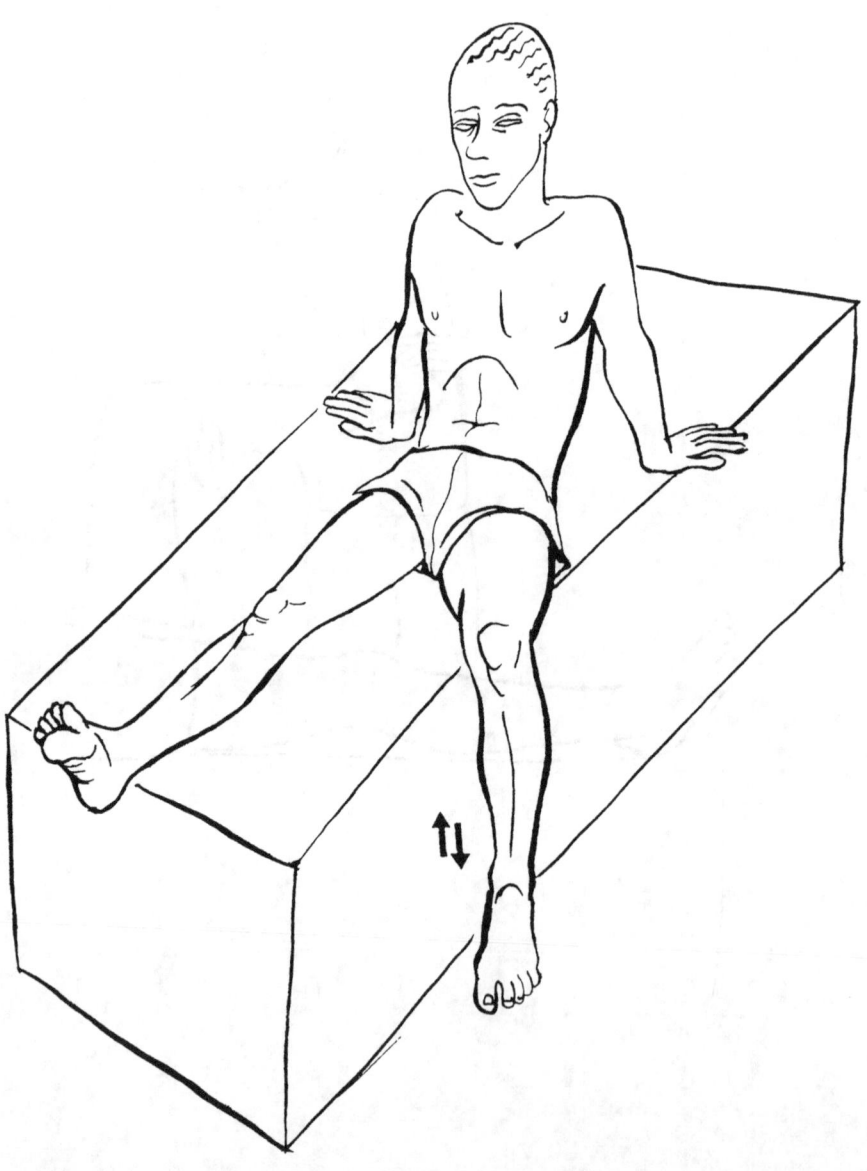

Nakajima Test

Description

The patient lies supine. The examiner holds the patient's distal lower leg with one hand and internally rotates the tibia. The examiner places the other hand over the patient's lateral femoral condyle while the thumb is placed behind the head of the fibula and pushes it forward. The examiner then slowly extends the knee while continuing to push the head of the fibula forward.

Interpretation

A positive test is one in which excessive movement of the tibia and fibula occurs, indicating subluxation of tibia and fibula.

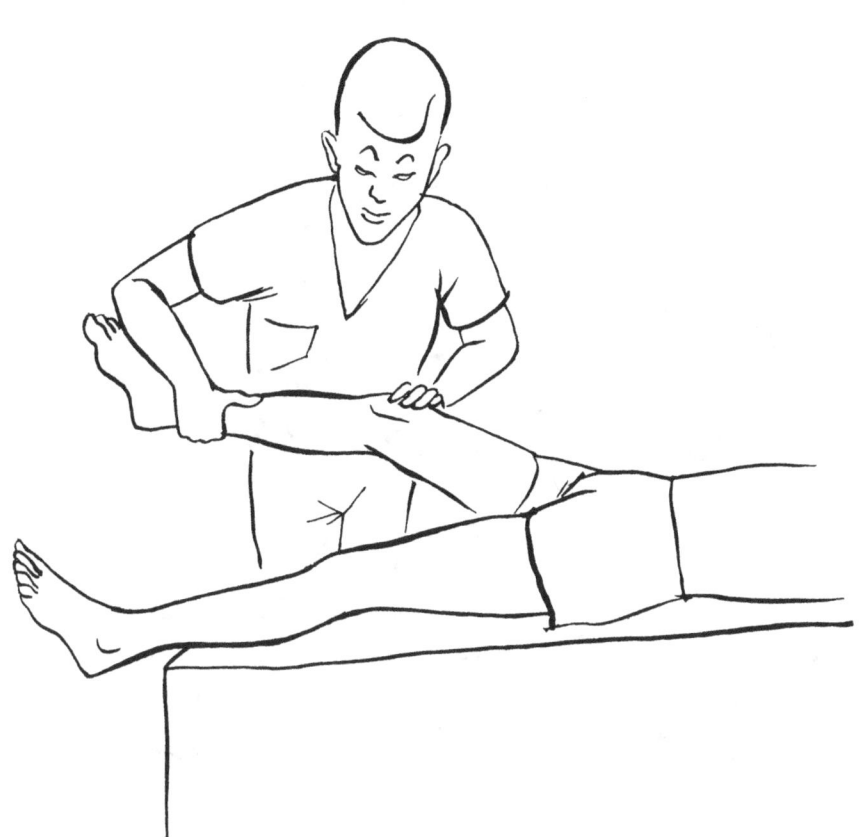

Martens Test

Description
The patient lies supine. The examiner stabilizes the patient's lower leg by holding the patient's ankle between the examiner's trunk and arm. With the hand of the stabilizing arm, the examiner grasps the proximal tibiofibula and applies valgus stress to the knee while pushing the femur posteriorly with the other hand.

Interpretation
A positive test is one in which excessive movement of the tibia and fibula occurs, indicating subluxation of tibia and fibula.

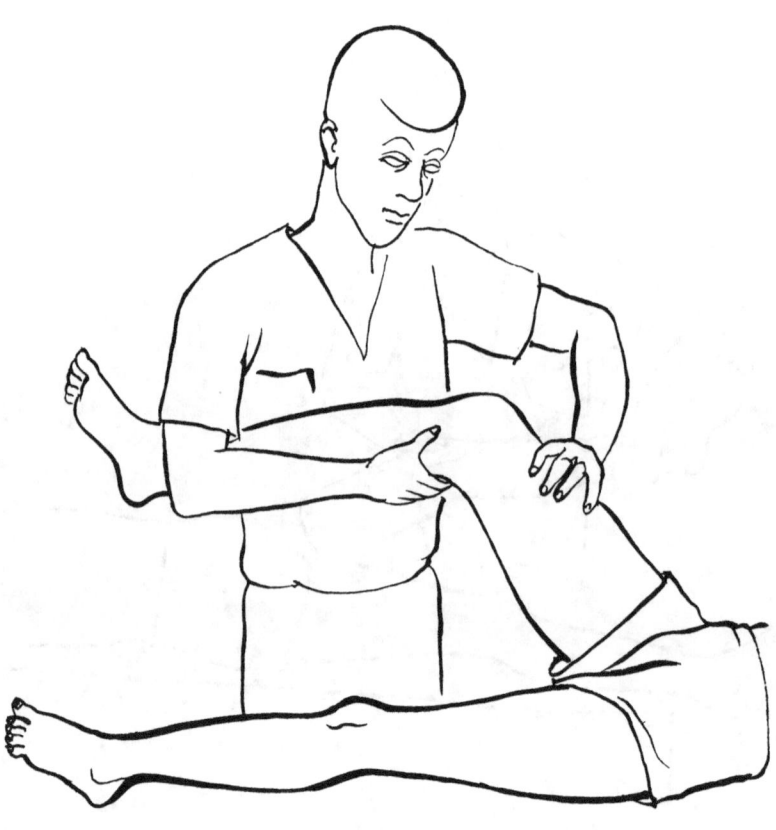

Apley Distraction Test

Description

The patient lies prone. The examiner flexes the patient's knee to 90°. The examiner stabilizes the patient's posterior thigh with the examiner's knee, grasps the patient's distal tibiofibula with both hands, and applies traction through the foot to the knee joint. Simultaneously, the examiner performs internal and external rotation of the tibia.

Interpretation

A positive test is one in which pain is elicited, indicating ligamentous damage.

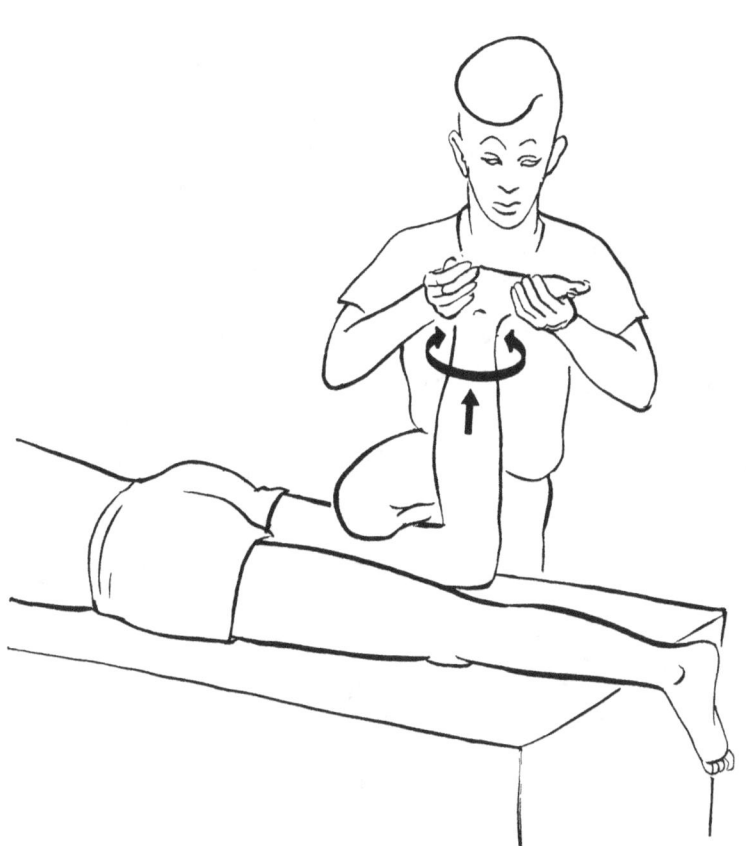

Lachman Test

Description

The patient sits on the table with the involved knee flexed to 20° and the hip in external rotation. The examiner stabilizes the patient's distal femur with one hand and with the other hand applies a firm anterior pressure on the proximal tibia.

Interpretation

A positive test is one in which excessive anterior tibial movement is produced with a soft end-feel, indicating anterior cruciate ligament injury.

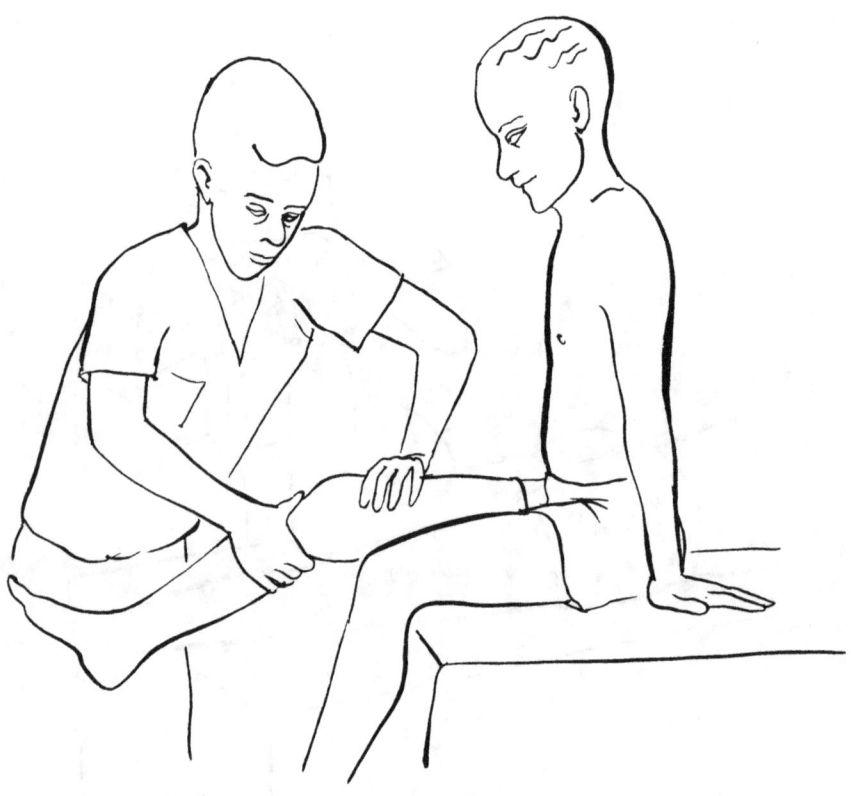

Dynamic Extension Test

Description

This is a dynamic Lachman Test. The patient lies supine with knee extended. The examiner places a closed fist under the patient's distal femur. After complete quadricep muscles relaxation, the patient is instructed to raise the leg, then let it fall back onto the examiner's fist and relax the muscles.

Interpretation

A positive test is one in which excessive anterior tibial movement is produced as the leg is rested back on the fist, indicating anterior cruciate ligament laxity.

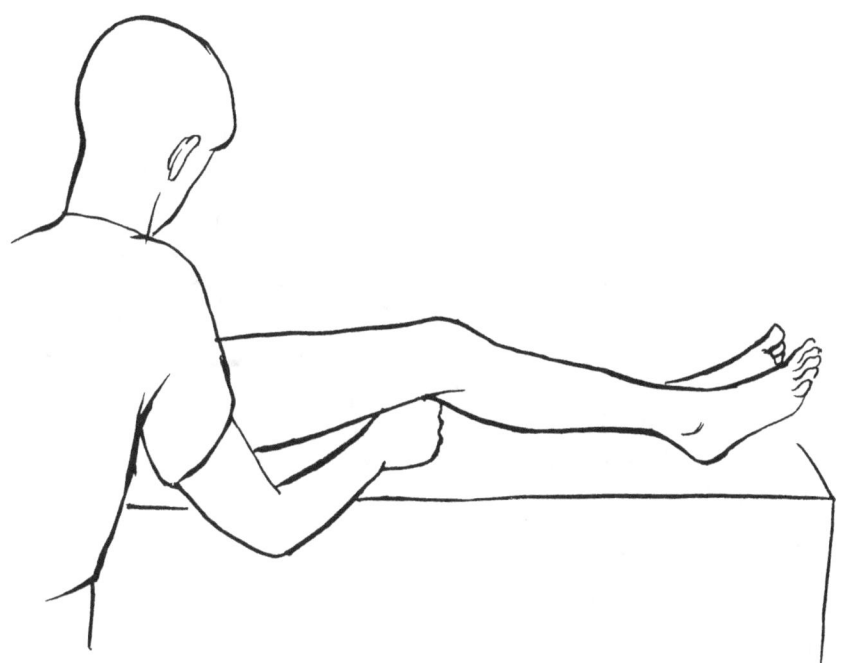

Anterior Drawer Test

Description

The patient sits with knee flexed to 90°. The examiner places the thumbs on the anteromedial and anterolateral joint lines with the fingers circling the proximal lower leg at the level of the gastrocnemius insertions. The examiner then applies a firm anterior pressure on the tibia.

Interpretation

A positive test is one in which the proximal tibia displaces anteriorly, indicating instability of the anterior cruciate ligament.

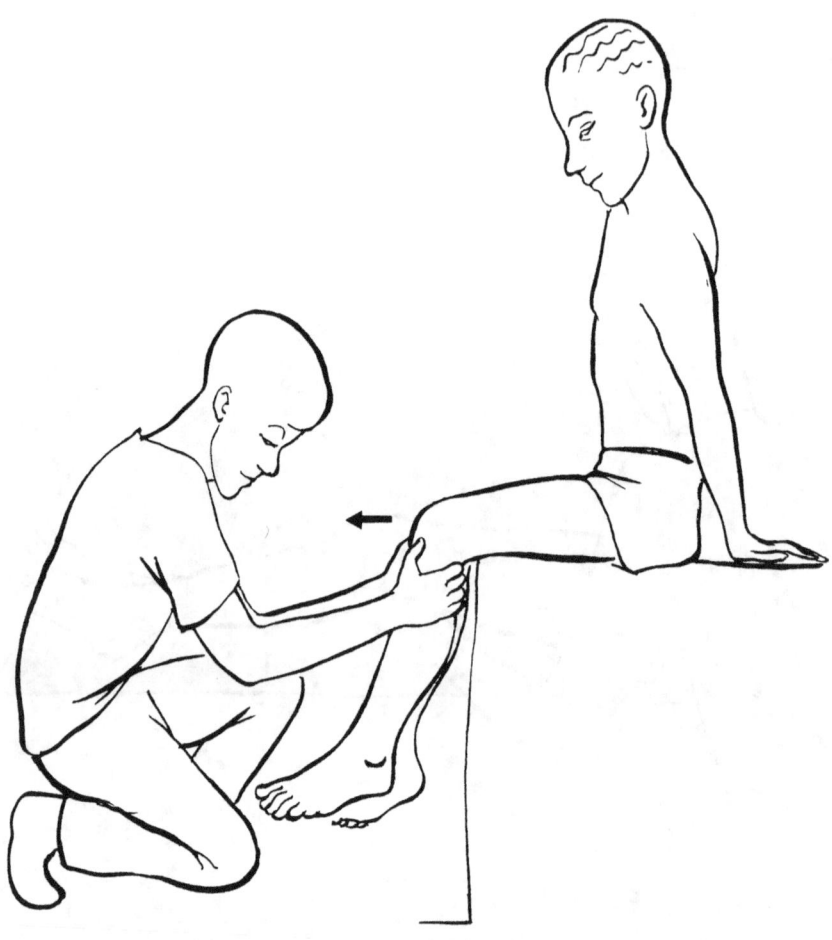

Hyperextension Recurvatum Test

Description

The patient lies supine. The examiner holds the patient's heels and lifts the legs above the table. The examiner views the patient's knees from the side and notes the degree of knee extension and external rotation of tibia on the femur.

Interpretation

A positive test is one in which the knee extends beyond a straight line into a position of recurvatum, indicating injury to the anterior cruciate ligament and posterior lateral corner of the knee.

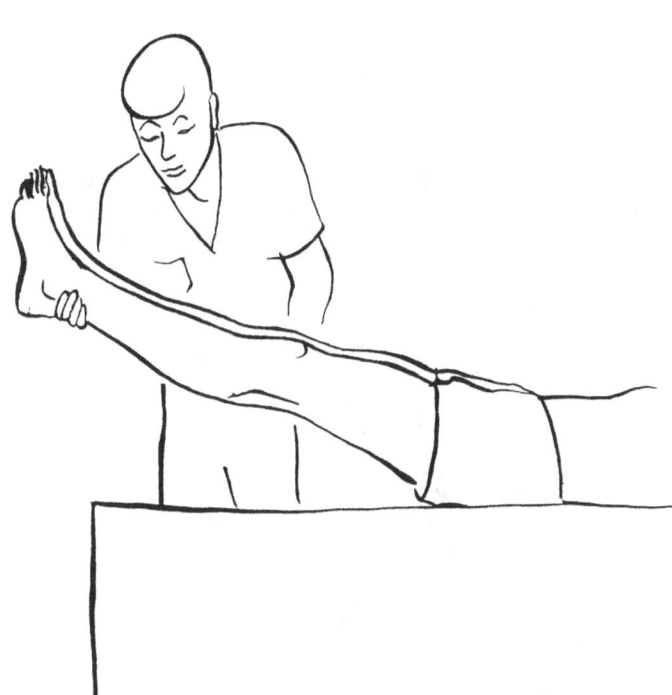

External Rotational Recurvatum Test

Description
The patient lies supine with quadricep and hamstring muscles relaxed. The examiner grasps the patient's great toes of both feet and raises the legs up from the table.

Interpretation
A positive test is one in which a knee goes into excessive recurvatum, indicating anterior cruciate ligament (ACL) deficiency. An excessive recurvatum with the tibial tubercle sagging posteriorly and relating externally indicates ACL insufficiency plus arcuate complex insufficiency.

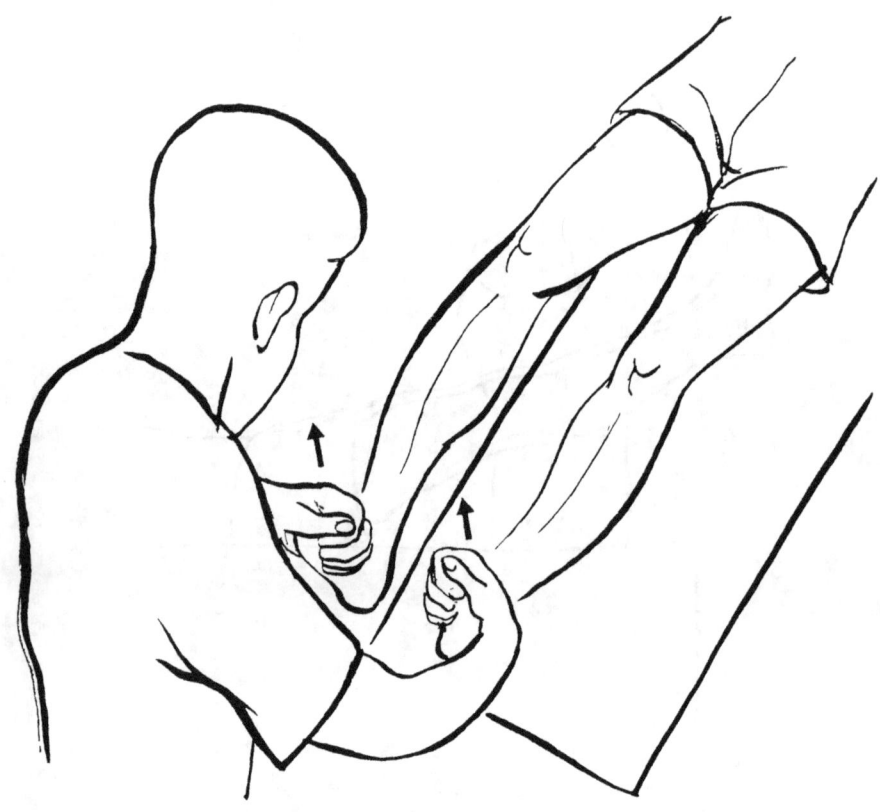

Flexion Rotation Drawer Test

Description

The patient lies supine. The examiner holds the patient's tibiofibula in neutral position with the knee flexed to approximately 20°. With the tibiofibula held in stable position, the thigh is permitted to fall posteriorly and rotate externally.

Interpretation

A positive test is one in which the femur moves posteriorly more than 3 mm, indicating anterior cruciate ligament laxity in both translation and rotation.

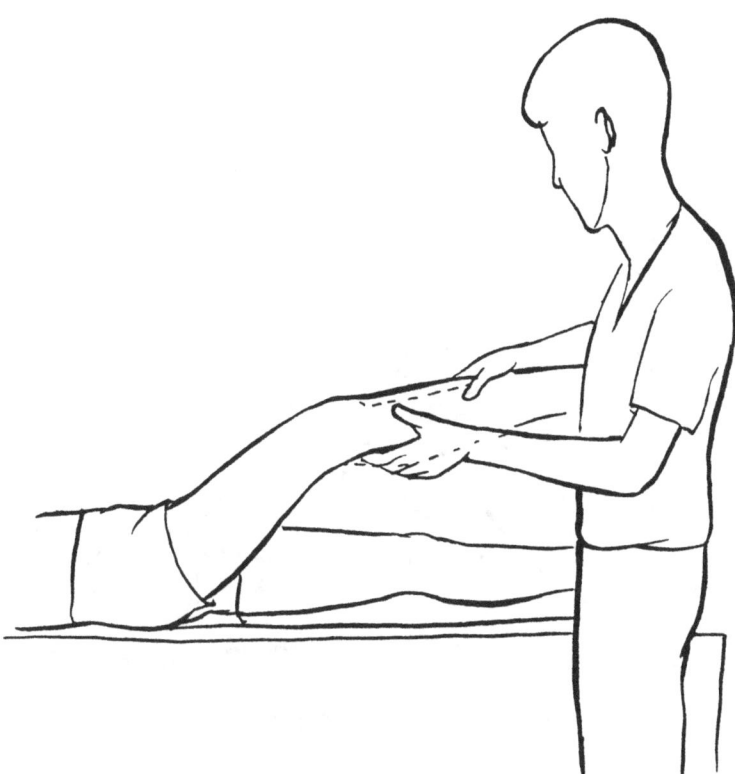

Posterior Drawer Test

Description

The patient lies supine with the involved knee flexed to 90°. The examiner places the thumbs on the anteromedial and anterolateral joint lines with the fingers circling the proximal lower leg at the level of the gastrocnemius insertions. The examiner then applies a firm posterior pressure on the tibia.

Interpretation

A positive test is one in which the proximal tibia displaces posteriorly, indicating instability of the posterior cruciate ligament.

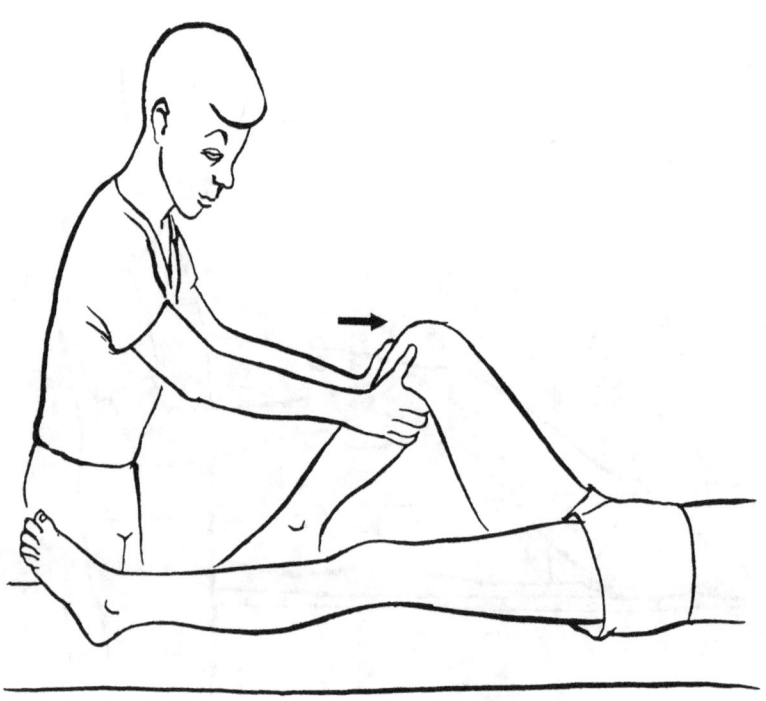

Abduction Stress Test

Description

The patient lies supine. The examiner grasps the patient's distal tibiofibula with one hand and with the other hand holds the proximal tibiofibula. The examiner then flexes the patient's knee to about 25° and applies a valgus stress. The examiner palpates the medial knee joint when applying the valgus stress.

Interpretation

A positive test is one in which the tibia excessively moves away from the femur, indicating medial instability of the knee due to medial collateral ligament injury.

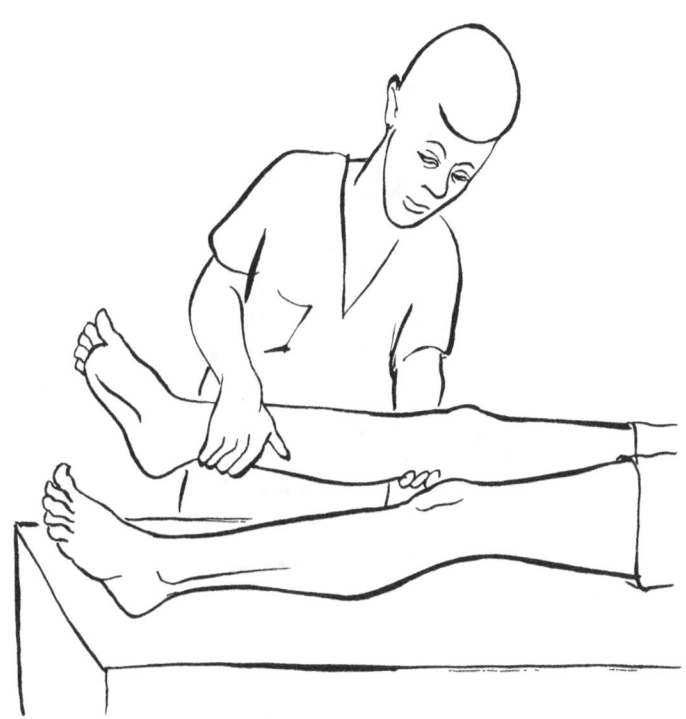

Adduction Stress Test

Description

The patient lies supine. The examiner grasps the patient's distal tibiofibula with one hand and with the other hand holds the distal femur. The examiner then flexes the patient's knee to about 25° and applies a varus stress. The examiner palpates the lateral knee joint when applying the varus stress.

Interpretation

A positive test is one in which the tibia excessively moves away from the femur, indicating lateral instability of the knee due to lateral collateral ligament injury.

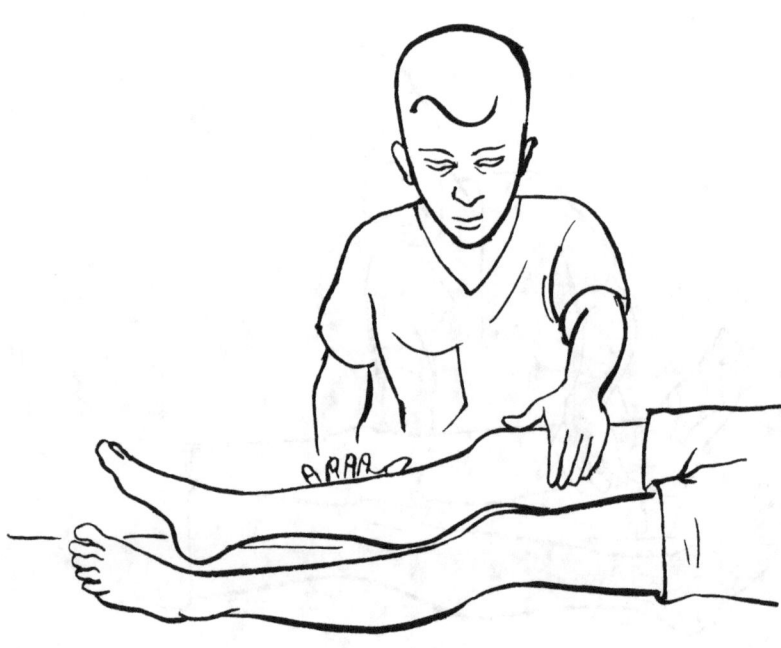

MacIntosh Test

Description

The patient lies supine with hips and knees extended. The examiner grasps the patient's distal tibiofibula with one hand and places the other hand over the distal, lateral aspect of the femur. The examiner applies a valgus stress to the knee while internally rotating the tibia. The examiner then flexes the patient's knee to approximately 60° to 70°.

Interpretation

A positive test is one in which a sudden jump is produced as the lateral tibial plateau suddenly subluxates at 20° to 40° of flexion and then falls back after this point, indicating anterolateral rotatory instability.

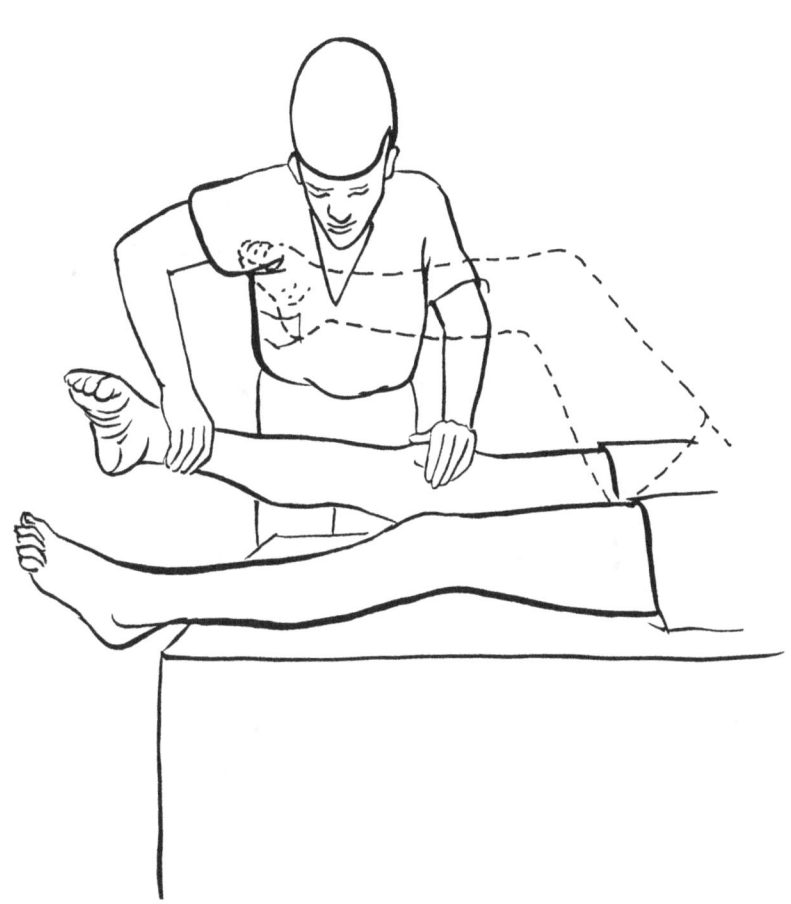

Pivot Jerk Test

Description

The patient lies on the uninvolved side. The examiner supports the patient's lower leg and flexes the hip to 45° and the knee to about 90° while at the same time internally rotating the tibia. The examiner then exerts a valgus stress to the knee with one hand and gradually extends the knee while maintaining the internal rotation and valgus stress.

Interpretation

A positive test is one in which a subluxation of the lateral femoral condyle on the tibia occurs at about 20° of knee flexion and with further extension a spontaneous relocation occurs, indicating anterolateral rotatory instability of the knee.

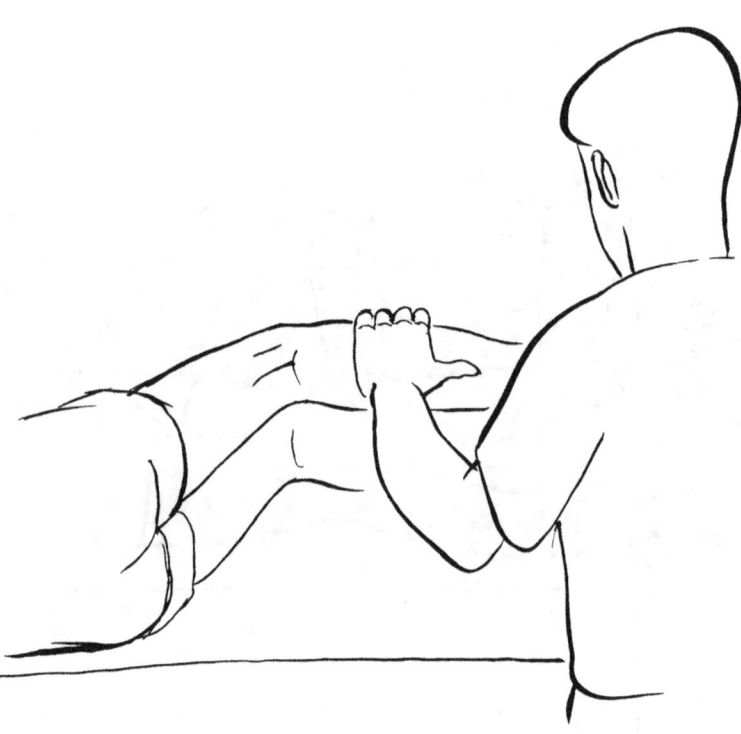

Slocum Test

Description

The patient lies supine with the involved knee flexed to 90° and hip flexed to 45°. The examiner holds the patient's proximal tibiofibula and internally rotates the patient's tibia to 30°. The examiner then applies an anterior force on the tibia.

Interpretation

A positive test is one in which the tibia moves primarily on the lateral side, indicating anterolateral instability of the knee.

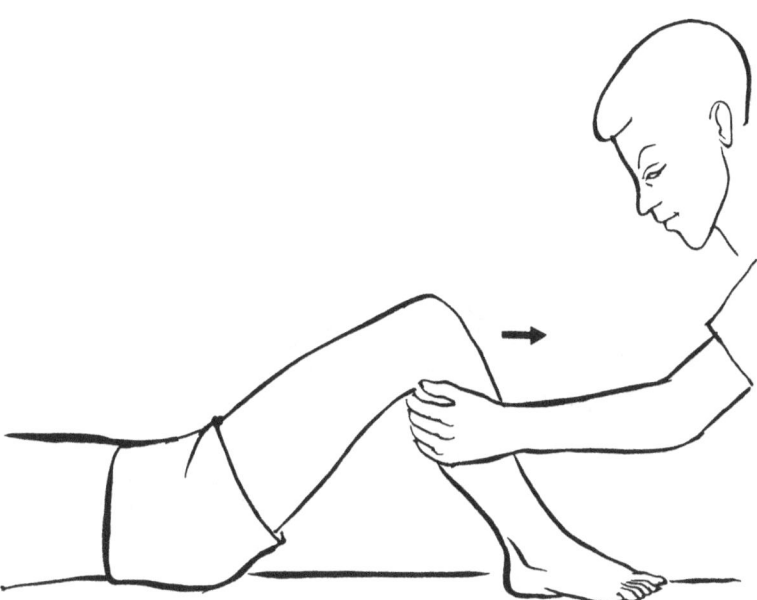

Slocum ALRI Test

Description

The patient lies on the uninvolved side with the uninvolved hip and knee flexed to 45°. The examiner grasps the patient's involved proximal tibiofibula with one hand and holds the distal femur with the other hand. The examiner moves the foot of the patient's involved leg to rest on the table in internal rotation with the knee in extension. The examiner then applies a valgus stress to the knee while flexing the knee.

Interpretation

A positive test is one in which the subluxation of the knee is reduced between 25° and 45° of flexion, indicating anterolateral rotatory instability.

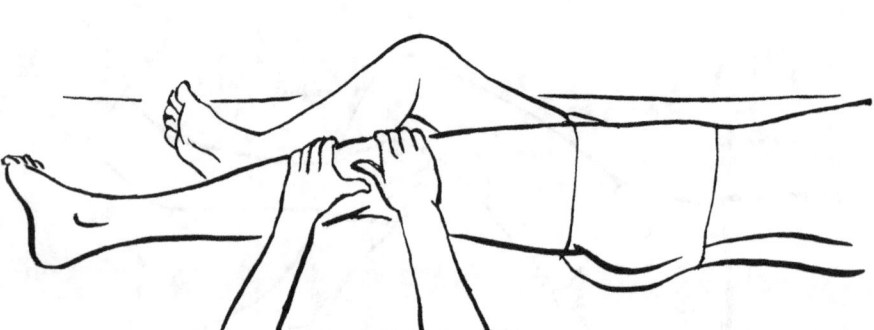

Losee Test

Description

The patient lies supine. The examiner holds the patient's distal tibiofibula with one hand. The examiner then externally rotates the leg and braces it against the abdomen. While the patient's hamstring muscles are relaxed, the examiner flexes the patient's knee to 30°. The examiner then positions the other hand so that the fingers lie over the patella and the thumb is hooked behind the fibular head. The examiner then extends the patient's knee while pushing the fibula anteriorly with the thumb and applies a valgus stress to the knee, allowing the tibia to rotate externally during extension.

Interpretation

A positive test is one in which the lateral tibial plateau subluxes anteriorly just before full extension of the knee, indicating anterolateral rotatory instability of the knee.

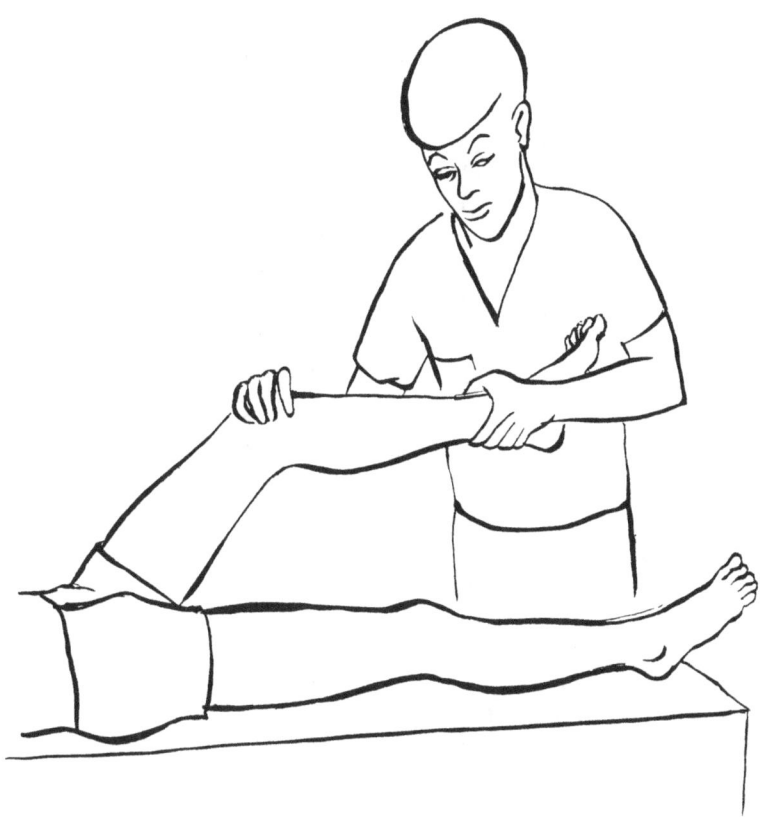

Cross-over Test

Description

The patient stands. The examiner secures the foot of the patient's involved leg by carefully stepping on it, then instructs the patient to cross the uninvolved leg in front of the involved leg. The patient is instructed to rotate the upper torso away from the involved leg as far as possible and then to contract the quadricep muscles.

Interpretation

A positive test is one in which the patient gets a feeling of the knee "giving way," indicating anterolateral instability of the knee.

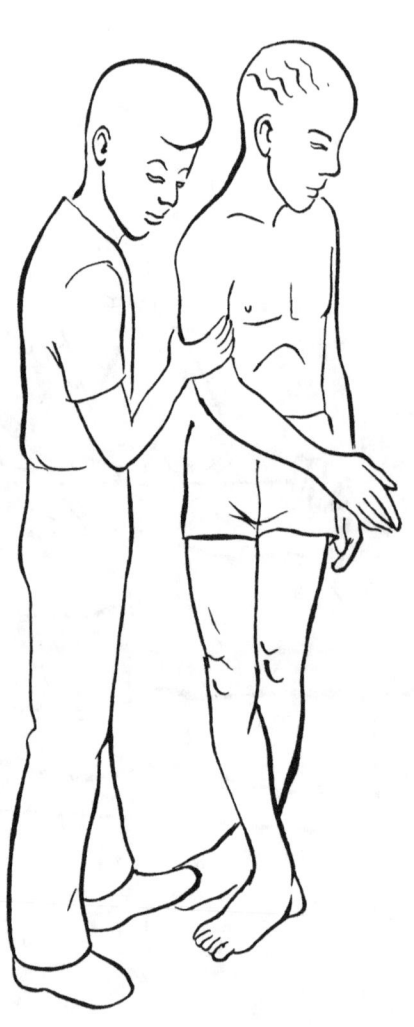

Pivot Shift Test

Description

The patient lies supine. The examiner supports the patient's tibiofibula proximally just behind the fibular head with one hand and with the other hand holds the bottom of the patient's foot. The examiner flexes the patient's knee to approximately 5° and then subluxes the tibia by internally rotating with both hands. The examiner then flexes the knee to about 90° with slight valgus stress.

Interpretation

A positive test is one in which a sudden shift of the tibia on the femur is experienced between 20° and 40° of flexion, indicating anterolateral instability of the knee.

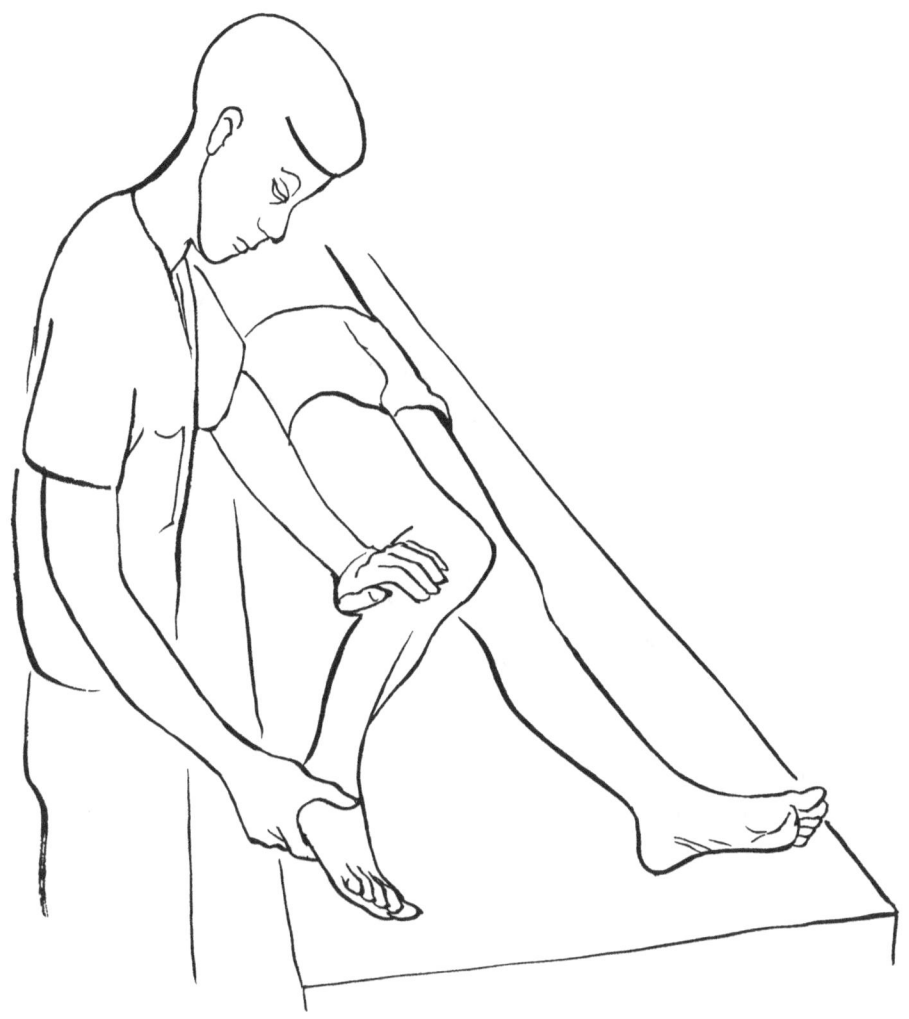

Arcuate Spin Test

Description

The patient lies supine. The examiner holds the patient's leg at the distal tibiofibula with one hand and with the other hand holds the proximal tibiofibula. The examiner flexes the patient's knee to 90°, applies force posteriorly at the proximal tibia, and externally rotates the tibia.

Interpretation

A positive test is one in which the tibia excessively externally rotates on the femur, indicating posterolateral instability.

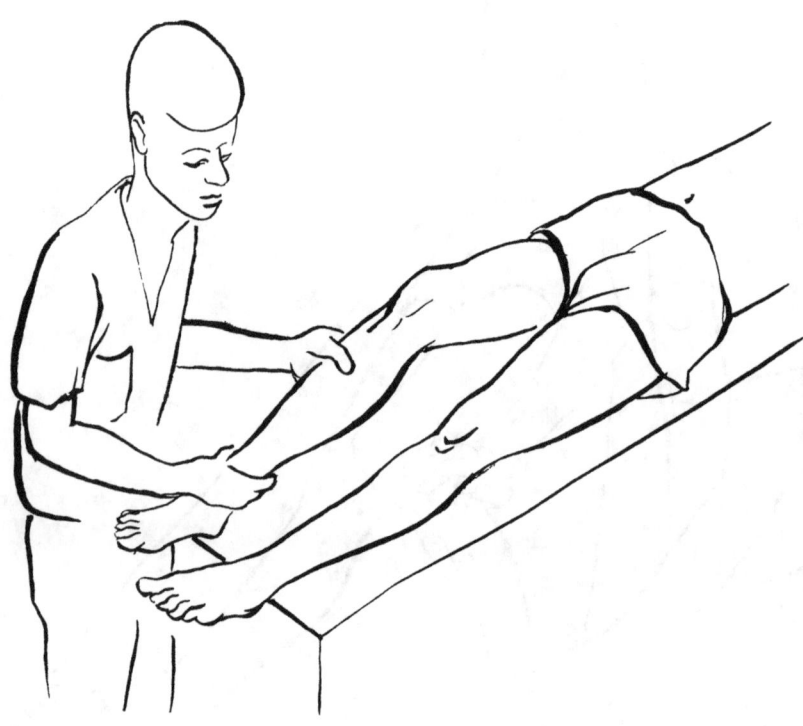

Jakob Test

Description

The patient lies supine with hamstring muscles relaxed. The examiner stands at the foot end of the patient, flexes the patient's knee to 70°-80° and supports the patient's foot against the examiner's pelvis. The examiner then places one hand over the proximal tibiofibula laterally and with the other hand holds the patient's ankle. The examiner externally rotates the patient's foot causing the lateral tibial plateau to sublux posteriorly. The knee is then taken into extension by its own weight while the examiner leans on the foot to impart a valgus stress to the knee through the leg.

Interpretation

A positive test is one in which, as the knee approaches 20° of flexion, the lateral tibial tubercle shifts anteriorly into the neutral rotation and reduces the subluxation, indicating a posterolateral rotatory instability of the knee.

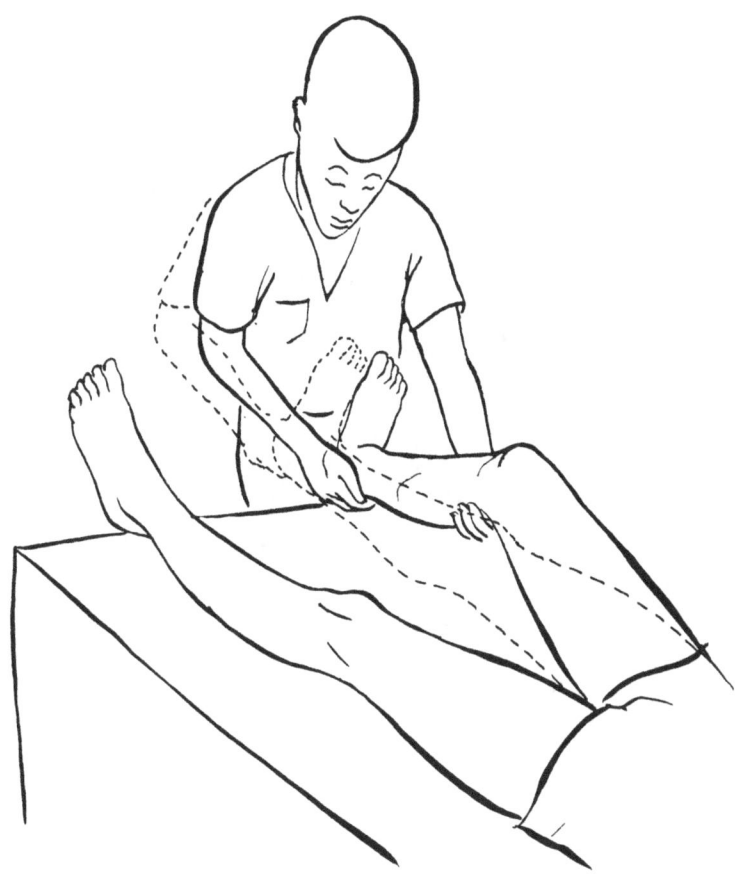

Q-Angle (Patellofemoral Angle) Test

Description

The patient lies supine with knees extended. The examiner draws one line along the axis of the mid-patella to the anterior superior iliac spine and a second line between the tibial tubercle and the mid-patella intersecting the first line. The examiner then measures the angle. The normal range for Q-angle is 15° for males and 20° for females.

Interpretation

A positive test is one in which the angle is high, indicating an increased potential for lateral subluxation of the patella. A low angle indicates an increased potential for medial subluxation of the patella from the femoral sulcus during muscle contraction.

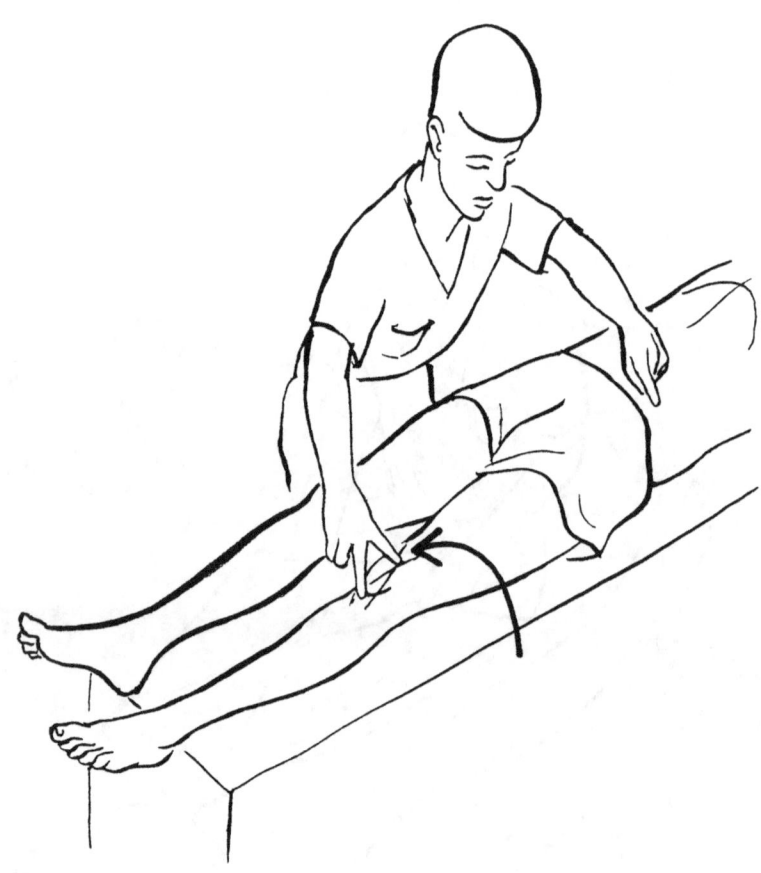

Wilson Test

Description

The patient lies supine with the involved knee and hip flexed to 90°. The examiner stabilizes the patient's knee at proximal tibiofibula with one hand and holds the distal tibiofibula with the other hand. The examiner internally rotates the tibia on the femur and then extends the knee slowly with the tibia maintained in the internal rotation.

Interpretation

A positive test is one in which pain is elicited at about 30° of knee flexion, indicating a lesion on the medial femoral condyle. The pain can often be immediately relieved by externally rotating the tibia while the same position of flexion-extension is maintained.

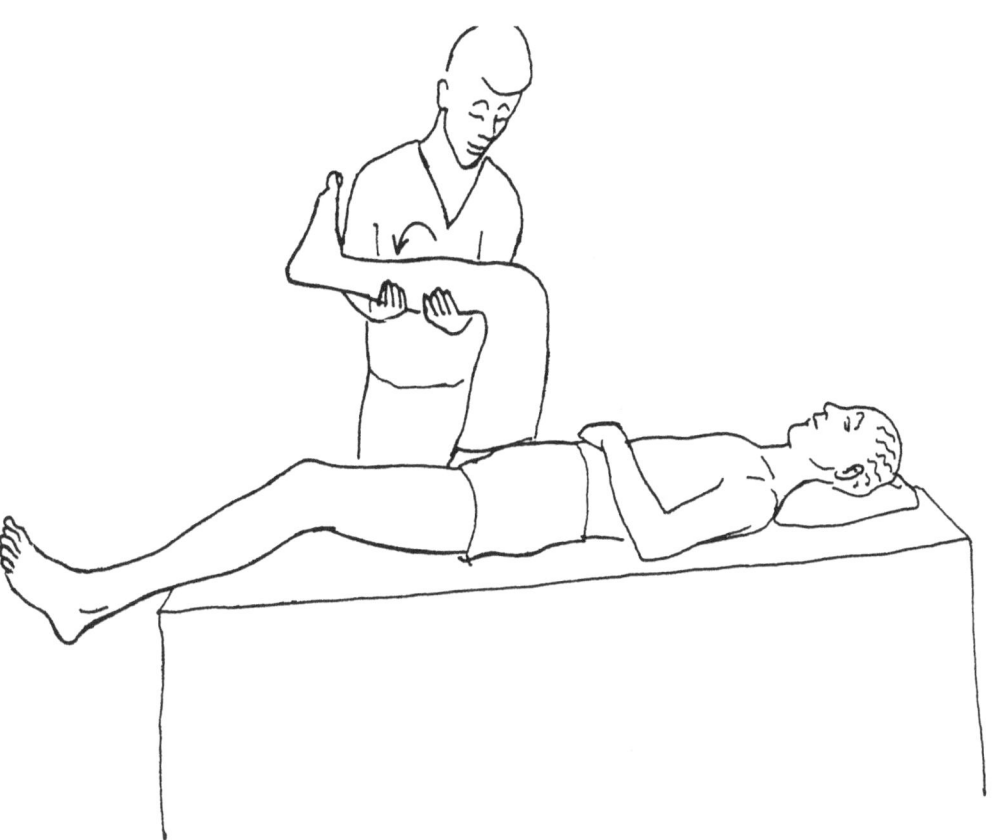

Section 6
Ankle and Foot

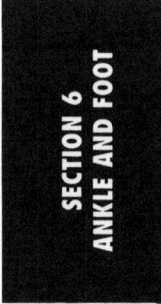

Modified Romberg Test

Description

The patient stands. The patient is instructed to first stand on the uninvolved foot with the eyes open and then with the eyes closed. The test is then repeated on the involved side.

Interpretation

A positive test is one in which the patient is unable to stand on the involved foot, indicating proprioceptive defect.

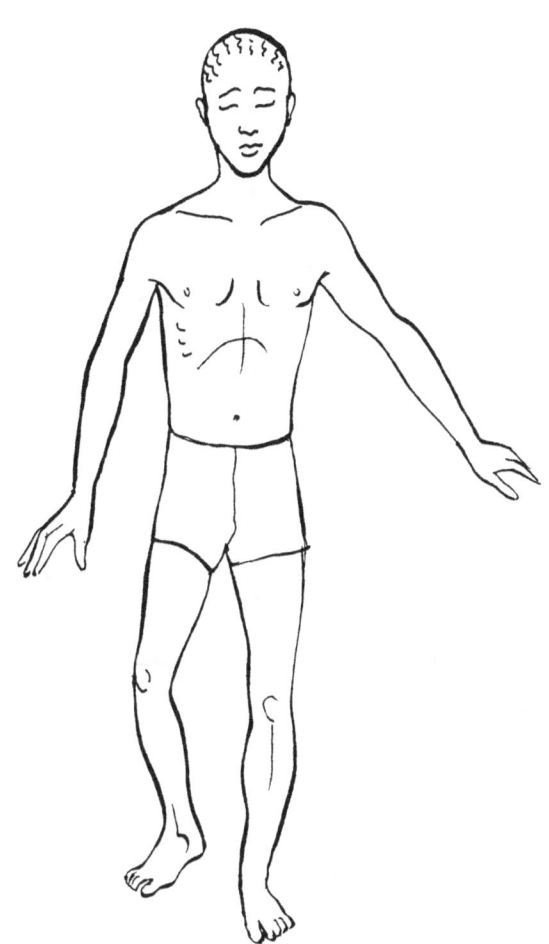

Thompson Test

Description

The patient lies prone or kneels on a chair. The examiner places the hand distal to the apex of the curve of the soleus. The examiner then squeezes the patient's calf at the middle third just below the place of the widest girth.

Interpretation

A positive test is one in which the ankle fails to plantar flex, indicating a complete rupture of the Achilles tendon.

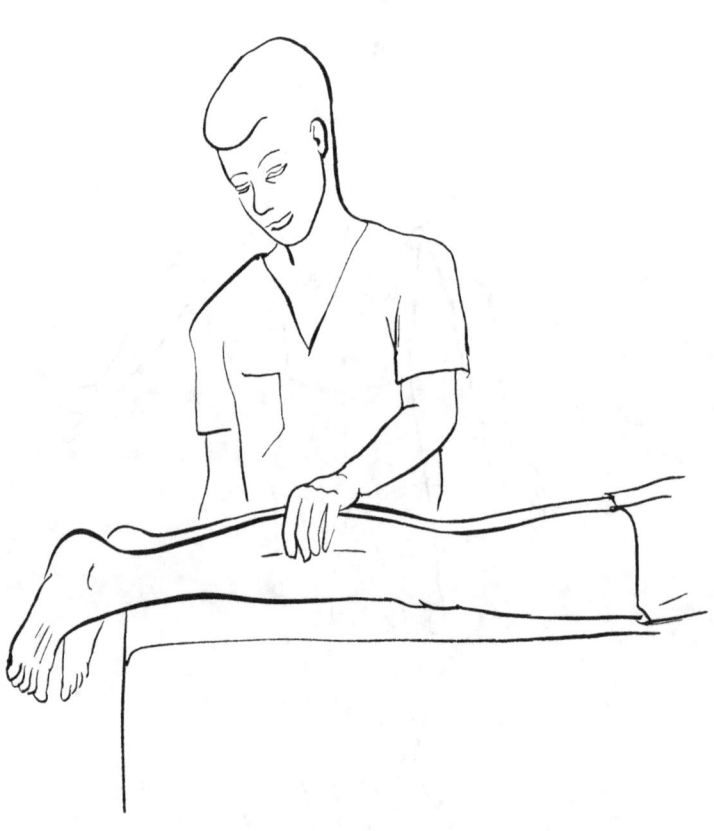

Homan Test

Description

The patient lies supine. The examiner stabilizes the patient's knee with one hand and with the other hand dorsiflexes the patient's foot.

Interpretation

A positive test is one which causes increased pain in the calf, indicating thrombophlebitis of the calf.

Comments

This test should be further confirmed by the Calf Compression Test.

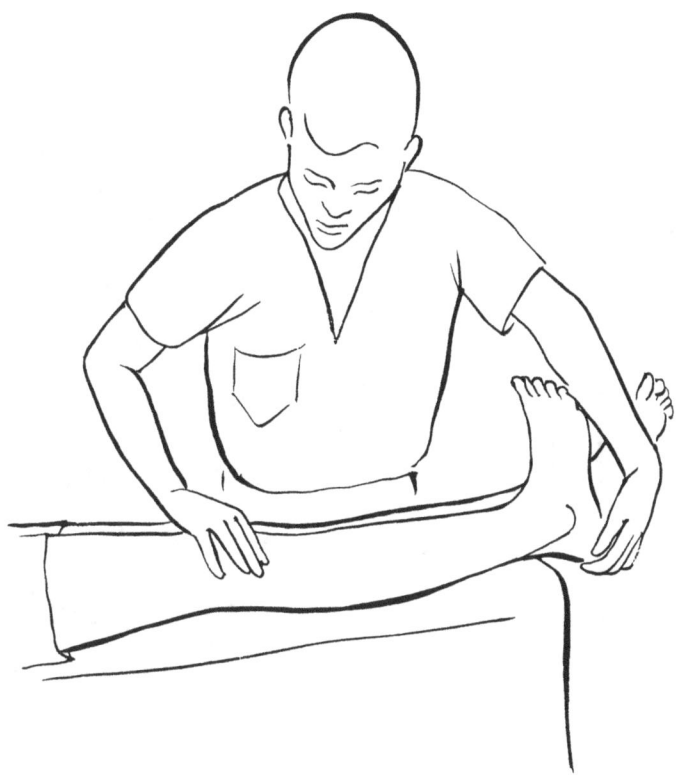

Calf Compression Test

Description

The patient sits on the edge of the table. The examiner supports the patient's foot in the neutral and slightly plantar flexed position with one hand. With the other hand the examiner compresses the patient's calf muscles.

Interpretation

A positive test is one which causes increased pain in the calf muscles, indicating thrombophlebitis of the calf.

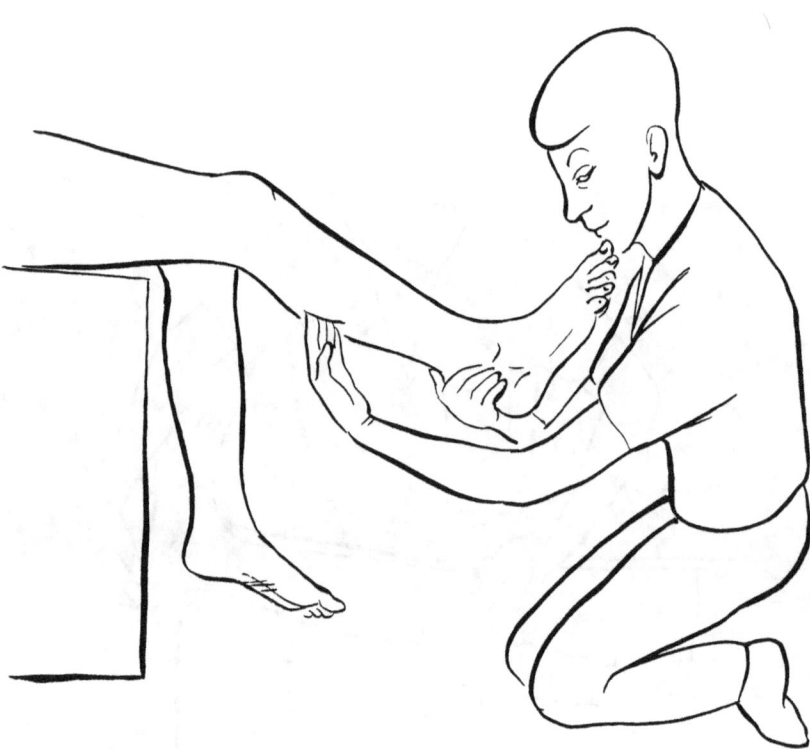

Talar Tilt Test

Description

The patient lies on the uninvolved side. The patient is instructed to flex the involved knee and plantar flex the ankle to relax the calf muscles. The examiner places one hand medially over the tibia while pressing the other hand lateral to the heel. The examiner notes the degree of talar tilt. The test is then repeated with the ankle in the neutral position.

Interpretation

A positive test is one in which the talar is displaced 10° or more, indicating anterior talofibular ligament dysfunction when the ankle is in the plantar flexed position, and calcaneofibular ligament dysfunction when the ankle is in the neutral position.

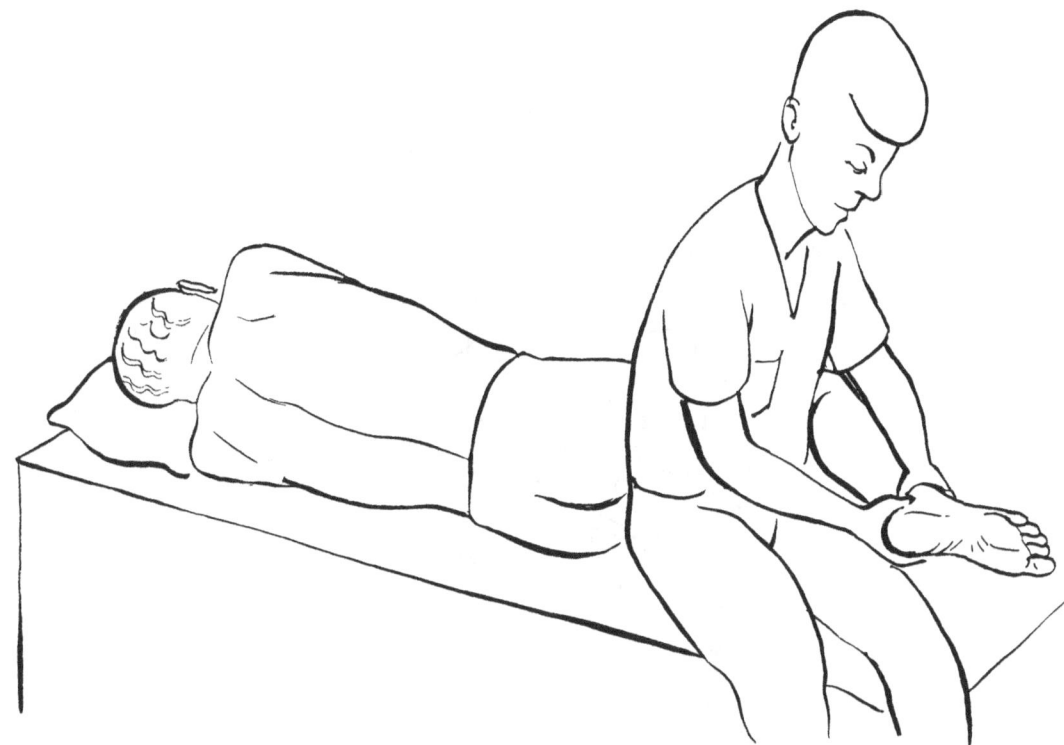

Inversion Stress Test

Description
The patient sits or lies supine. The examiner holds the patient's distal tibiofibula with one hand and with the other hand holds the patient's foot. The examiner then inverts the foot.

Interpretation
A positive test is one in which the ankle moves excessively medially, indicating the anterior talofibular or calcaneofibular ligament laxity.

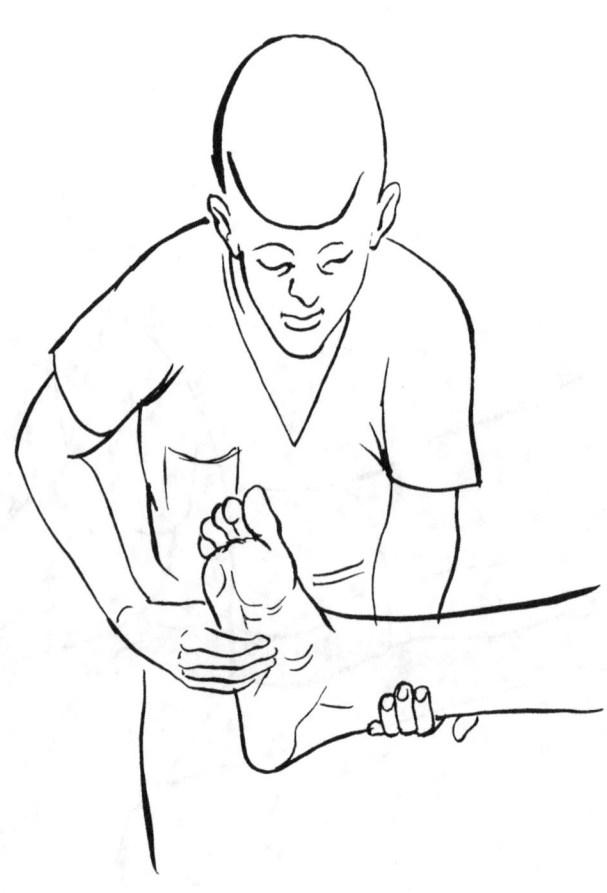

Anterior Drawer Test

Description

The patient sits on the table with knee flexed to relax the calf muscles. The examiner stabilizes the patient's distal tibiofibula with one hand and with the other hand holds the patient's heel, then gently pulls the patient's heel anteriorly.

Interpretation

A positive test is one in which the foot moves anteriorly more than 3 mm and moves with crepitation, indicating a torn anterior talofibular ligament.

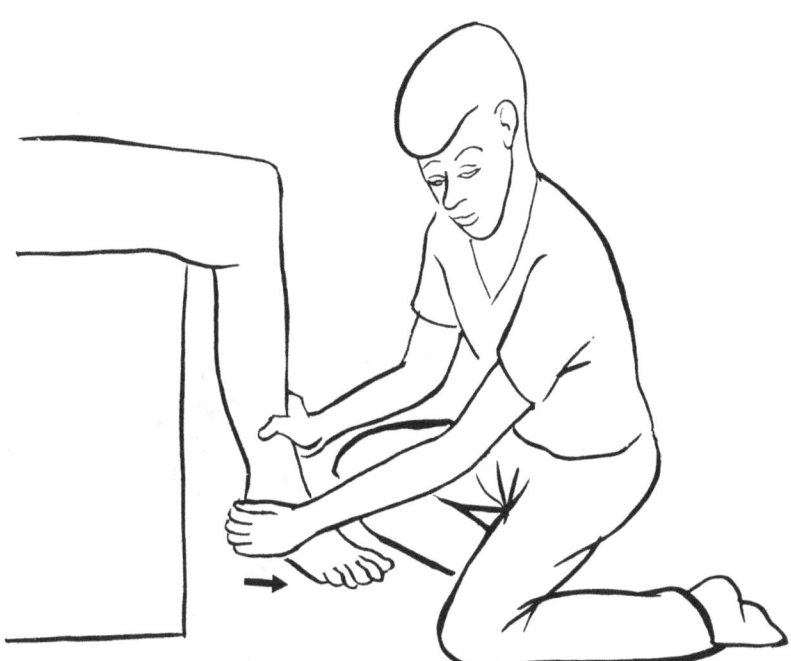

Posterior Drawer Test

Description

The patient lies supine with knee slightly flexed to relax the calf muscles. The examiner stabilizes the patient's distal tibiofibula with one hand and with the other hand holds the patient's talus. The examiner gently pushes the talus posteriorly.

Interpretation

A positive test is one in which the ankle moves excessively posteriorly, indicating a torn posterior talofibular ligament.

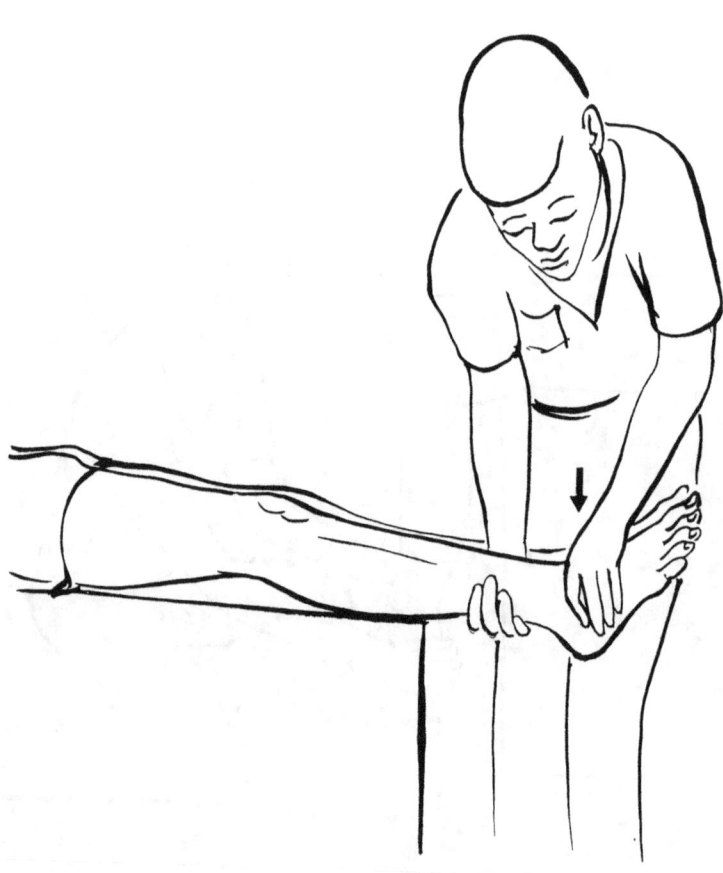

Eversion Stress Test

Description

The patient sits or lies supine. The examiner stabilizes the patient's distal tibiofibula with one hand and with the other hand holds the patient's foot. The examiner then everts the foot.

Interpretation

A positive test is one in which the ankle moves excessively laterally, indicating deltoid ligament laxity.

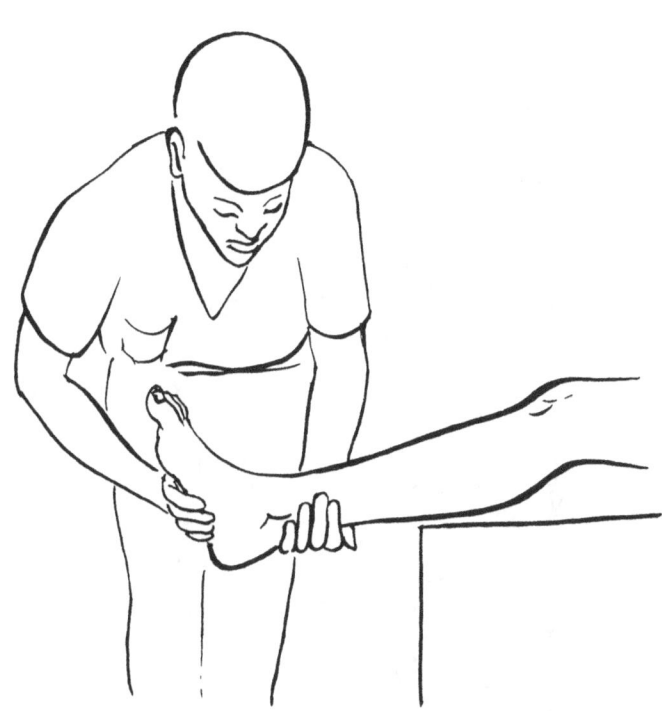

Kleiger Test

Description

The patient sits with knee flexed to 90°, the foot relaxed and non-weight bearing. The examiner holds the patient's proximal tibiofibula with one hand and with the other hand grasps the patient's foot and rotates it externally.

Interpretation

A positive test is one which produces pain medially and laterally and the examiner feels the talus being displaced from the medial malleolus, indicating a torn deltoid ligament.

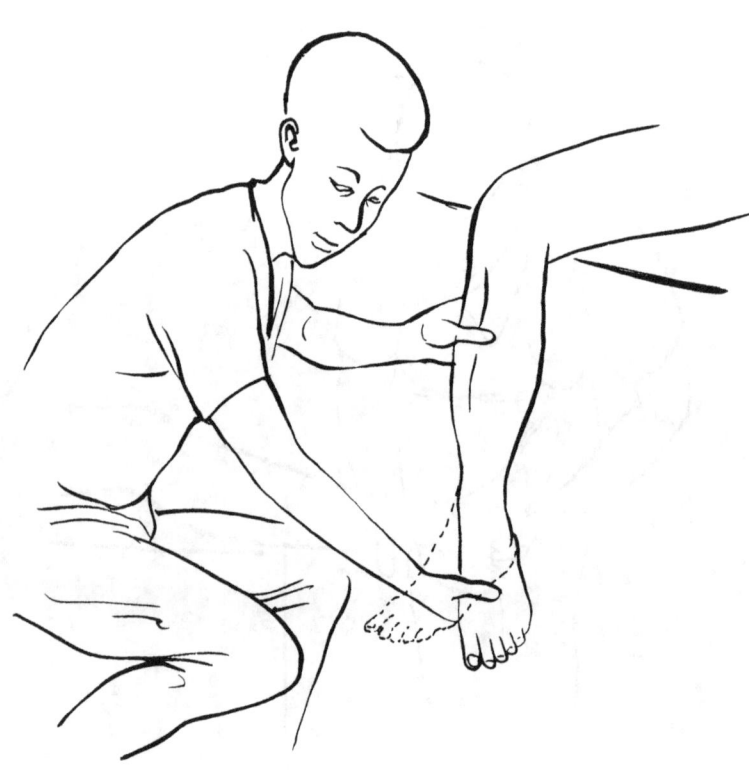

Swing Test

Description

The patient sits with the knees flexed to 90°; the feet are kept non-weight bearing and relaxed. The examiner holds the dorsal aspect of the patient's feet and keeps the feet parallel to the floor. The examiner palpates the anterior portion of the talus with the thumbs. The examiner then passively plantar flexes and dorsiflexes the feet, one at a time, and compares the quality of movement.

Interpretation

A positive test is one in which resistance to normal dorsiflexion is felt, indicating posterior tibiotalar subluxation.

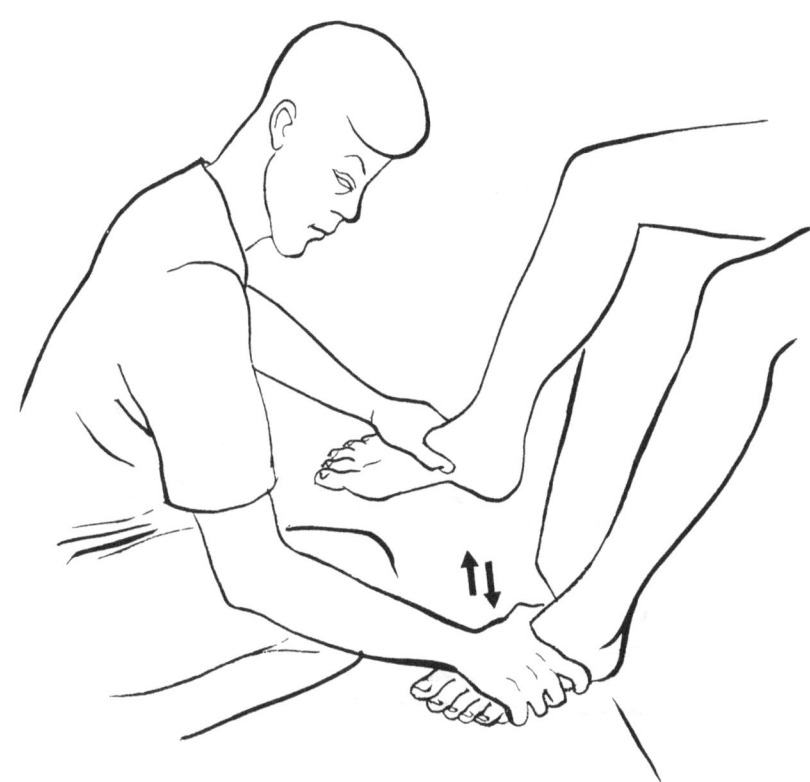

Tinel Test

Description

The patient sits with foot resting on the table. The examiner taps the posterior tibial nerve proximal at its entrance to the tarsal tunnel just proximal to the medial malleolus.

Interpretation

A positive test is one which reproduces symptoms of tingling and/or pain in the medial arch or the plantar aspect of the foot, indicating medial tarsal tunnel syndrome.

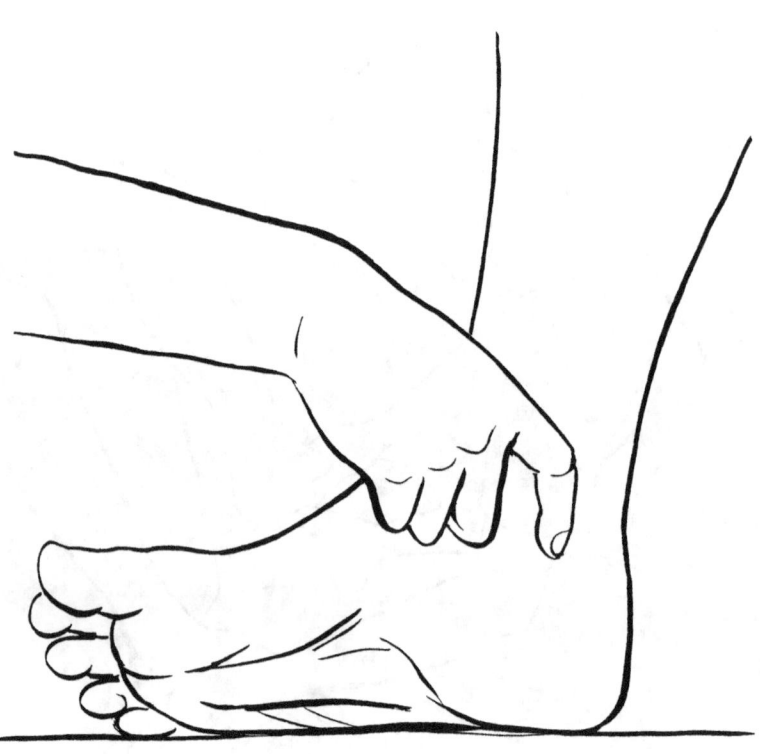

Hyperpronation Test

Description

The patient sits or lies supine. The examiner stabilizes the patient's distal tibiofibula with one hand and with the other hand holds the patient's foot. The examiner then moves the patient's foot in excessive pronation at the subtalar joint and maintains this position for 30 to 60 seconds.

Interpretation

A positive test is one which reproduces symptoms of tingling and/or pain in the medial arch or the plantar aspect of the foot, indicating medial tarsal tunnel syndrome.

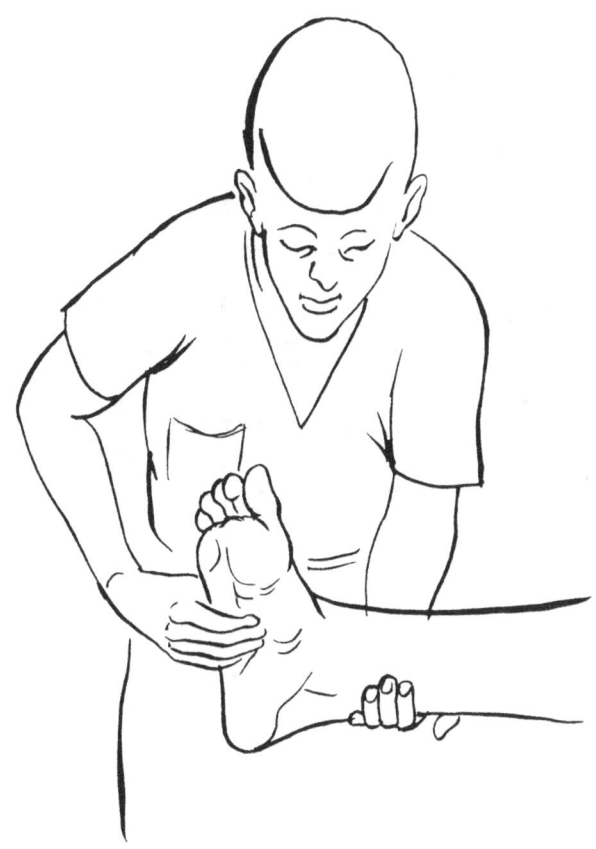

Squeeze Test

Description
The patient lies supine with foot in the neutral position and relaxed. The examiner grasps the patient's forefoot and squeezes the metatarsal area.

Interpretation
A positive test is one which causes increased pain in the forefoot, indicating metatarsalgia or neuroma of the forefoot.

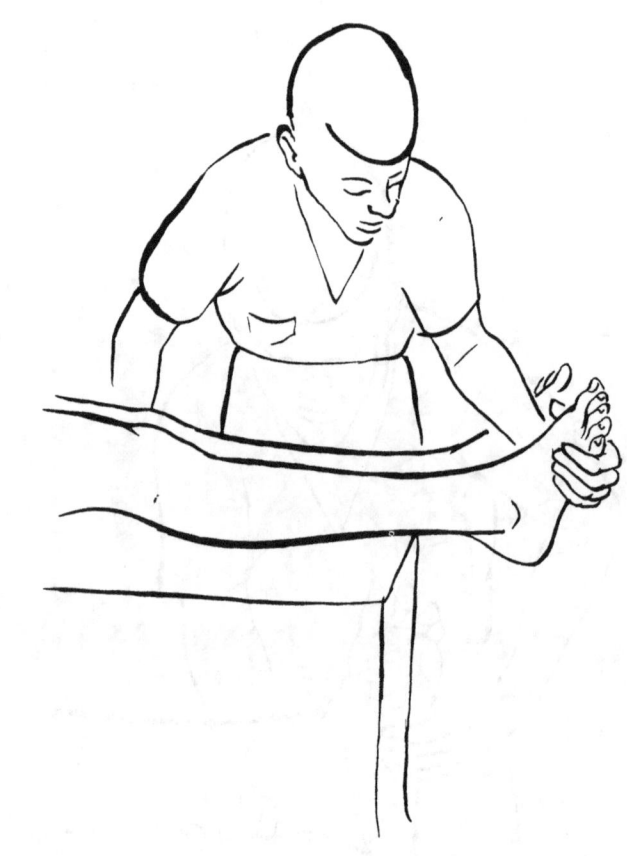

Strunsky Test

Description

The patient lies supine with feet slightly plantar flexed and relaxed. The examiner grasps the patient's toes and quickly flexes them.

Interpretation

A positive test is one which increases the sharp pain in the forefoot, indicating metatarsalgia of the metatarsophalangeal joints.

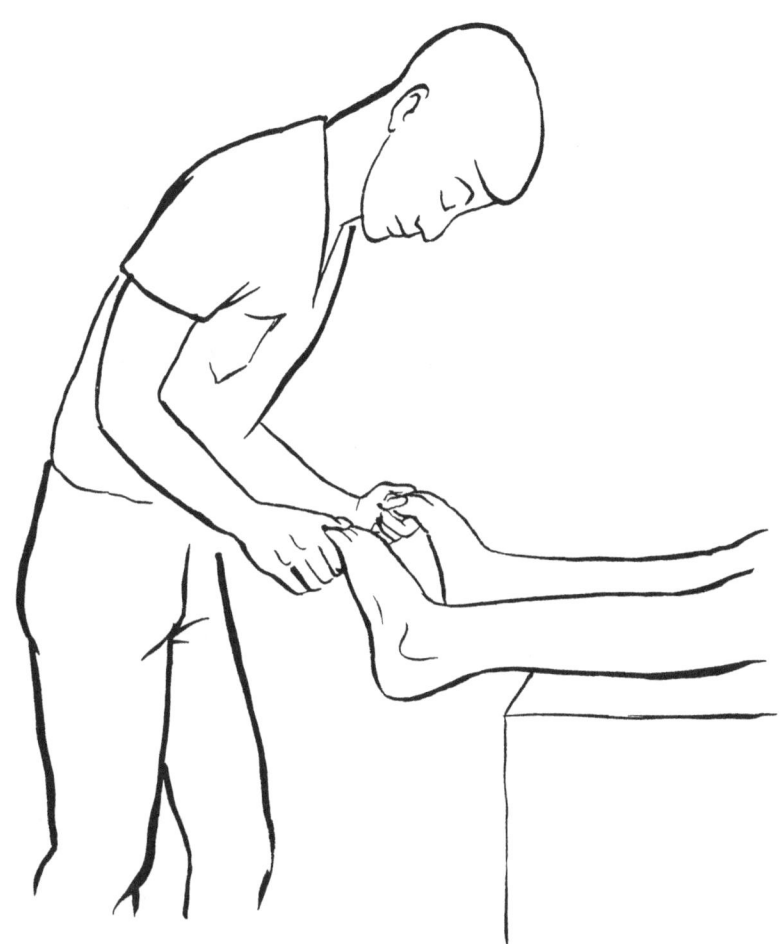

Section 7
Temporomandibular

Jaw Reflex Test

Description

The patient sits or stands with mouth slightly open. The examiner places the thumb of one hand over the patient's chin and with the other hand gently taps the thumb with a reflex hammer.

Interpretation

A positive test is one in which the mouth does not close (absent or diminished reflex), indicating a pathology along the fifth cranial nerve, i.e., the trigeminal nerve. A brisk reflex may indicate upper motor neuron lesion.

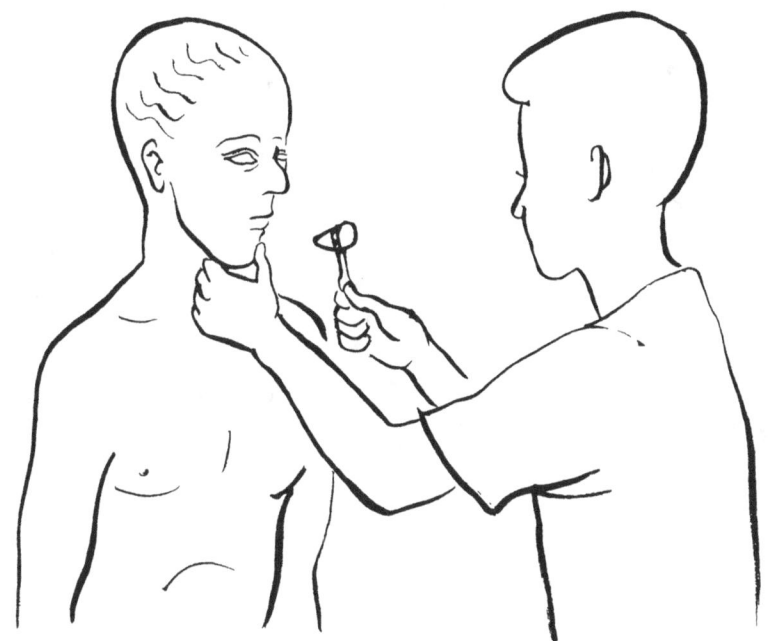

Chvostek Test

Description
The patient sits or stands. The examiner taps on the patient's facial nerve in the area of the parotid gland overlying the masseter muscle.

Interpretation
A positive test is one in which the facial muscles contract in a twitch, indicating a low calcium level in the blood.

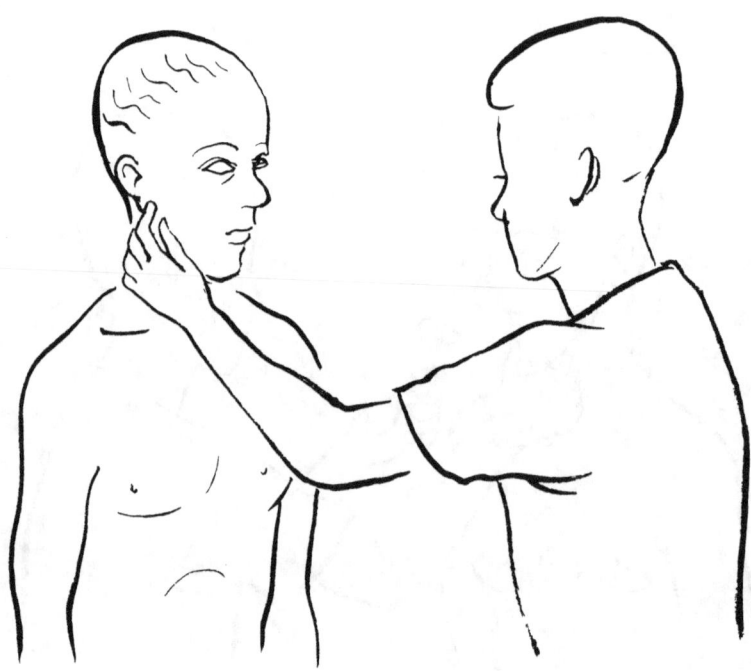

Loading Test

Description

The patient sits in a chair. The examiner instructs the patient to chew or bite forcefully on a cotton roll placed between the molars on the uninvolved side.

Interpretation

A positive test is one in which pain is elicited in the involved temporomandibular joint, indicating an anteriorly dislocated disc.

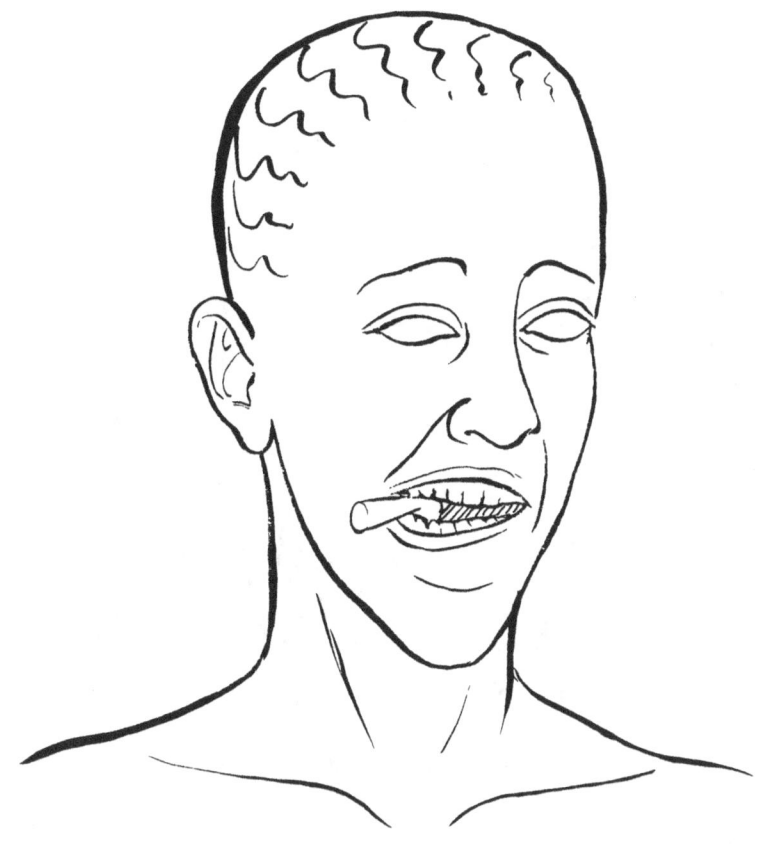

Palpation Test

Description
The patient sits in a chair. The examiner stands in front of the patient and places the little fingers in the patient's ears with the finger nails pointed posteriorly. The patient is then instructed to open and close the mouth several times while the examiner exerts pressure anteriorly.

Interpretation
A positive test is one in which pain is elicited as the pressure is applied during opening and closing of the mouth, compressing the tissue, indicating synovitis of the temporomandibular joint.

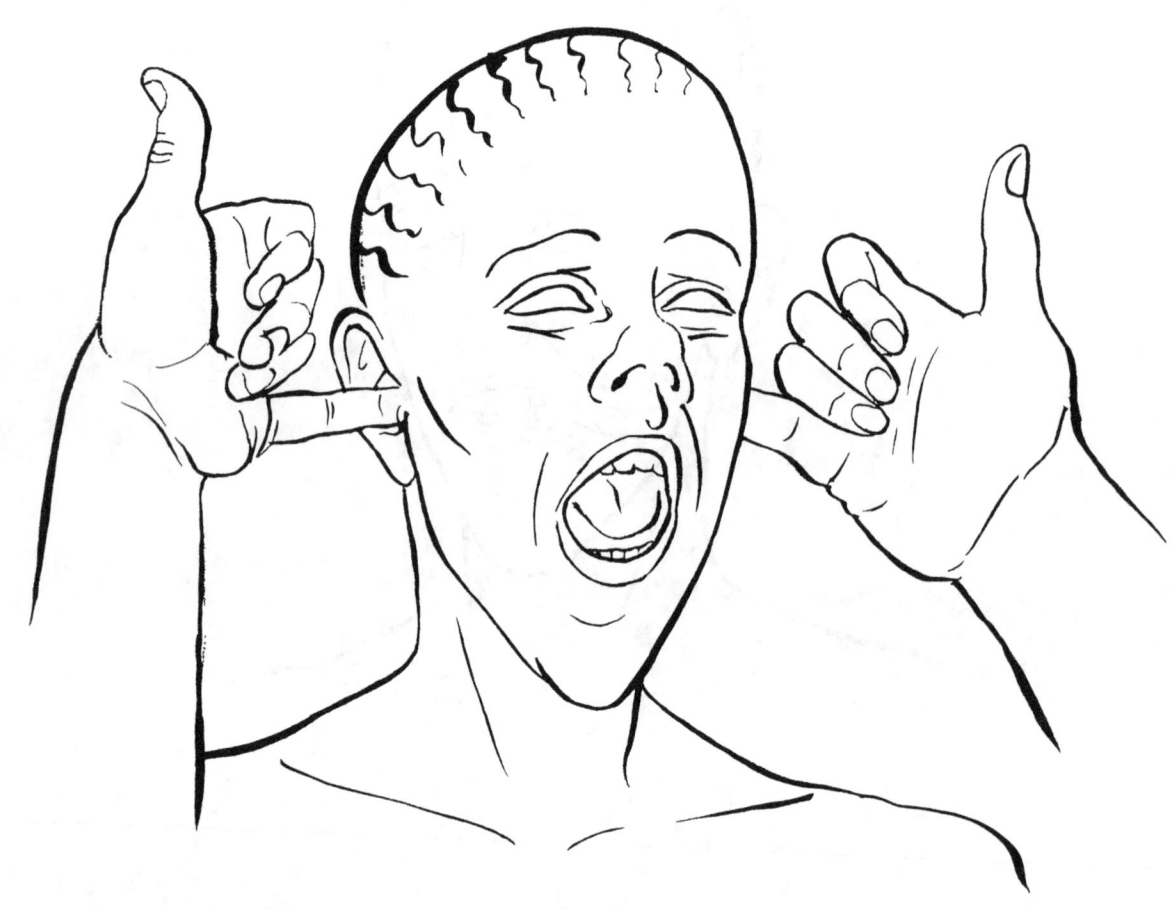

Section 8
Cervical

Swallowing Test

Description
The patient sits. The patient is then instructed to swallow.

Interpretation
A positive test is one in which the patient experiences difficulty or pain upon swallowing, indicating possible cervical spine pathology such as bony protuberances, bony osteophytes, or soft tissue swelling due to hematomas, infection, or tumors in the anterior portion of the cervical spine.

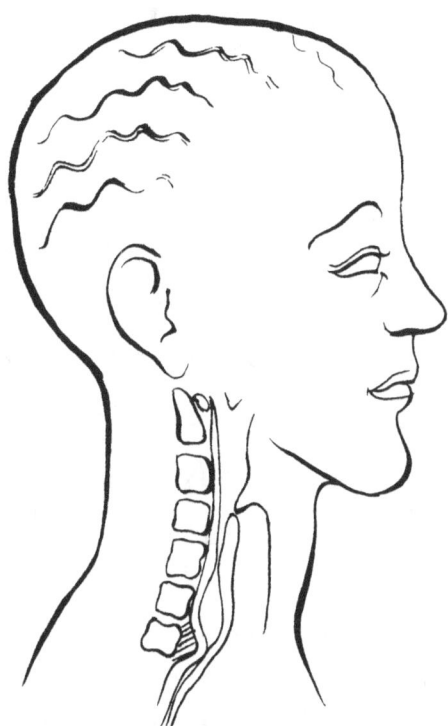

Temperature Test

Description

The patient sits. The examiner alternatively applies hot and cold test tubes just behind the patient's ears on each side.

Interpretation

A positive test is one which causes vertigo, indicating an inner ear infection.

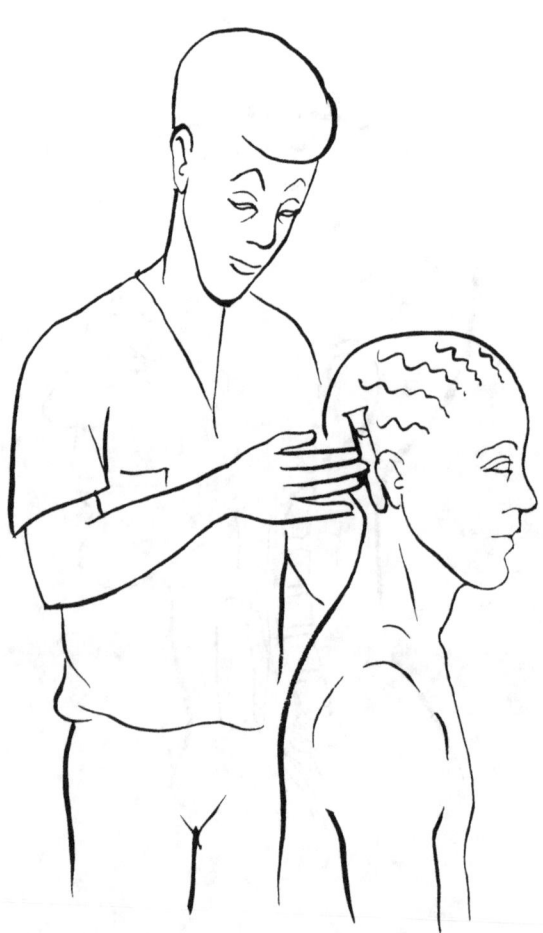

Vertebral Artery Test

Description

The patient lies supine with eyes open. The examiner supports the patient's shoulder with one hand and with the other hand passively extends the patient's head and rotates it to the opposite side. The examiner maintains this position for 10 to 15 seconds and observes the patient's eye movement, looking for asymmetric pupil changes. The patient may report any unusual sensations such as dizziness, giddiness, light-headedness, or visual changes. The test is then repeated on the other side.

Interpretation

A positive test is one in which the patient has nystagmus of the eyes or asymmetric pupils or experiences unusual changes, indicating vertebrobasilar insufficiency.

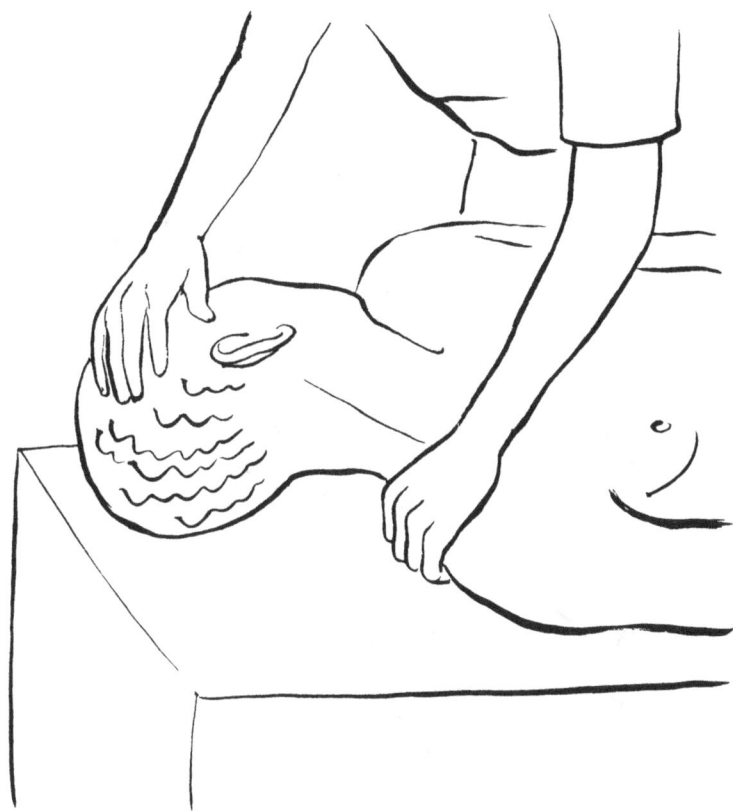

Dizziness Test

Description

The patient lies supine. The examiner passively rotates the patient's head as far as possible, first to the right and then to the left. The patient is then instructed to rotate the shoulders as far to the right as possible and as far to the left as possible while keeping the eyes open and looking straight ahead.

Interpretation

A positive test is one which causes dizziness while the head and shoulders are rotated, indicating vertebral artery dysfunction. If the dizziness is experienced only when the head is rotated, the semicircular canals of the inner ears are involved.

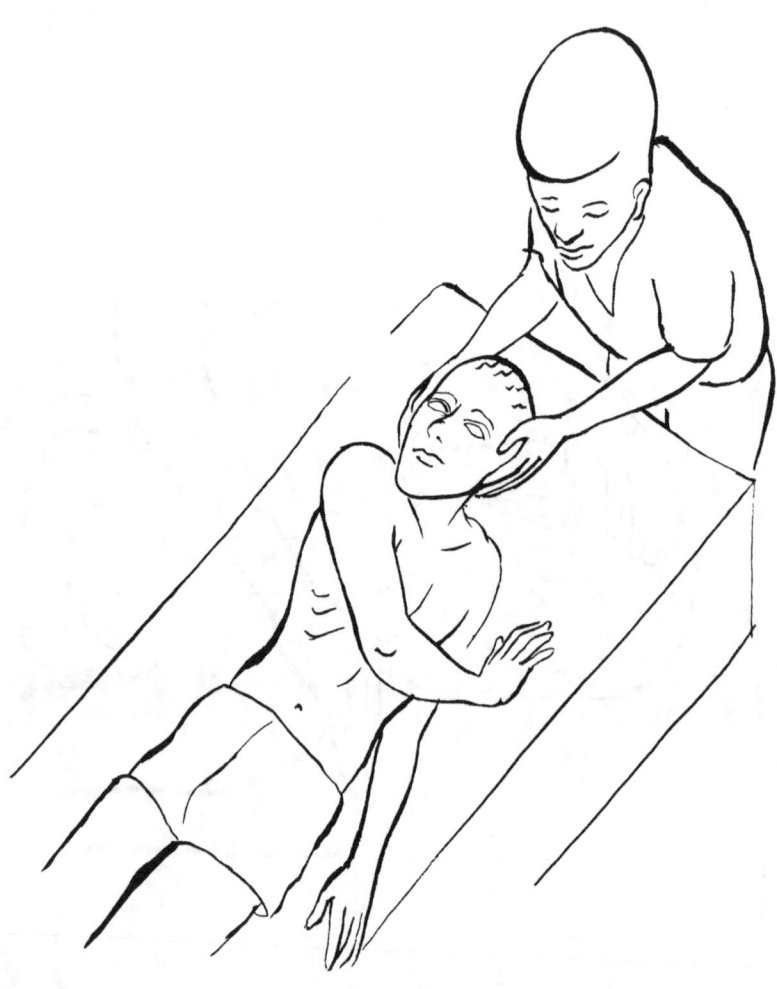

Sharp-Purser Test

Description
The patient sits. The examiner places one hand over the patient's forehead and the thumb of the other hand over the spinous process of the axis. The patient is then instructed to slowly flex the head while the examiner presses backward with the hand placed over the patient's forehead.

Interpretation
A positive test is one in which the patient's head slides backward during the movement and may be accompanied by a "clunk," indicating subluxation of the atlas on the axis.

Comments
This test should be performed with extreme caution.

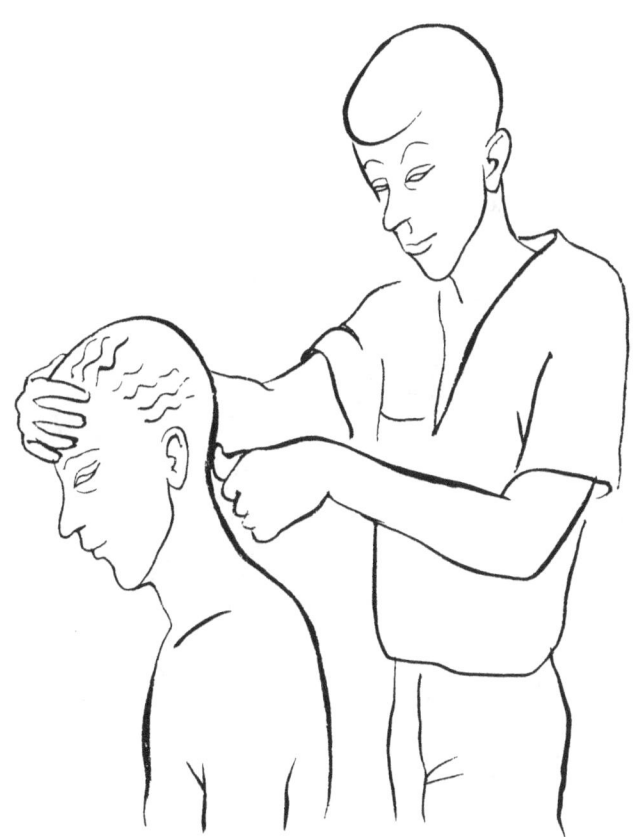

Alar Odontoid Integrity Test

Description
The patient lies supine. The examiner stands at the head of the patient and rests the patient's head on the examiner's abdomen. The examiner cradles the patient's head with both hands and places fingers on the upper cervical spine on each side of the midline. The examiner then slowly side bends the patient's cervical spine just a few degrees.

Interpretation
A positive test is one in which the spinous processes do not move as the patient's cervical spine is being side bent, indicating either odontoid fracture or alar ligament rupture.

Comments
This test should be performed with extreme caution.

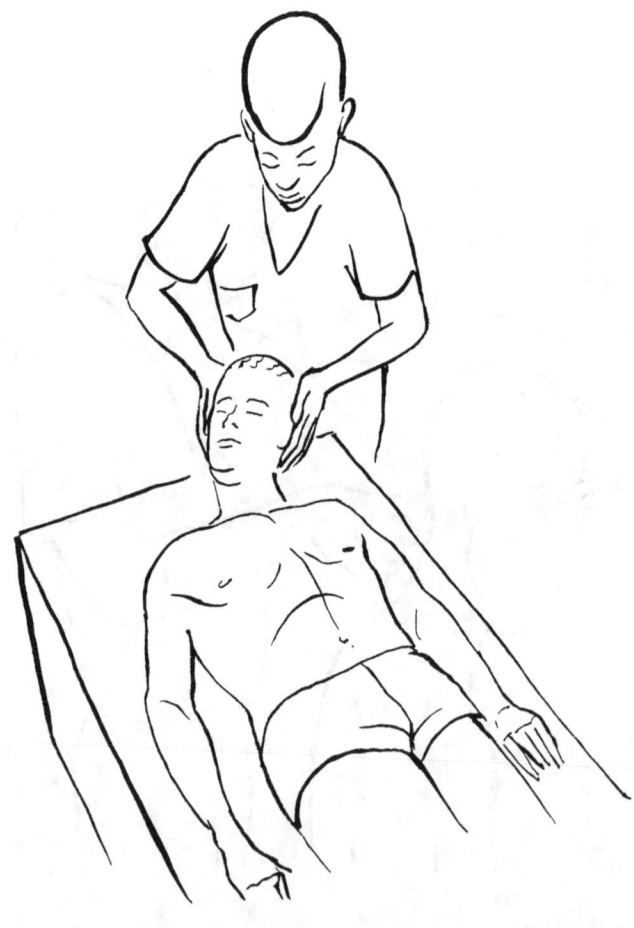

O'Donoghue Test

Description

The patient sits in a chair. The patient is instructed to perform range of motion of the cervical spine in all planes while the examiner resists the motion. The examiner then passively moves the patient's cervical spine through range of motion in all planes.

Interpretation

A positive test is one which causes increased pain during resisted range of motion, indicating muscle strain, while increased pain during passive range of motion indicates ligamentous sprain.

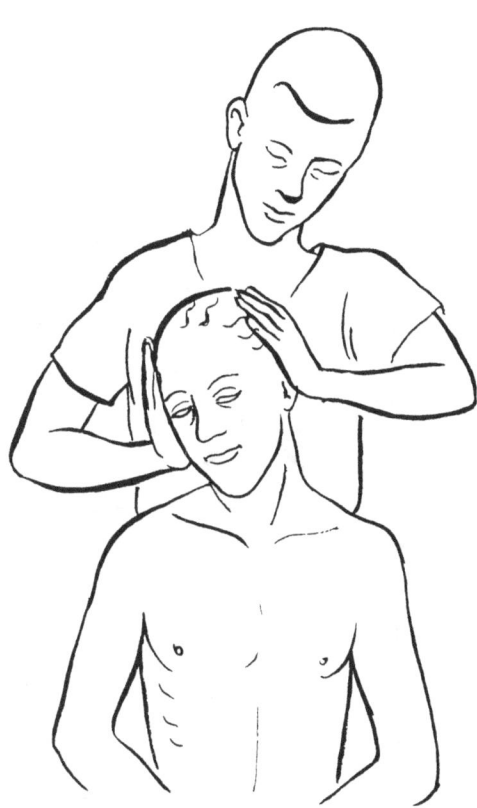

Adson Test

Description
The patient stands or sits. The examiner holds the patient's arm in slight abduction and monitors the radial pulse. The patient is then instructed to take and hold a deep breath, extend the neck, and turn the chin toward the side being tested while the examiner externally rotates and extends the patient's shoulder. The patient is then instructed to turn the head toward the opposite side.

Interpretation
A positive test is one in which the radial pulse disappears and other symptoms are produced indicating thoracic outlet syndrome.

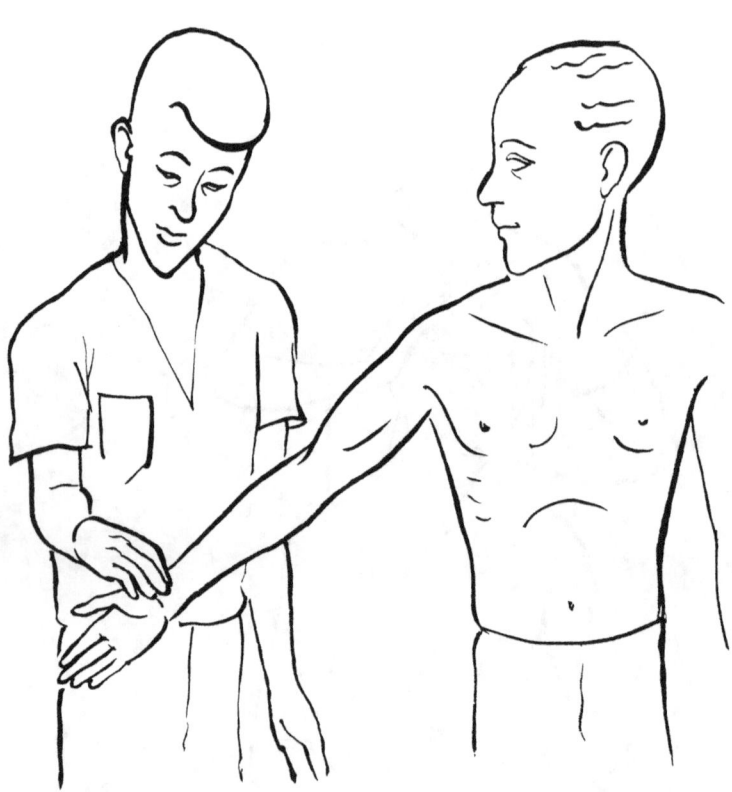

Allen Test

Description

The patient stands or sits. The examiner flexes the patient's elbow to 90° while the patient's shoulder is abducted to 90° and externally rotated. The examiner monitors the radial pulse and instructs the patient to rotate the head away from the test side.

Interpretation

A positive test is one in which the pulse disappears and other symptoms are produced indicating thoracic outlet syndrome.

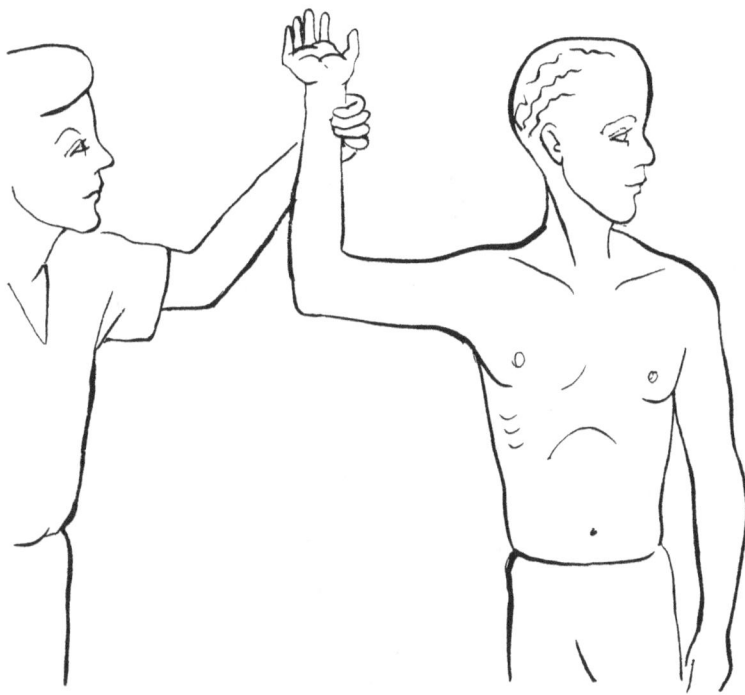

Roos Test

Description

The patient stands. The patient is instructed to abduct the shoulders to 90°, externally rotate the shoulders, and flex the elbows to 90°. The patient is then instructed to open and close the hands slowly for 3 minutes while maintaining this position.

Interpretation

A positive test is one in which the patient is either unable to maintain the starting position for 3 minutes or experiences pain, heaviness in the arms, or tingling/numbness in the hands, indicating thoracic outlet syndrome.

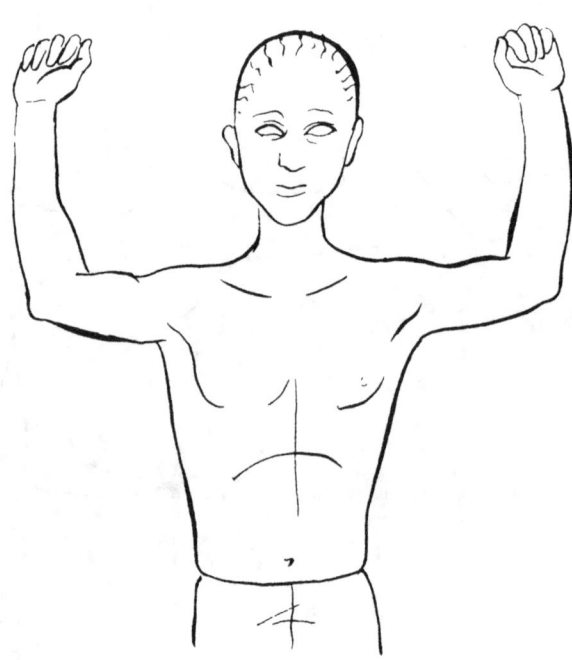

Wright Test

Description

The patient sits. The examiner holds the patient's arm at approximately 45° of shoulder abduction and monitors the radial pulse. While monitoring the radial pulse, the examiner moves the patient's arm in hyperabduction.

Interpretation

A positive test is one in which the radial pulse disappears on hyperabduction of the arm, indicating thoracic outlet syndrome.

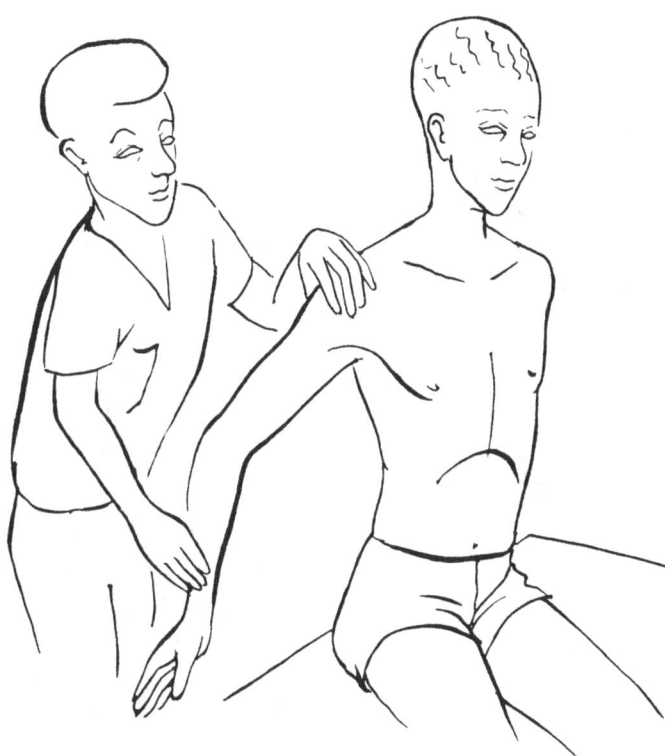

Hyperabduction Test

Description
The patient sits. The examiner holds the patient's arm in hyperabduction and external rotation, and monitors the radial pulse.

Interpretation
A positive test is one in which pain is produced in the arm and the radial pulse disappears, indicating thoracic outlet syndrome.

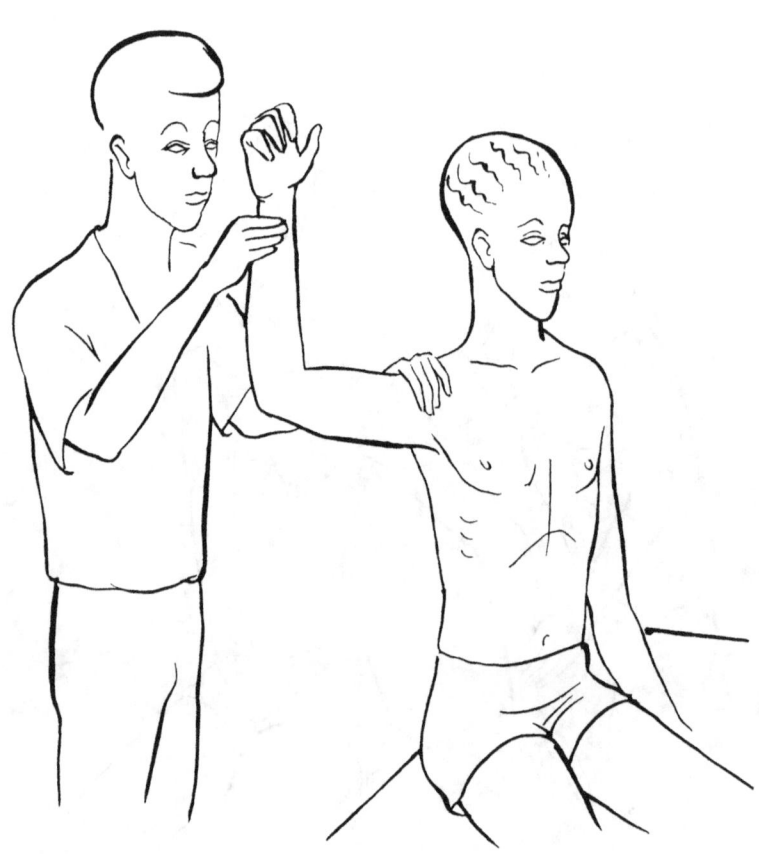

Costoclavicular Test

Description

The patient sits. The examiner moves the patient's shoulder to about 45° abduction. The patient is instructed to adduct the scapula. The examiner monitors the patient's radial pulse and extends the patient's shoulder.

Interpretation

A positive test is one in which the radial pulse decreases and other symptoms are produced indicating thoracic outlet syndrome.

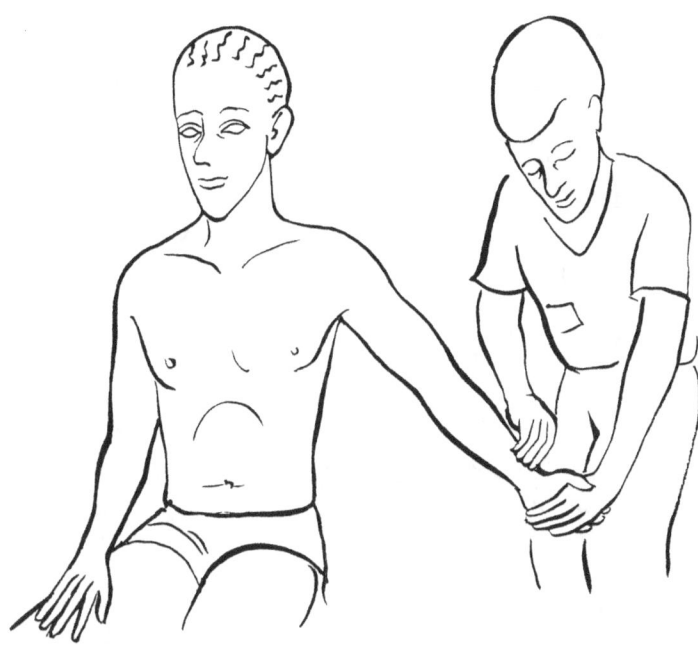

Halstead Test

Description

The patient sits or stands. The examiner monitors the patient's radial pulse and applies a downward force on the arm. The patient is then instructed to extend and rotate the head away from the test side.

Interpretation

A positive test is one in which the radial pulse disappears, indicating thoracic outlet syndrome.

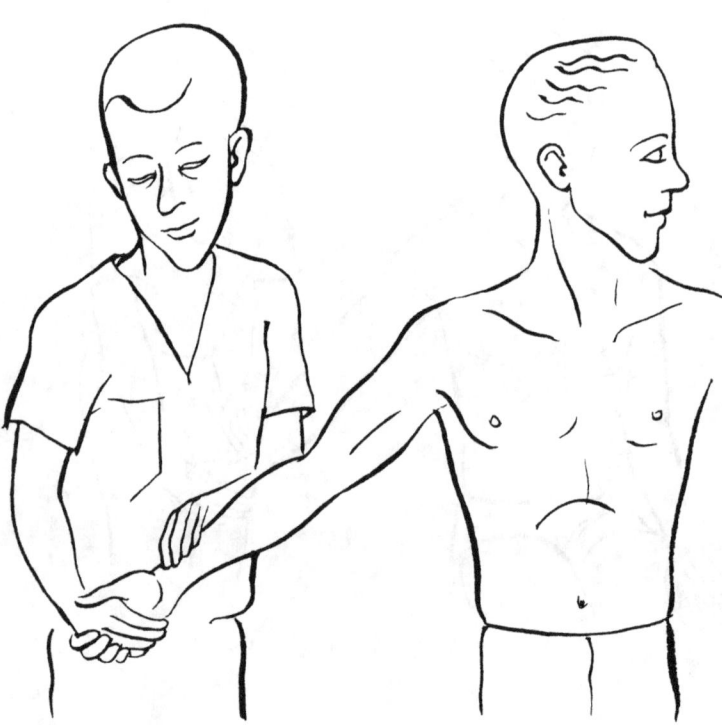

Compression Test

Description

The patient either lies supine or sits in a chair. The examiner stands at the head of the patient if the patient is lying or stands behind the patient if the patient is sitting and presses inferiorly on top of the patient's head.

Interpretation

A positive test is one which increases the patient's symptoms, indicating foraminal encroachment or facet joint pressure.

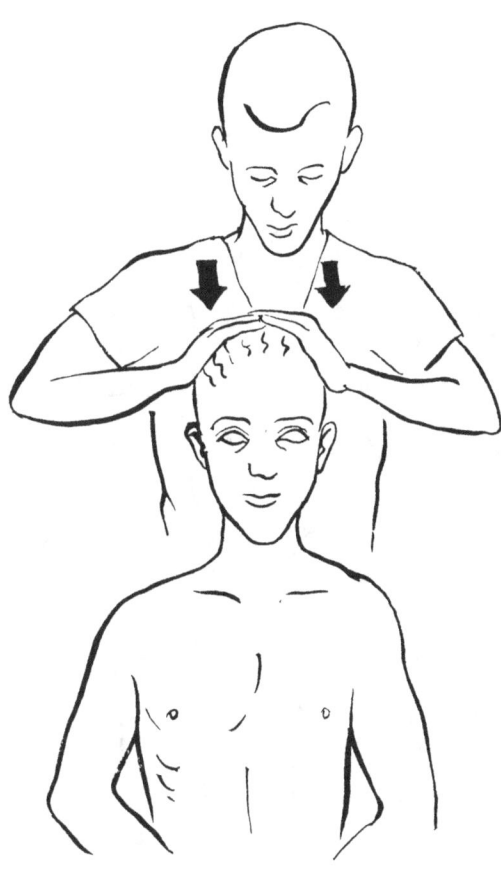

Foraminal Compression Test

Description
The patient sits in a chair. The examiner stands behind the patient and rotates the patient's neck while firmly pushing down the head.

Description
A positive test is one in which localized pain is produced in the cervical area, indicating foraminal encroachment.

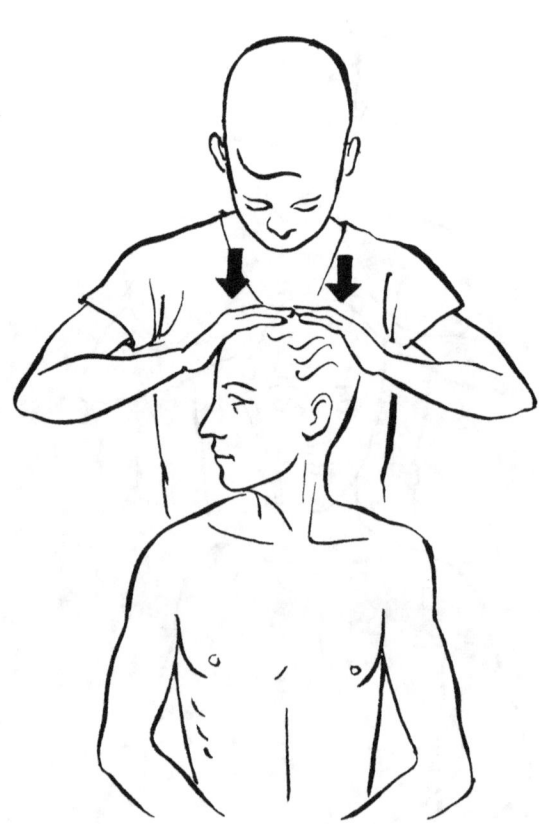

Jackson Compression Test

Description

The patient sits in a chair. The examiner stands behind the patient. The examiner side bends the patient's neck and exerts firm inferior pressure on the head.

Interpretation

A positive test is one in which localized pain is produced in the cervical area, indicating foraminal encroachment.

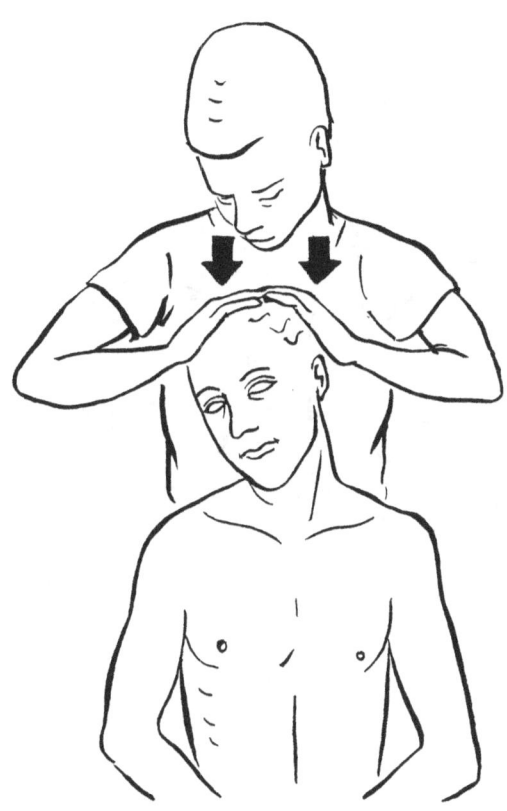

Maximal Foraminal Compression Test

Description
The patient sits in a chair. The patient is instructed to approximate the chin to the shoulder, and then to extend the neck.

Interpretation
A positive test is one in which pain is produced on the concave side, indicating nerve root or facet involvement. Pain on the convex side indicates muscle strain.

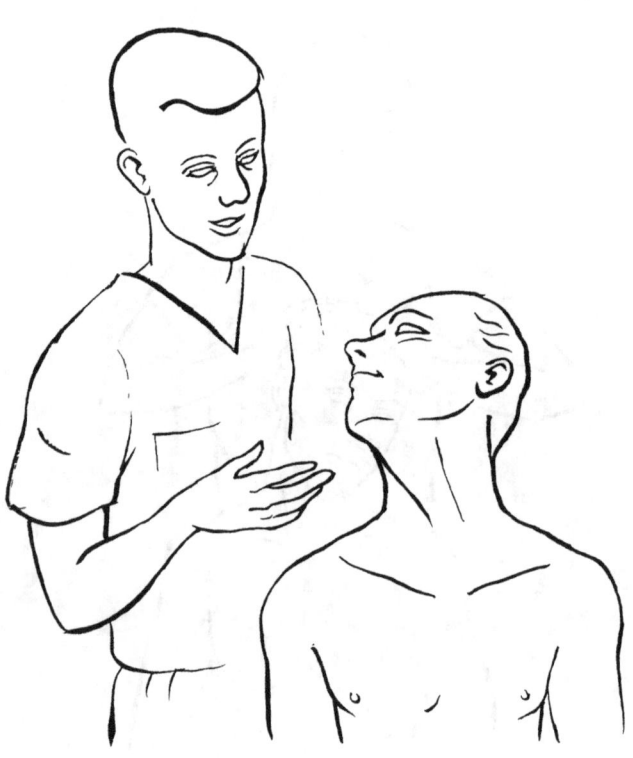

Slump Test

Description

The patient sits on the edge of the table with legs hanging downward and hands resting in the lap. This position should not produce any pain. The examiner stands to the side being tested. The patient is instructed to slump the thoracic and lumbar spine into flexion while the cervical spine is kept neutral. The patient is then instructed to flex the head and neck and the examiner applies over pressure to the upper trunk. While maintaining full spinal flexion, the patient is instructed to fully extend the knee and the examiner holds the knee. The patient is then instructed to actively dorsiflex the foot while the examiner applies an over pressure.

Interpretation

A positive test is one in which pain is produced at each step of the test, indicating thecal or intrathecal pathology.

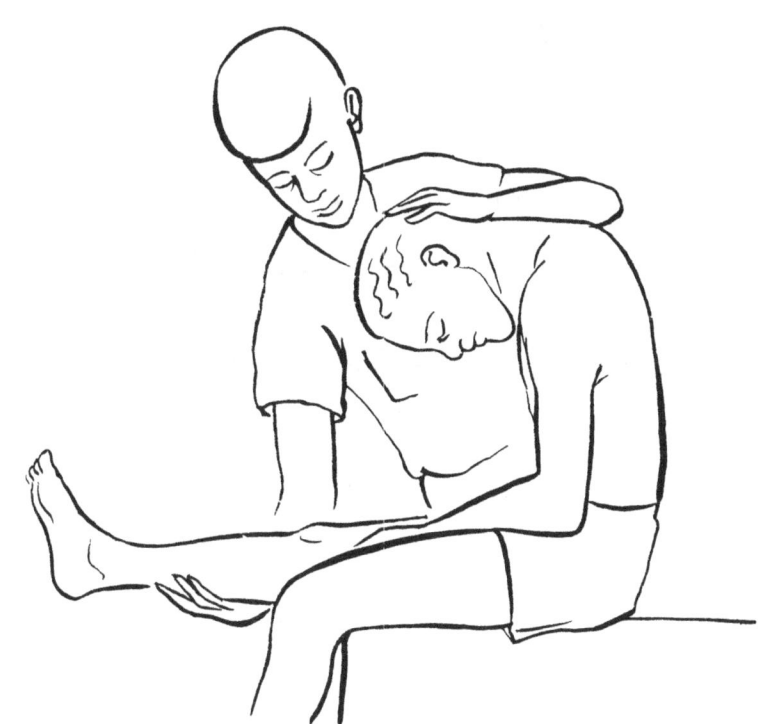

Milgram Test

Description

The patient lies supine. The patient is then instructed to raise both legs straight about two inches high and to hold this position as long as possible. The patient should be able to hold this position for at least 30 seconds.

Interpretation

A positive test is one in which the patient is unable to hold this position for 30 seconds, or is unable to lift legs at all, or experiences pain as the maneuver is attempted, indicating thecal, intrathecal or extrathecal pathology.

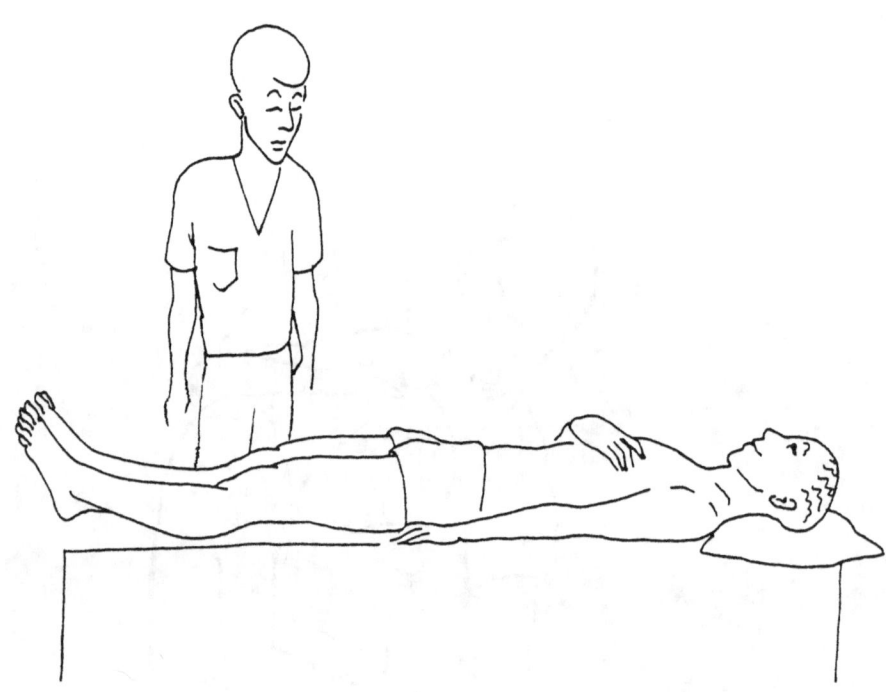

Naffziger Test

Description

The patient lies supine. The examiner gently compresses the patient's jugular veins with both hands for about 10 seconds until the patient's face begins to flush. The patient is then asked to cough.

Interpretation

A positive test is one in which coughing causes pain, indicating intrathecal pathology.

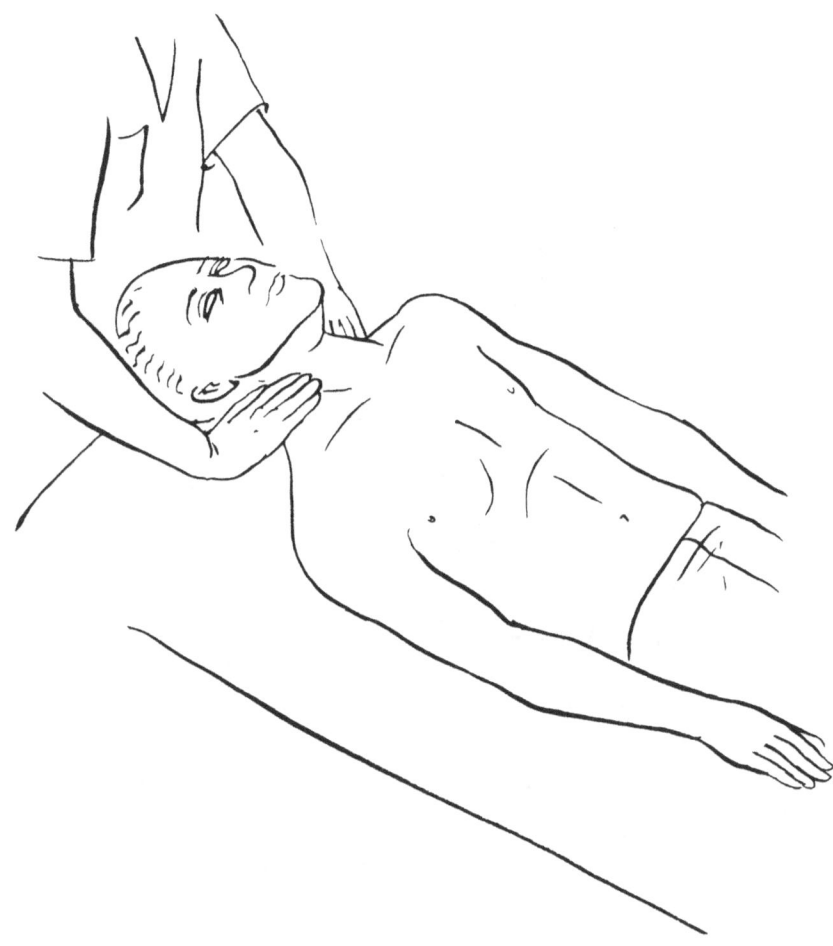

Valsalva Test

Description
The patient sits in a chair with feet resting on the floor. The patient is then instructed to bear down as if the patient were trying to move the bowel.

Interpretation
A positive test is one in which bearing down causes pain in the cervical spine or down the arms, indicating thecal or intrathecal pathology.

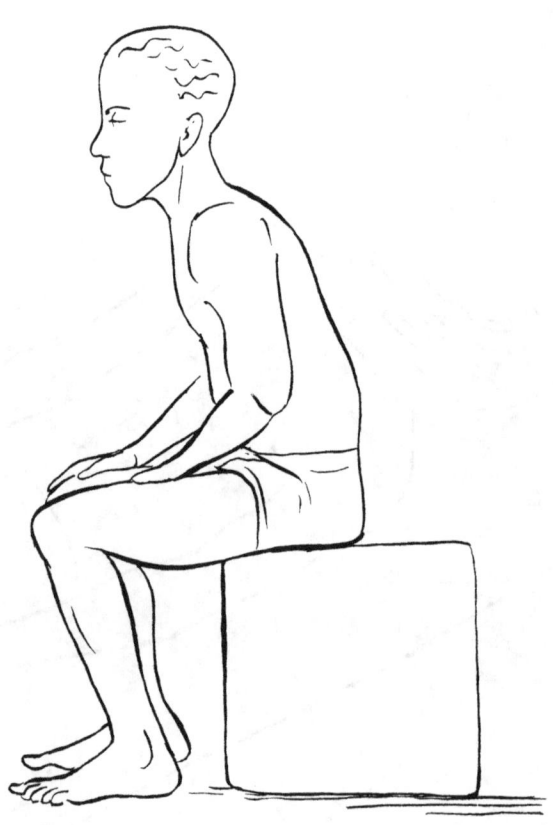

Upper Limb Tension Test

Description

The patient lies supine. The examiner holds the patient's hand with one hand and moves the patient's arm in slight hyperabduction with external rotation at the glenohumeral joint and the elbow slightly flexed. With the other hand the examiner stabilizes the patient's shoulder, maintaining the shoulder girdle in a depressed position. The patient is then instructed to side bend the neck in the opposite direction. The examiner extends the patient's elbow joint with the wrist in extension and the forearm in supination.

Interpretation

A positive test is one which produces pain in the arm, indicating irritation of the cervical nerve roots or the dura sheath.

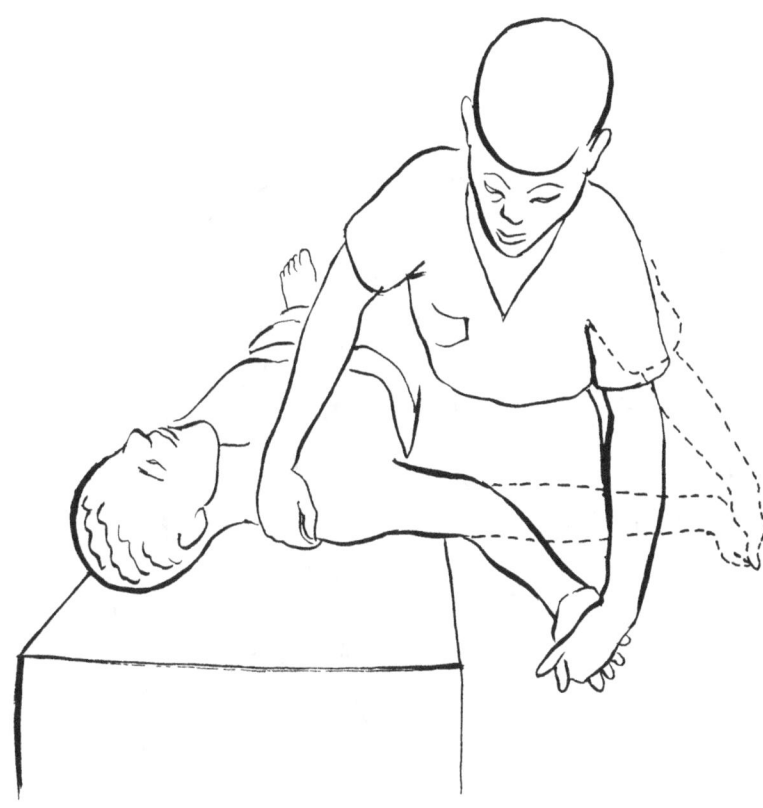

Brachial Plexus Tension Test

Description

The patient lies supine. The examiner supports the patient's shoulder with one hand. With the other hand the examiner holds the patient's hand, then externally rotates the patient's shoulder and supinates the forearm to the point which does not elicit pain. The patient is then instructed to flex the elbow.

Interpretation

A positive test is one in which the symptoms are reproduced, indicating nerve root compression, probably at C5 level. The symptoms are increased with flexion of the cervical spine.

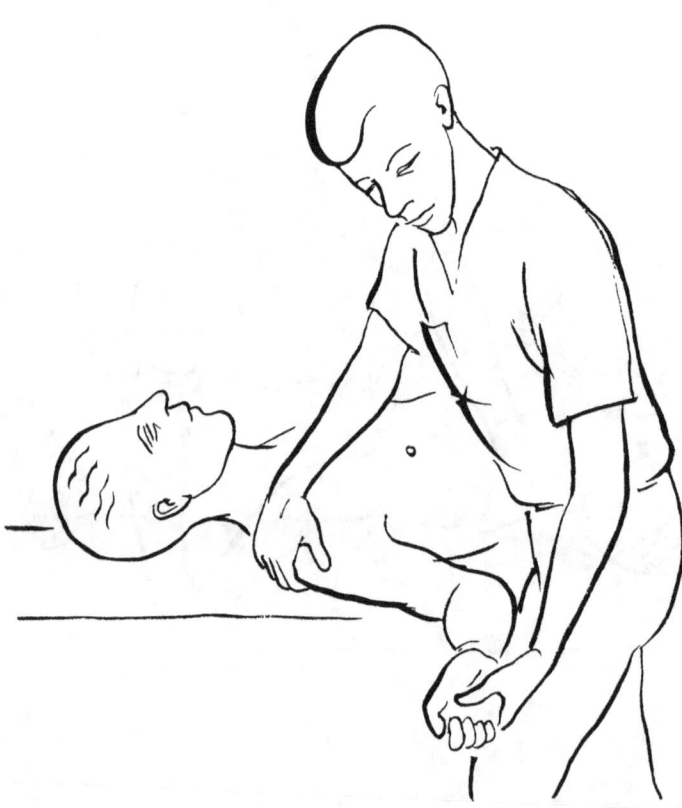

Shoulder Abduction Test

Description

The patient sits. The examiner then instructs the patient to elevate the arm through abduction so that the hand rests on top of the patient's head.

Interpretation

A positive test is one which decreases the symptoms, indicating a cervical extradural compression usually at C5-C6 level.

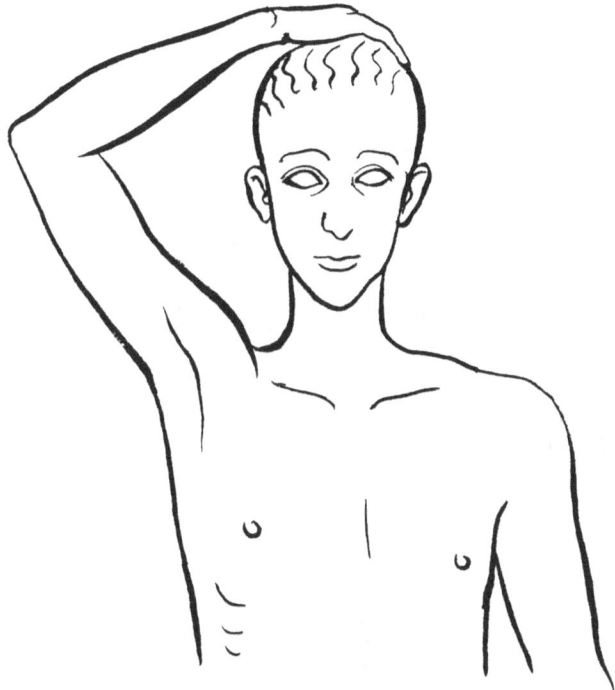

Shoulder Depression Test

Description

The patient sits. The examiner stabilizes the patient's shoulder with one hand and applies downward pressure. With the other hand the examiner side bends the patient's head to the opposite side.

Interpretation

A positive test is one in which pain is increased, indicating nerve root compression or dural adhesions to the nerve root or joint capsule.

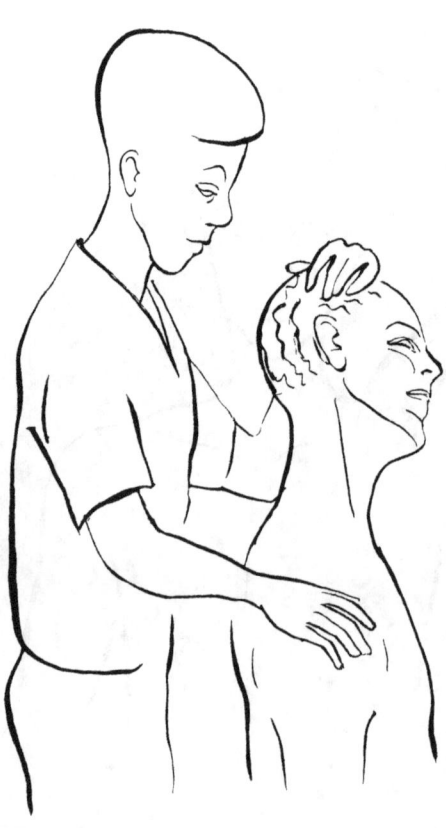

Kerning Test

Description

The patient lies supine with both hands placed behind the head. The examiner raises the patient's leg straight with knee in the extended position. The patient is then instructed to flex the head onto the chest.

Interpretation

A positive test is one in which the patient experiences pain in the cervical/lumbar spine or down the legs, indicating meningeal irritation, nerve root involvement, or irritation of the dura.

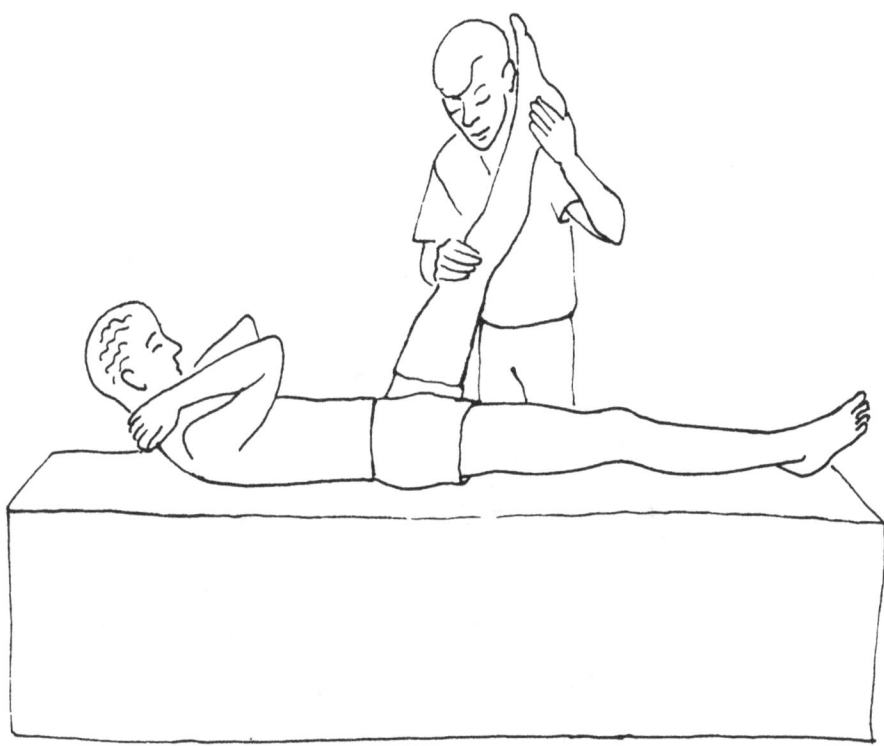

Distraction Test

Description
The patient either lies supine or sits in a chair. The examiner stands at the head of the patient if the patient is lying or stands behind the patient if the patient is sitting. The examiner cups one hand under the patient's jaw and places the other hand on the base of the occiput, then applies long axis distraction to the cervical spine.

Interpretation
A positive test is one which relieves the patient's symptoms, indicating a spinal nerve root entrapment.

Comments
This test is not a completely reliable test since it also relieves facet joint and disc pain.

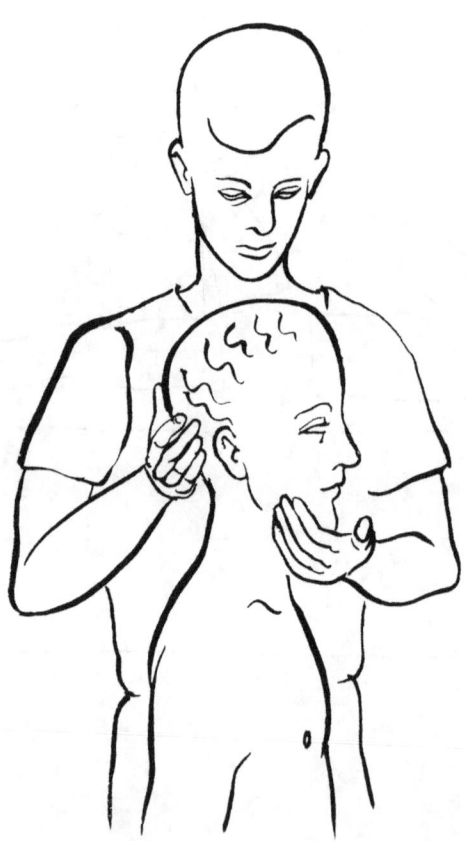

Biceps Reflex Test

Description

The patient sits or stands. The examiner places the patient's arm over his/her opposite arm. With the examiner's hand supporting the patient's arm under the elbow's medial side, the examiner places his/her thumb on the tendon of the biceps in the cubital fossa. When the patient's arm is totally relaxed, the examiner taps his/her thumbnail with a reflex hammer.

Interpretation

The reflex is compared to the opposite side. The reflex is noted as either normal, hypo, hyper, or absent. A positive test is one which is either hypo, hyper, or absent, indicating a C5 neurologic level dysfunction.

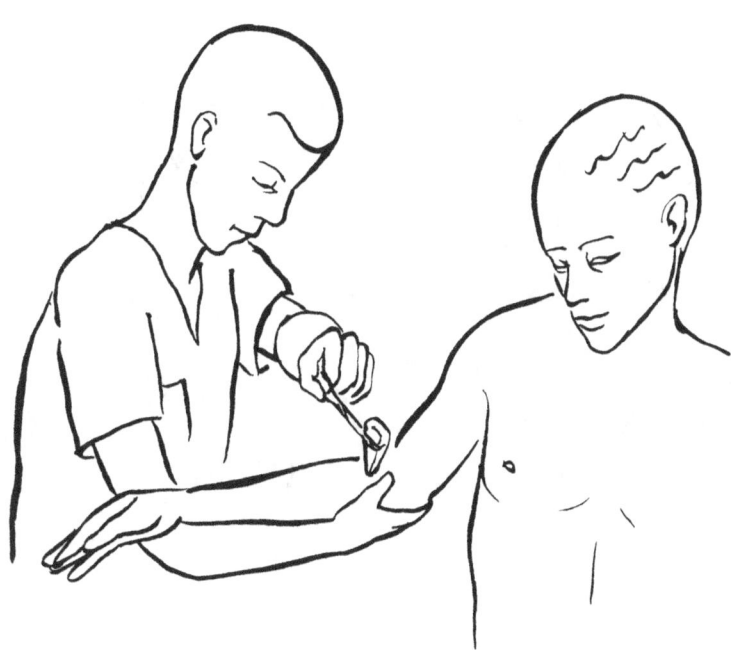

Brachioradialis Reflex Test

Description

The patient sits or stands. The examiner places the patient's arm over his/her opposite arm. When the patient's arm is totally relaxed, the examiner taps the brachioradialis tendon at the distal end of the radius with a reflex hammer.

Interpretation

The reflex is compared to the opposite side. The reflex is noted as either normal, hypo, hyper, or absent. A positive test is one which is either hypo, hyper, or absent, indicating a C6 neurologic level dysfunction.

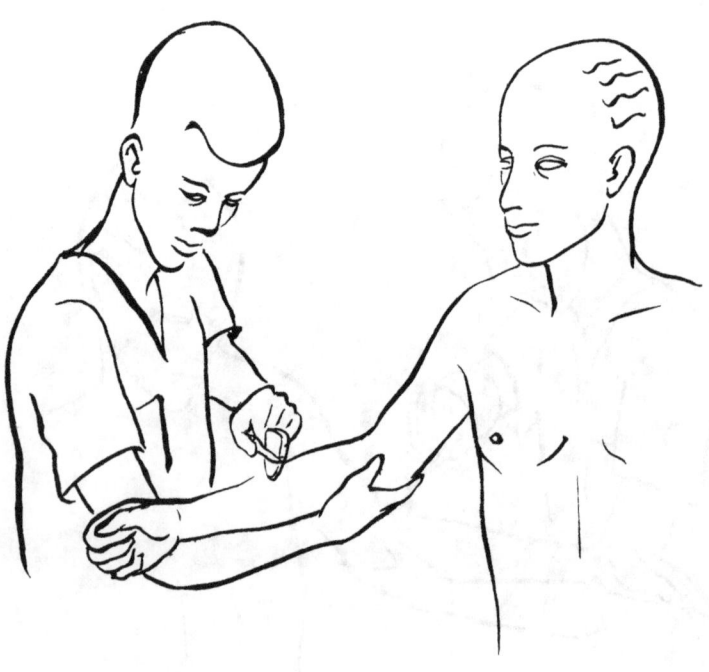

Triceps Reflex Test

Description

The patient sits or stands. The examiner places the patient's arm over his/her opposite arm. When the patient's arm is totally relaxed, the examiner taps the triceps tendon where it crosses the olecranon fossa with a reflex hammer.

Interpretation

The reflex is compared to the opposite side. The reflex is noted as either normal, hypo, hyper, or absent. A positive test is one which is either hypo, hyper, or absent, indicating a C7 neurologic level dysfunction.

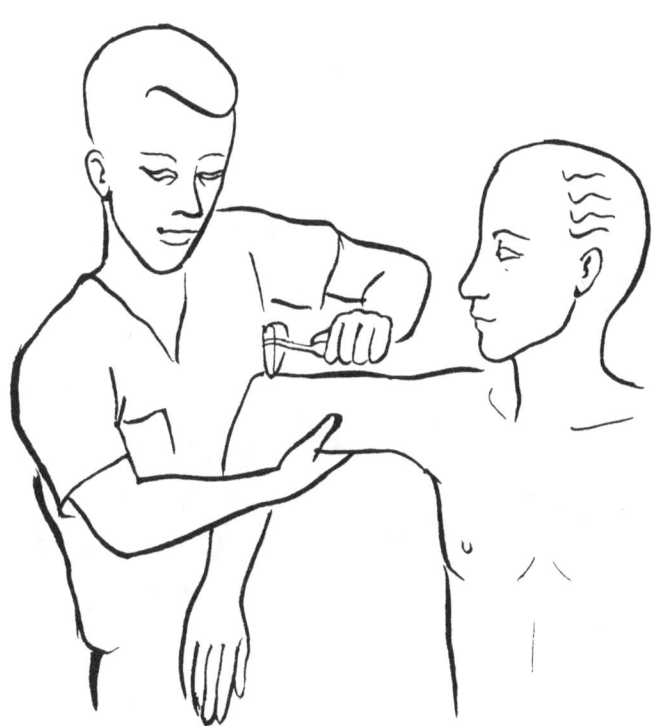

Babinski Reflex Test

Description

The patient lies supine. The examiner uses a blunt instrument and draws across the sole of the foot, starting at the heel, moving along the lateral aspect, and crossing the ball of the foot.

Interpretation

A positive test is one which consists of extension of the great toe, usually associated with fanning of the other toes, indicating an upper motor neuron lesion.

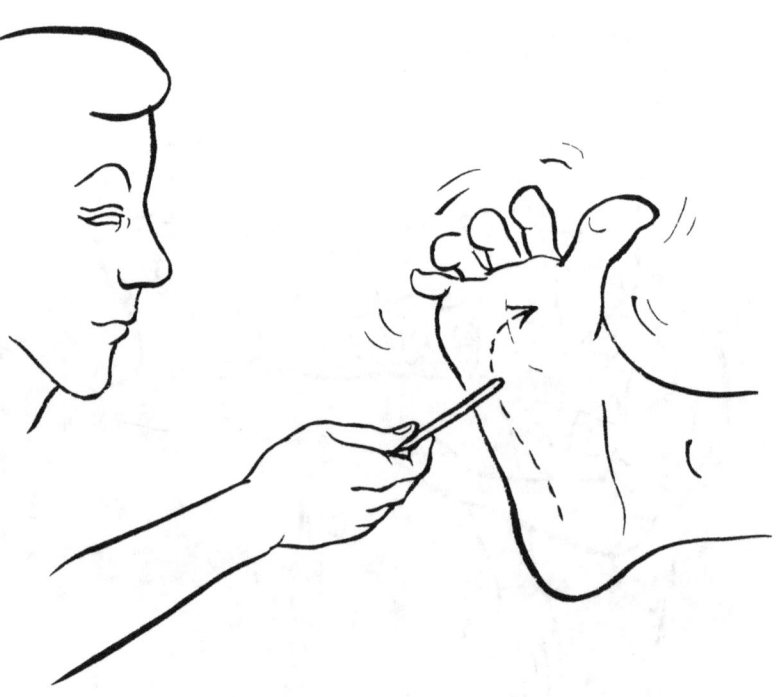

Section 9
Thoracic

Abdominal Reflex Test

Description

The patient lies supine. The examiner strikes each quadrant of the patient's abdomen with the sharp end of a reflex hammer.

Interpretation

A positive test is one in which the umbilicus does not move, indicating an upper motor neuron lesion. An absence of either upper or lower quadrant reflex indicates a lower motor neuron lesion at T7-T10 and T10-L1, respectively.

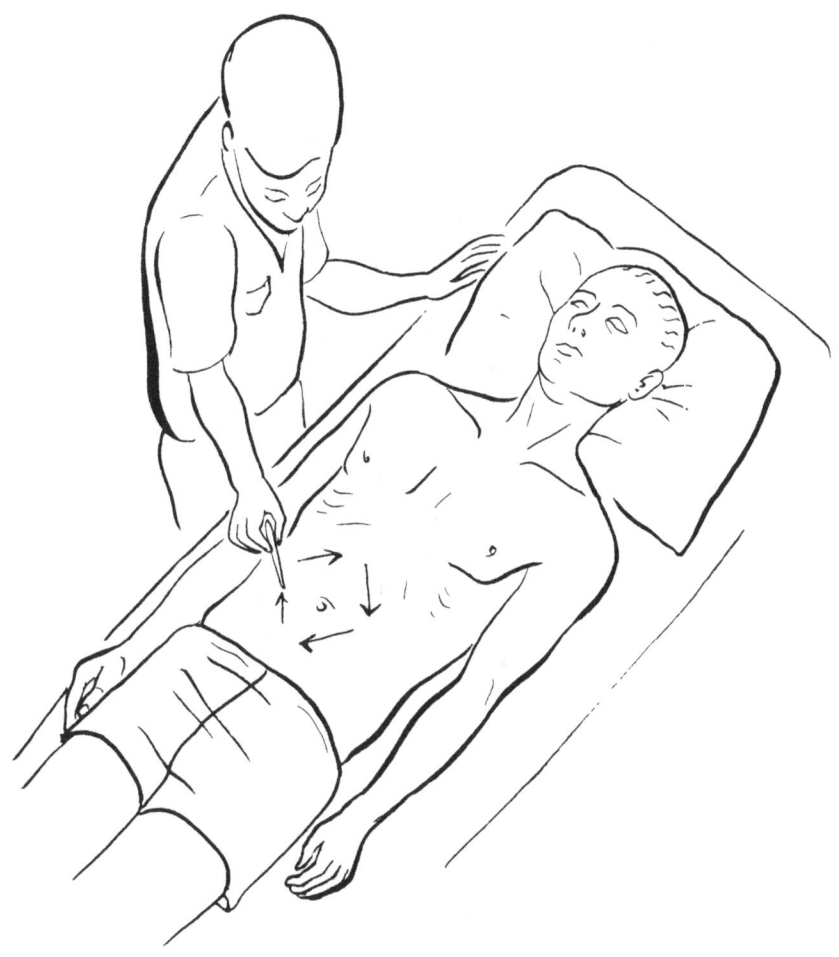

Scapular Approximation Test

Description

The patient sits. The patient is then instructed to approximate the two scapulas.

Interpretation

A positive test is one in which pain is elicited on scapular approximation, indicating either first and second thoracic nerve root compression or a lower thoracic disc lesion.

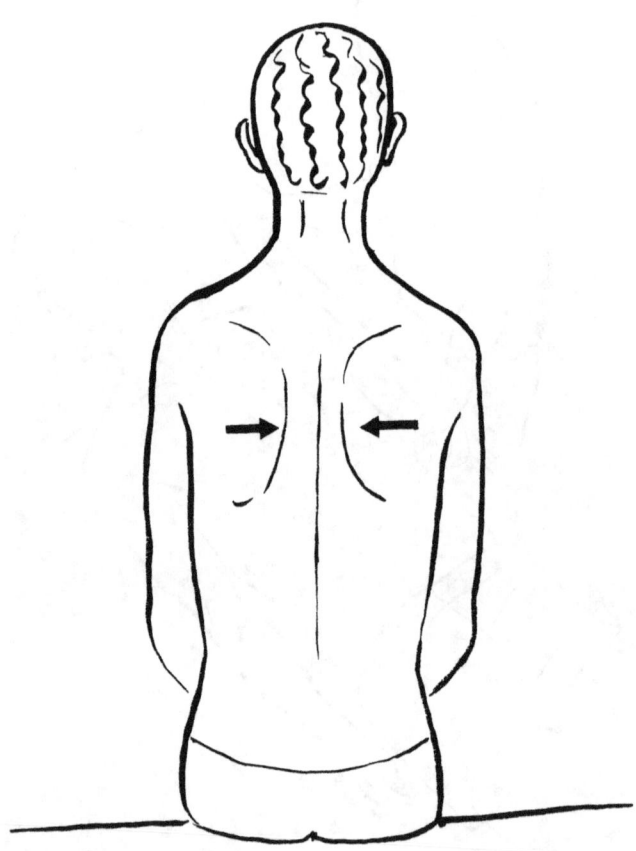

First Thoracic Stretch Test

Description

The patient sits. The patient is instructed to abduct the shoulder to 90° while keeping the elbow fully extended, and then to flex the elbow to 90°. This position does not produce any pain. The patient is then instructed to fully flex the elbow and to put the hand behind the neck.

Interpretation

A positive test is one in which pain is elicited in the scapular area or in the arm, indicating first thoracic nerve root compression.

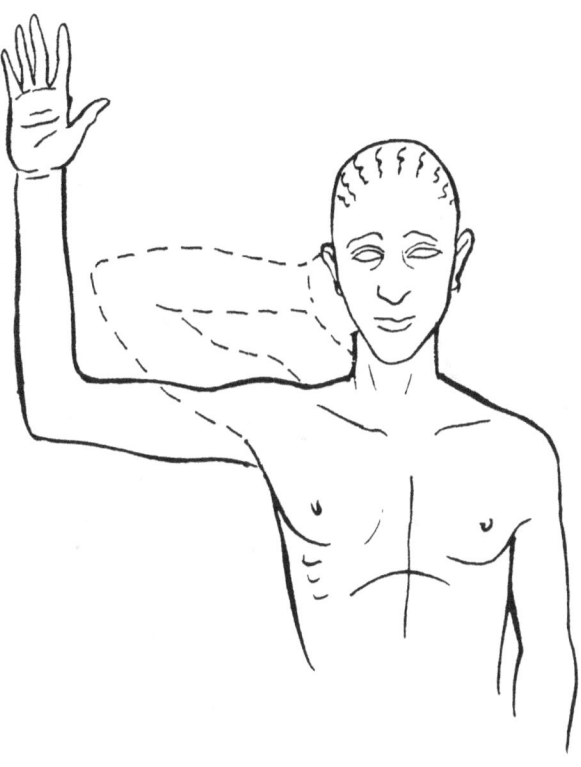

Beevor Test

Description

The patient lies supine with arms crossed on the chest. The patient is then instructed to do a quarter sit-up and to hold the position. The examiner observes the patient's umbilicus.

Interpretation

A positive test is one in which the umbilicus is drawn up, down, or to the side, indicating a weak segmental portion of the rectus abdominis and paraspinal muscles.

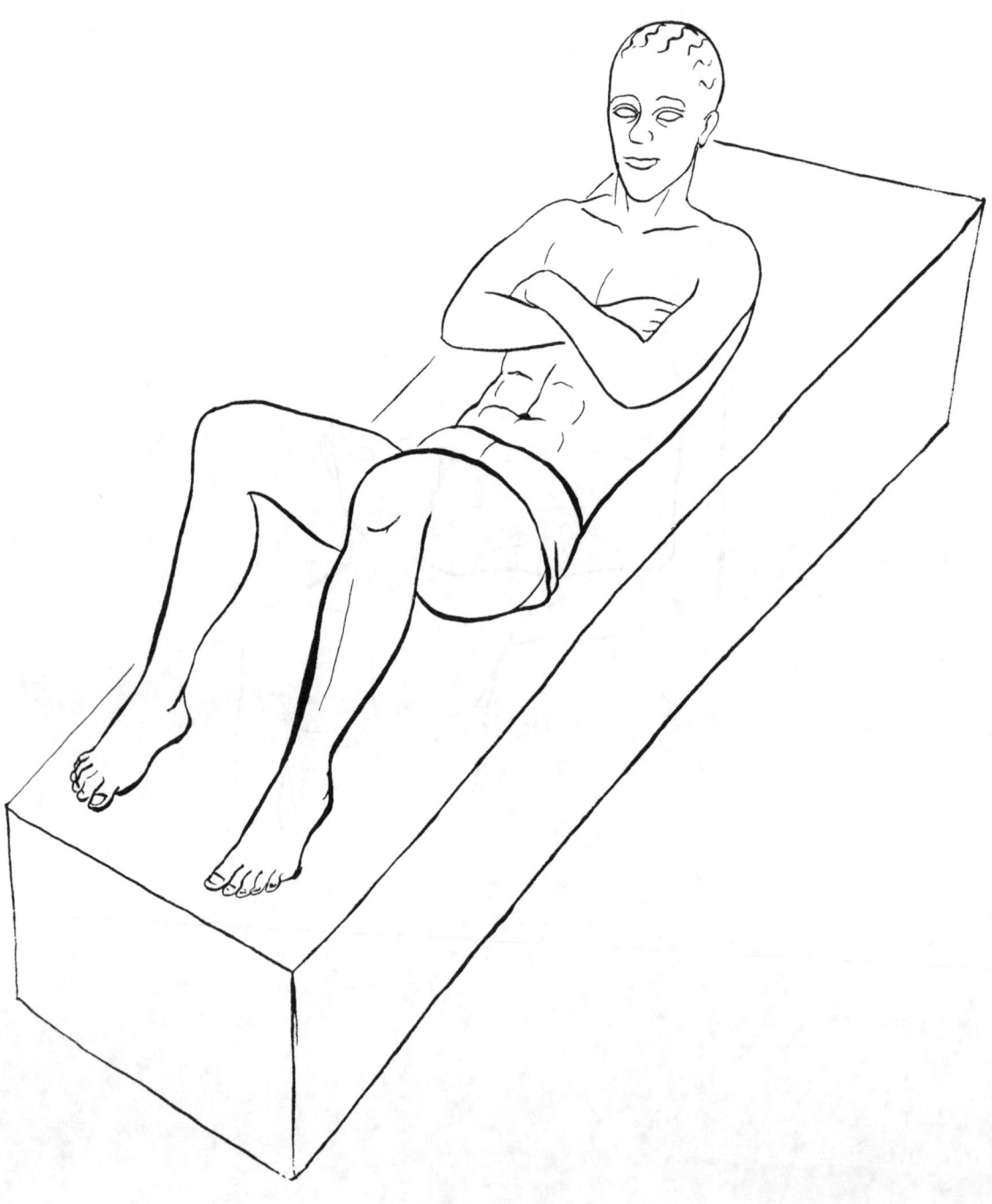

Section 10
Lumbar

Fabere/Patrick Test

Description

The patient lies supine. The examiner stabilizes the patient's pelvis with one hand. With the other hand the examiner places the foot of the patient's involved side on the opposite knee. In this way, the hip joint is flexed, abducted, and externally rotated. The examiner then lowers the involved leg toward the table.

Interpretation

A positive test is one in which pain is produced in the posterior and lateral sides of the hip, indicating sacroiliac joint and low lumbar dysfunction. Pain in the anterior hip indicates hip dysfunction.

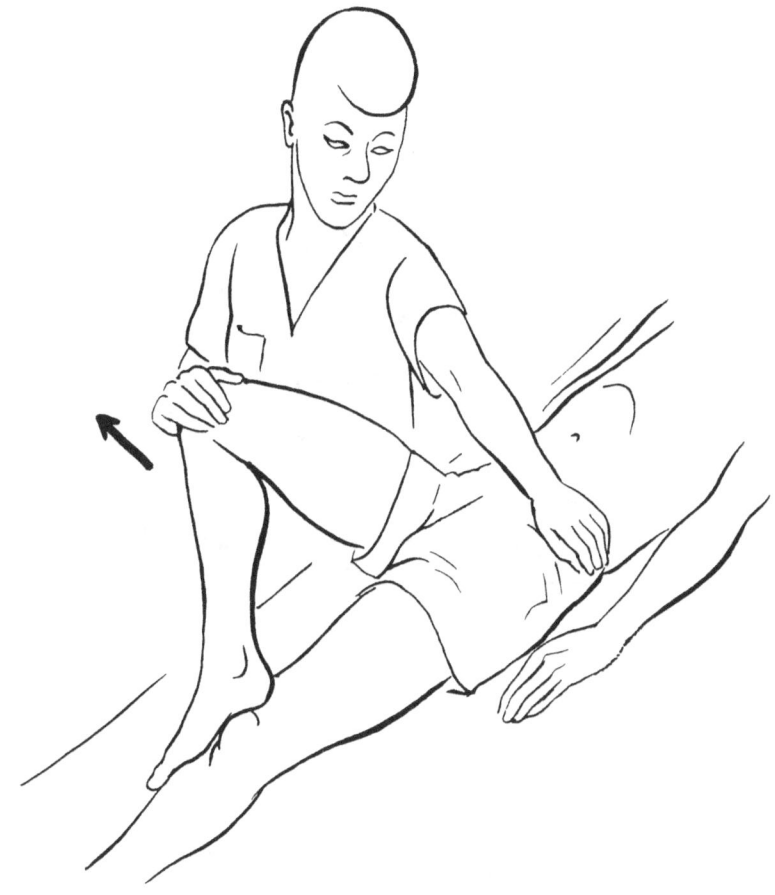

FADIR Test

Description

The patient lies supine. The examiner grasps the patient's knee with both hands and flexes the patient's hip, adducts it, and then internally rotates the hip.

Interpretation

A positive test is one which causes pain in the posterior and lateral side of the pelvis, indicating sacroiliac joint and/or lumbar dysfunction. Anterior pain indicates hip dysfunction.

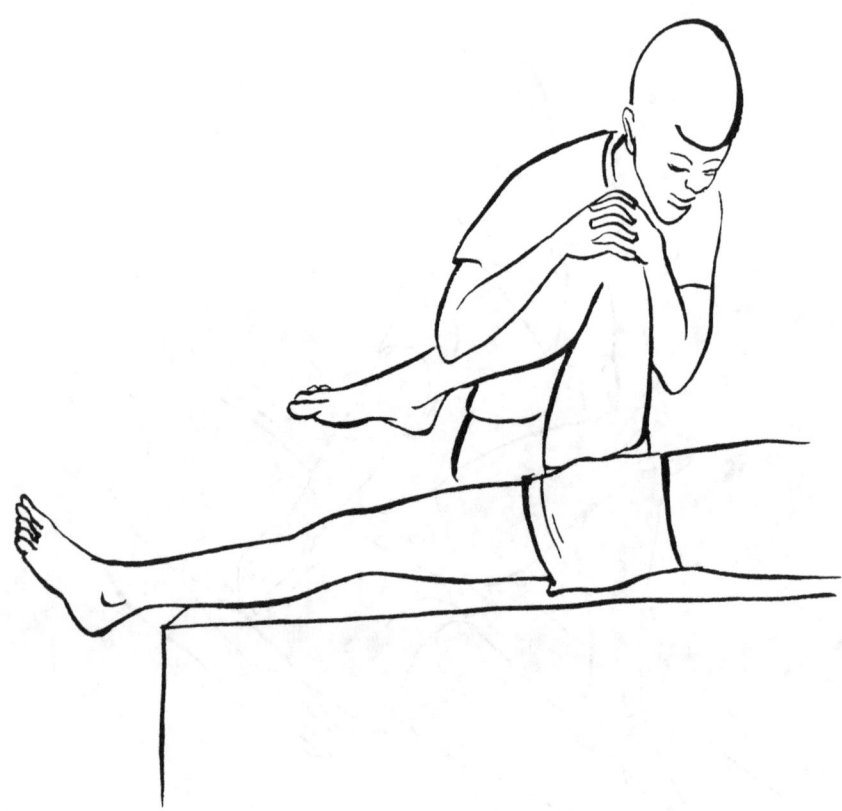

Balance Test

Description

The patient stands with hands resting on the iliac crests. The patient is then instructed to stand on one foot while resting the other foot over the opposite thigh. The test is then repeated on the other leg.

Interpretation

A positive test is one in which pain is produced, indicating balance problems that may initiate pain.

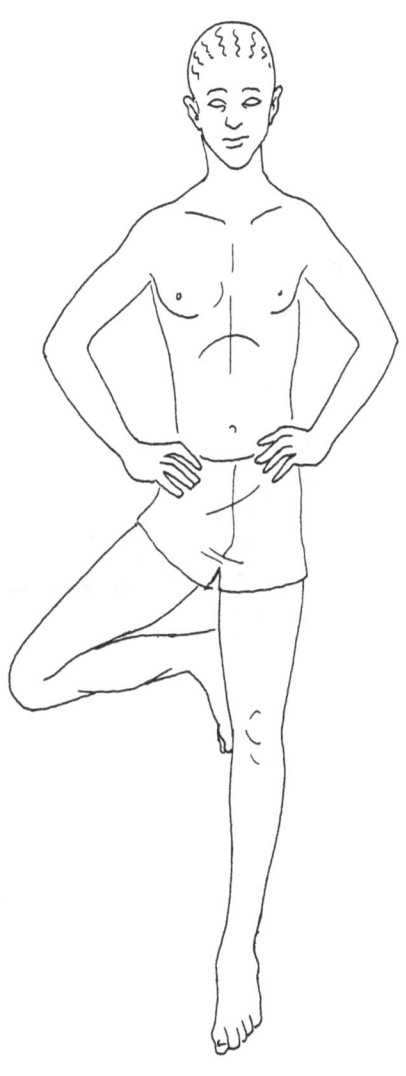

Thomas Test

Description
The patient lies supine with both knees and hips extended. The patient is instructed to flex the uninvolved hip toward the chest as far as possible and to hold the leg in this position.

Interpretation
A positive test is one in which the extended contralateral hip becomes flexed, indicating a fixed flexion contracture of that hip.

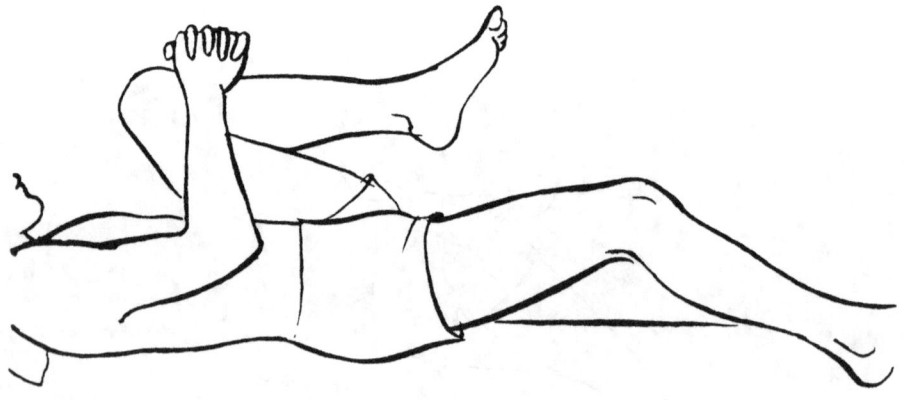

Squat Test

Description

The patient stands. The examiner stands in front of the patient and holds the patient's hands. The patient is instructed to first squat on the heels and then return to standing position.

Interpretation

A positive test is one in which changes in the symptoms are produced, indicating dysfunction of the peripheral joints.

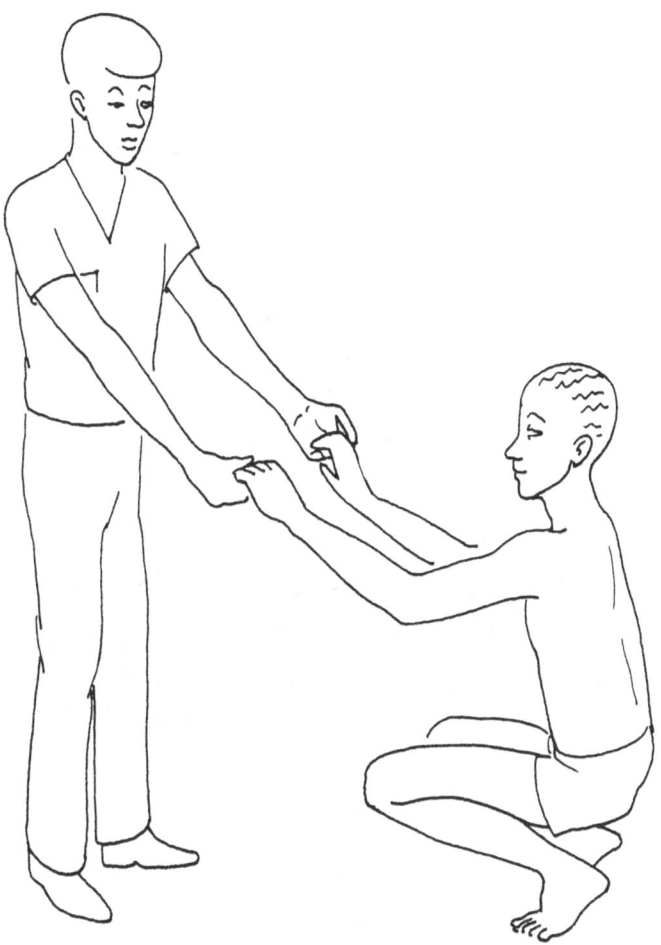

Yeoman Test

Description
The patient lies prone. The examiner grasps the patient's distal tibiofibula with one hand and flexes the patient's knee. The examiner grasps the bent knee with the other hand and then extends the hip. The test is repeated on the other leg.

Interpretation
A positive test is one in which pain is produced in the lumbar spine during both parts of the test, indicating a lumbar dysfunction, while pain on one side indicates sacroiliac dysfunction.

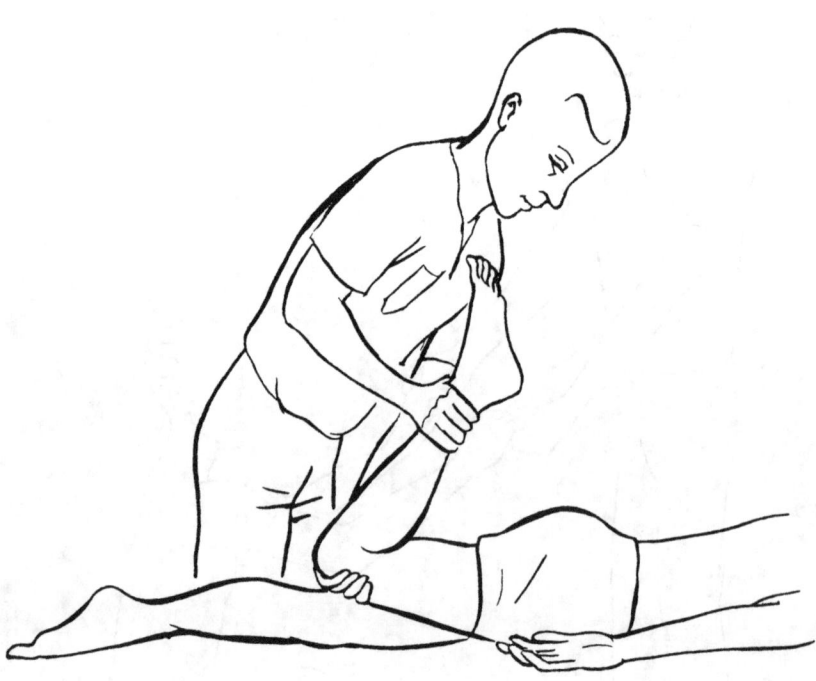

Pheasant Test

Description

The patient lies prone. The examiner gently applies pressure to the posterior aspect of the lumbar spine with one hand and with the other hand passively flexes the patient's knees to the buttocks.

Interpretation

A positive test is one in which pain is produced in the leg, indicating an unstable spinal segment.

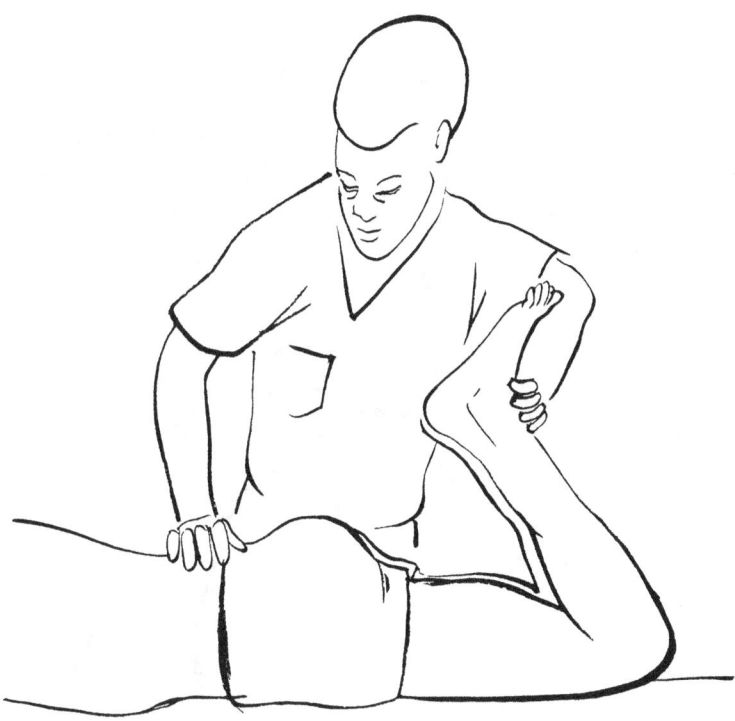

Skin Rolling Test

Description

The patient lies prone. The examiner rolls the patient's skin over the lumbar and thoracic spine area with both hands.

Interpretation

A positive test is one in which tightness is felt and pain is produced, indicating pathological changes such as abnormal amount of fat tissue fluid, tension, localized swelling, and nodules in the subcutaneous tissue.

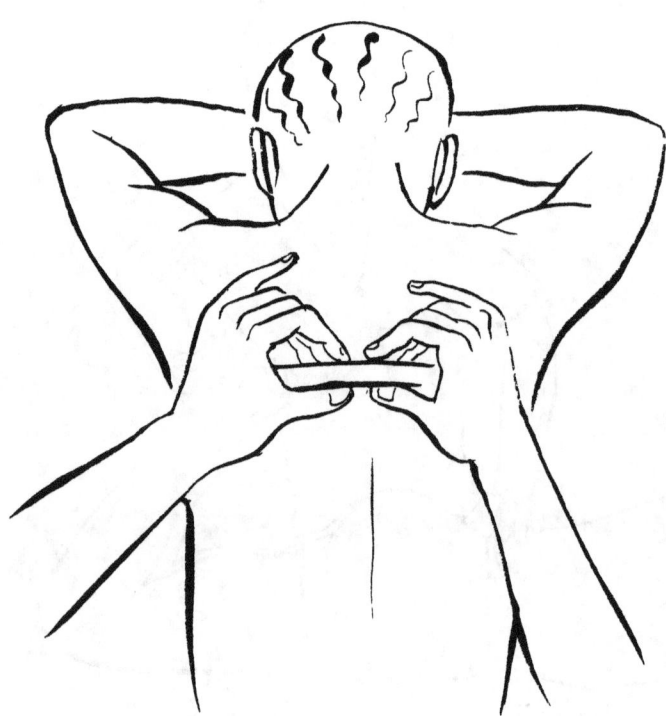

Schober Test

Description

The patient sits on the treatment table. The examiner marks a point midway between the "dimples of the pelvis" at the level of S2, a second point 0.5 cm below and a third point 10 cm above the first marked point. The examiner then measures the distance between the three points. The patient is then instructed to bend forward and the examiner again measures the distance.

Interpretation

The difference between the two measurements is an indication of flexion occurring in the lumbar spine.

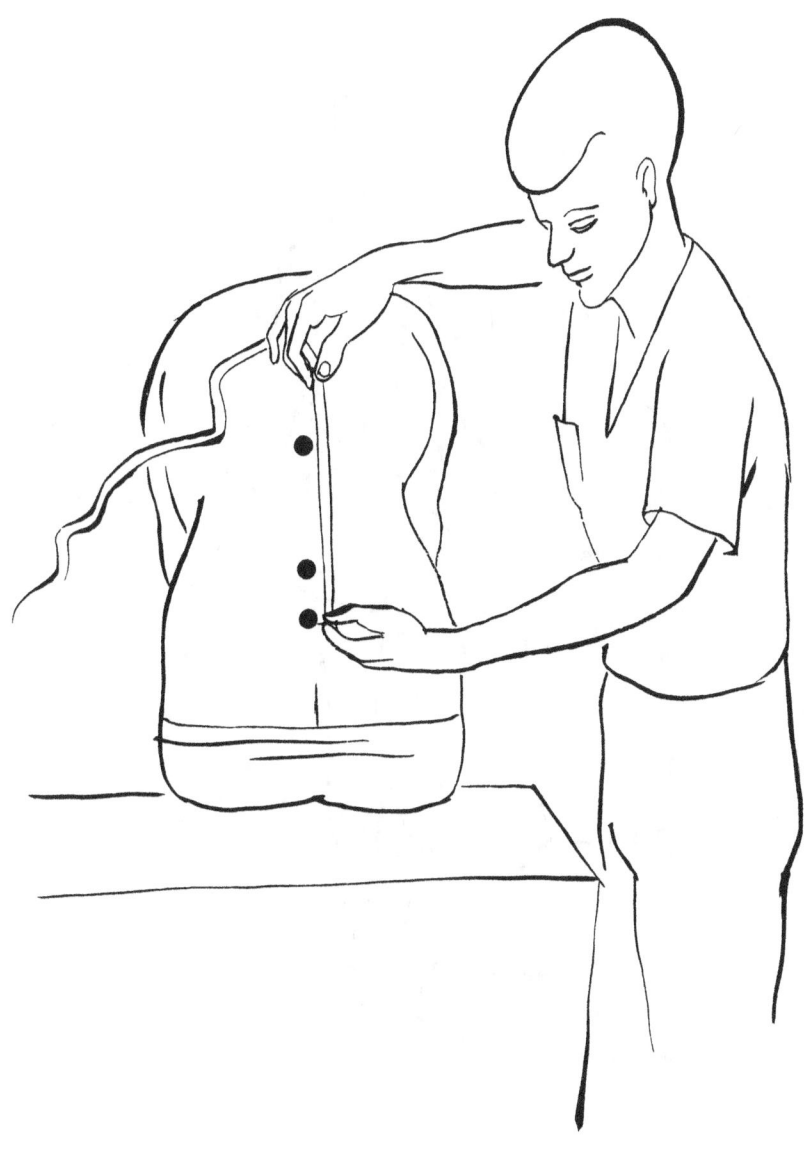

Weight Shift Test

Description

The patient stands. The examiner places the thumbs on the patient's lumbar paraspinals. The patient is then instructed to shift the weight from one foot to the other.

Interpretation

A positive test is one in which the muscles do not feel relaxed on the side of the stance foot, indicating muscle guarding and muscle spasm.

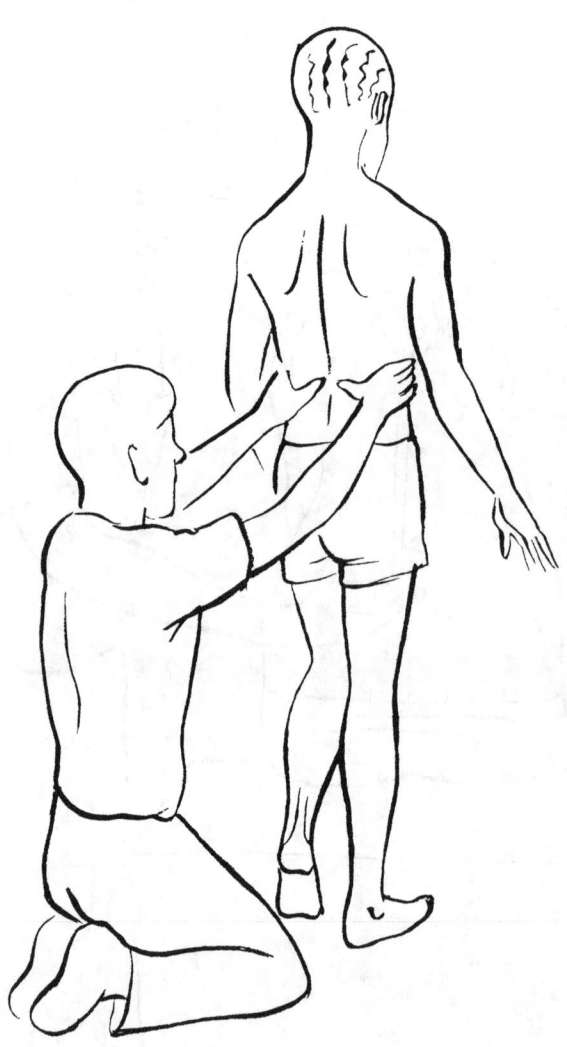

Flip Test

Description

The patient lies supine. The examiner performs a straight leg raise test (refer to page 245). The patient is then placed in sitting position and the examiner performs a sitting straight leg raising test (refer to page 247).

Interpretation

A positive test is one in which both tests produce pain in the sciatic nerve distribution, indicating low lumbar spine dysfunction.

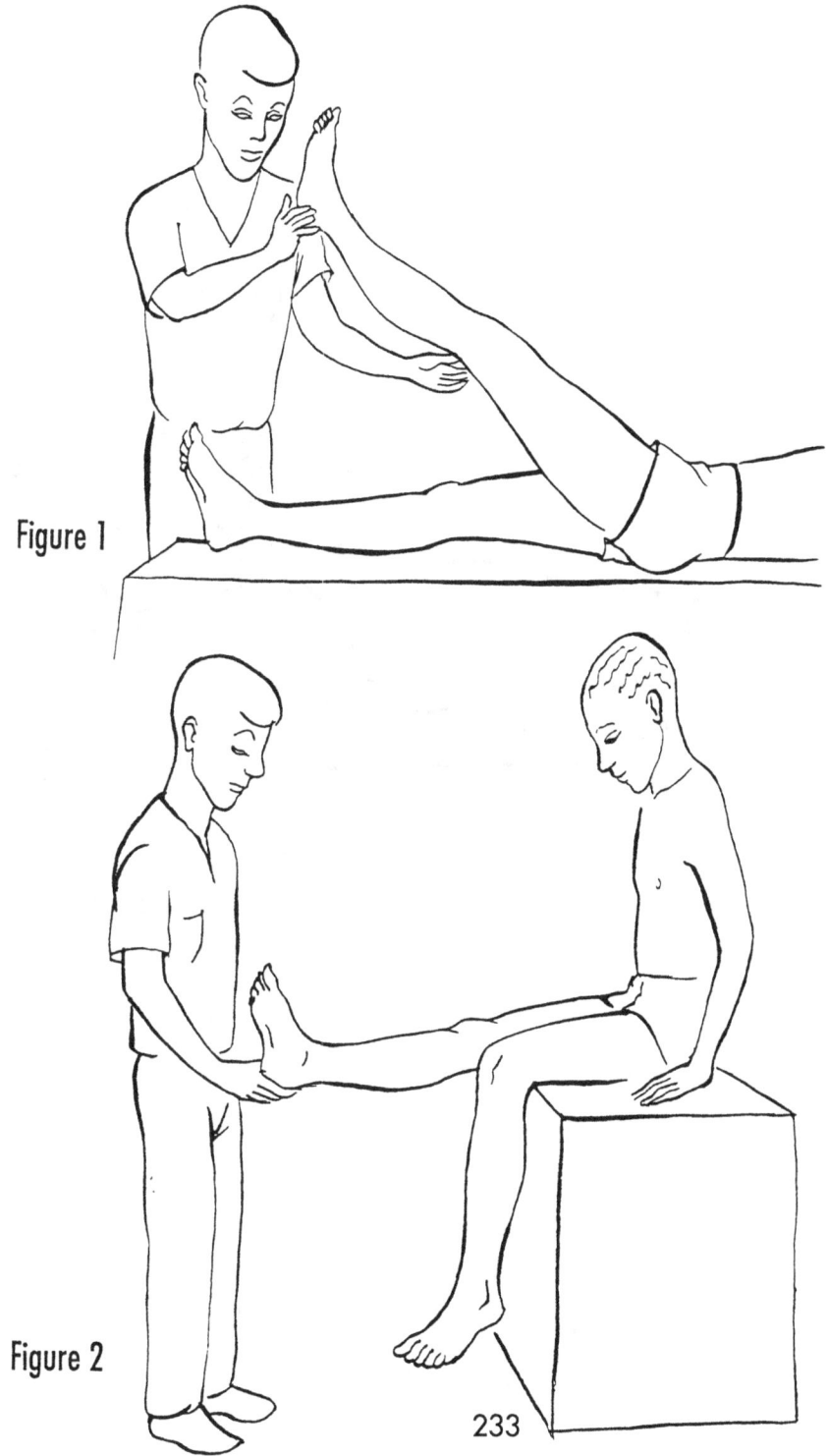

Figure 1

Figure 2

Brudzinski Test

Description

The patient lies supine. The examiner stands at the head of the patient and cradles the patient's head with both hands. The examiner then passively flexes the patient's neck while holding the chest down.

Interpretation

A positive test is one in which the patient flexes both hips as the neck is flexed, indicating nerve root involvement associated with meningeal irritation.

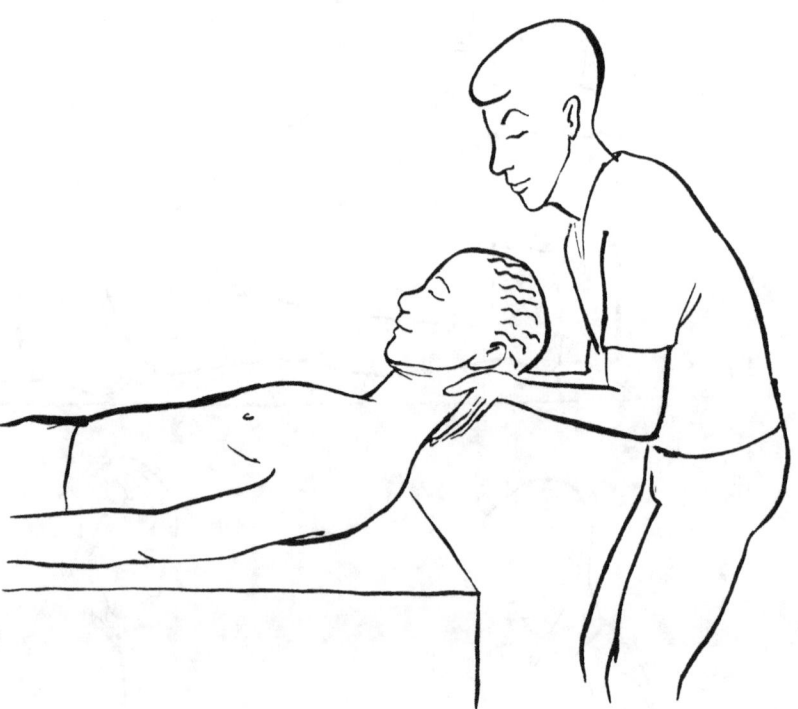

Slump Test

Description

The patient sits on the edge of the table with legs hanging downward and hands resting in the lap. This position should not produce any pain. The examiner stands to the side being tested. The patient is instructed to slump the thoracic and lumbar spine into flexion while the cervical spine is kept neutral. The patient is then instructed to flex the head and neck and the examiner applies over pressure to the upper trunk. While maintaining full spinal flexion, the patient is instructed to fully extend the knee and the examiner holds the knee. The patient is then instructed to actively dorsiflex the foot while the examiner applies an over pressure.

Interpretation

A positive test is one in which pain is produced at each step of the test, indicating thecal or intrathecal pathology.

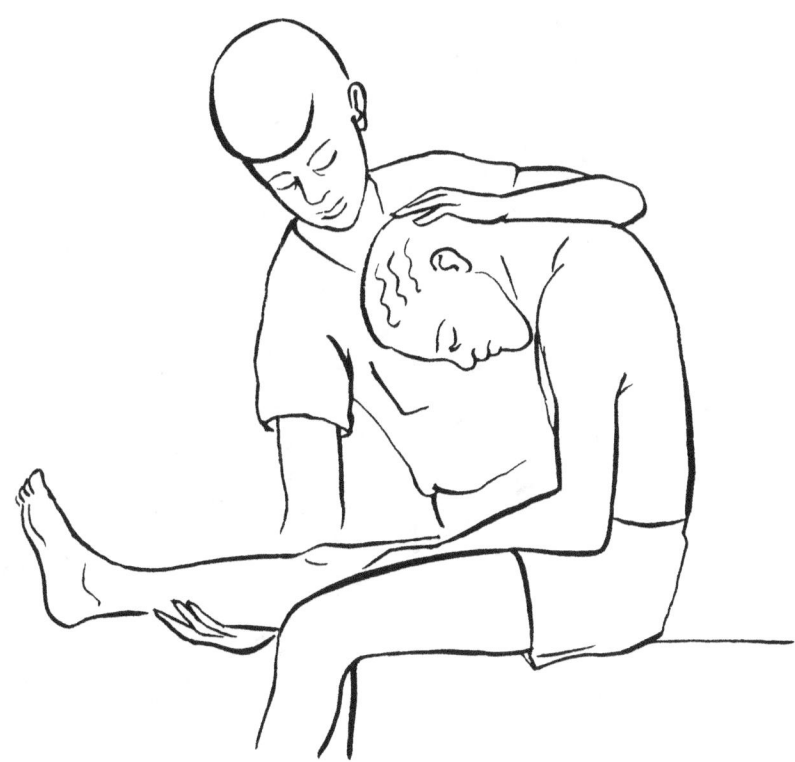

Naffziger Test

Description

The patient lies supine. The examiner gently compresses the patient's jugular veins with both hands for about 10 seconds until the patient's face begins to flush. The patient is then asked to cough.

Interpretation

A positive test is one in which coughing causes pain, indicating intrathecal pathology.

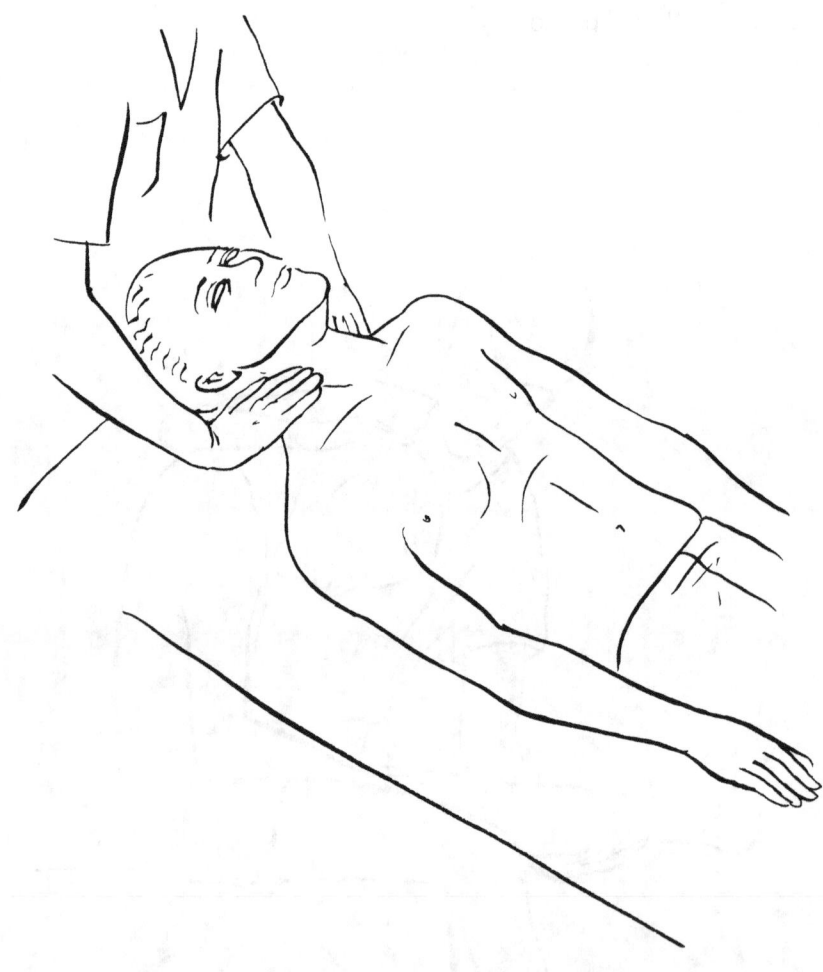

Milgram Test

Description

The patient lies supine. The patient is then instructed to raise both legs straight two inches high and to hold this position as long as possible. The patient should be able to hold this position for at least 30 seconds.

Interpretation

A positive test is one in which the patient is unable to hold this position for 30 seconds, or unable to lift the legs at all, or experiences pain as the maneuver is attempted, indicating thecal, intrathecal, or extrathecal pathology.

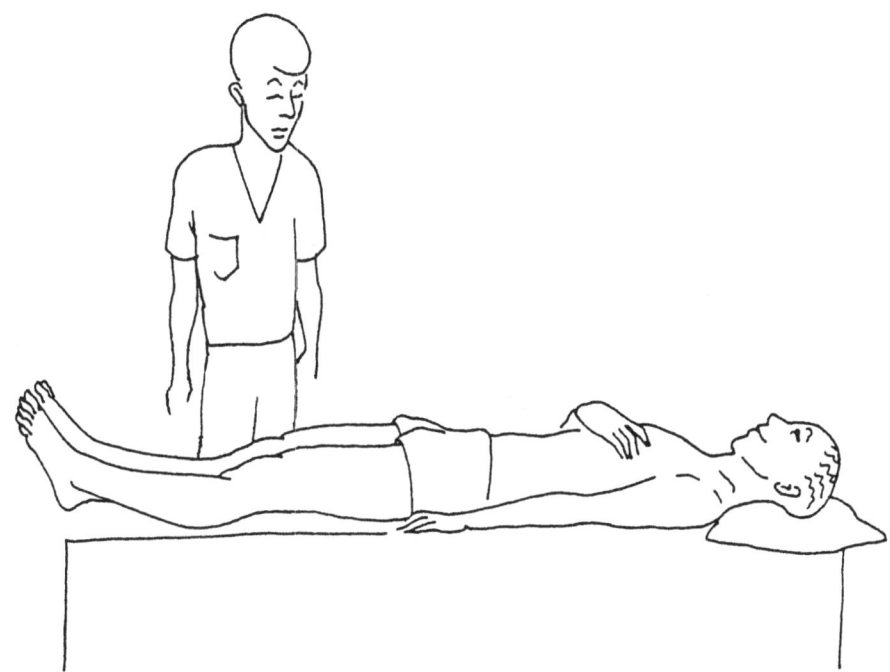

Kerning Test

Description

The patient lies supine with both hands placed behind the head. The examiner raises the patient's leg straight with knee in extended position. The patient is then instructed to flex the head onto the chest.

Interpretation

A positive test is one in which the patient experiences pain in the lower back or down the leg, indicating meningeal irritation, nerve root involvement, or irritation of the dural coverings of the nerve root.

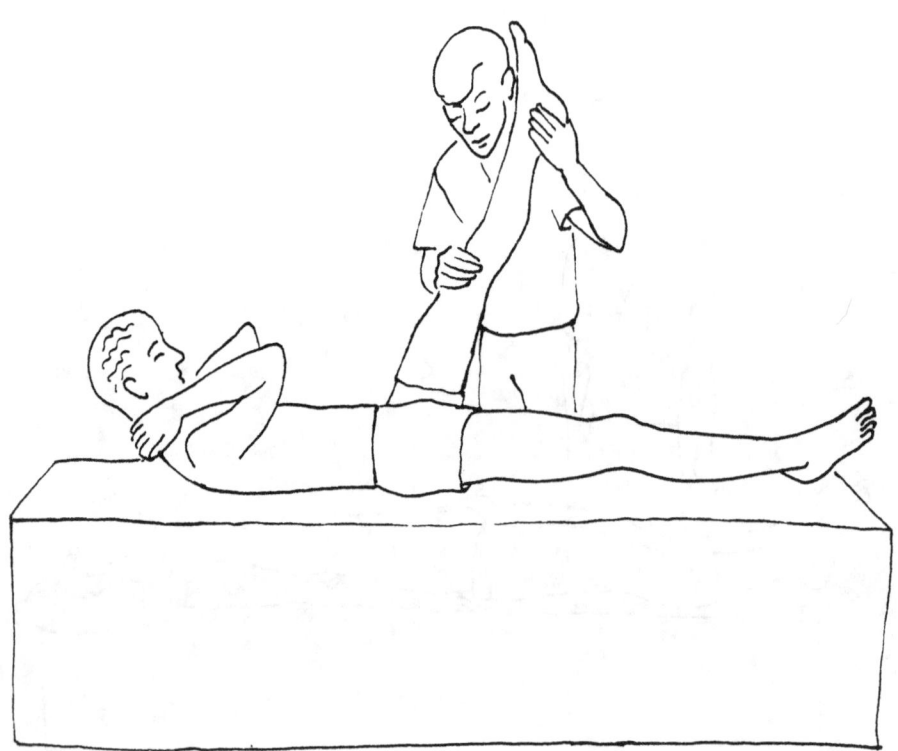

Prone Knee-Bending Test

Description

The patient lies prone. The examiner holds the patient's distal tibiofibula and passively flexes the patient's knee as far as possible (at least 90° of flexion), ensuring that the patient's hip is not rotated. The flexed knee position is maintained for 45-60 seconds.

Interpretation

A positive test is one in which pain is produced in the lumbar area, indicating L2-L3 nerve root lesion. Pain in the anterior thigh indicates tight quadricep muscles.

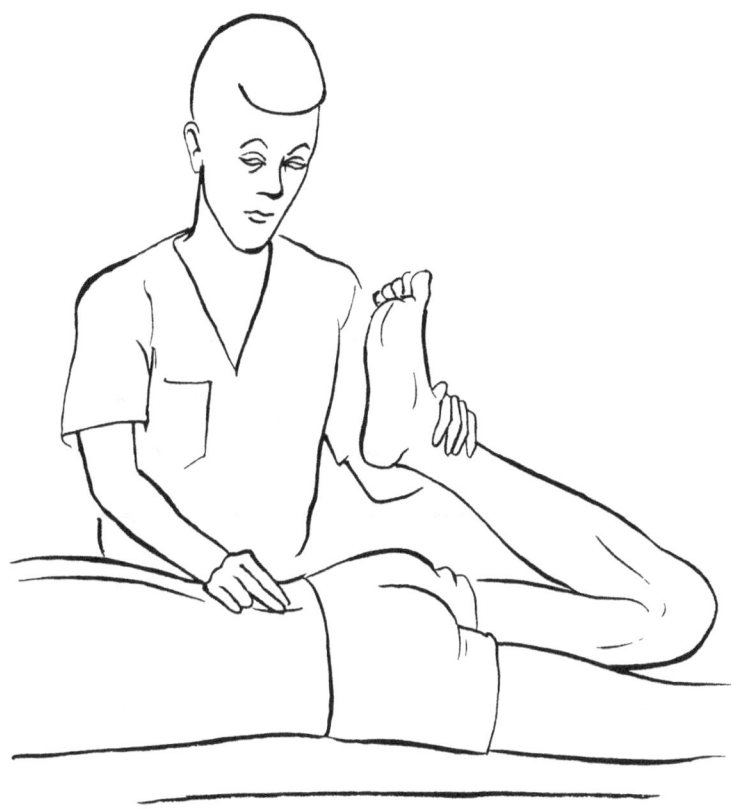

Femoral Nerve Stretch Test

Description

The patient lies prone. The examiner grasps the patient's distal tibiofibula and passively flexes the patient's knee and hyperextends the hip.

Interpretation

A positive test is one in which pain is produced in the femoral nerve distribution of the anterior thigh, indicating femoral nerve entrapment.

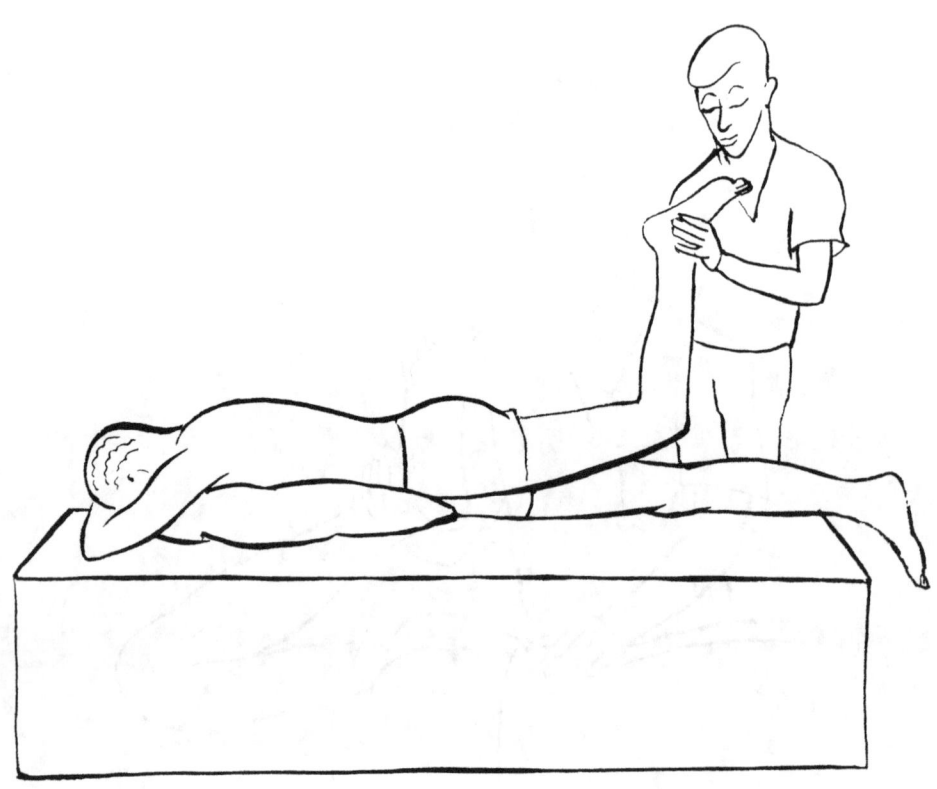

Sciatic Tension Test

Description

The patient sits on the edge of the table with legs hanging down. The examiner flexes the patient's involved leg at hip and knee to about 90°. The examiner holds the distal tibiofibula with one hand and with the other hand presses in the popliteal space.

Interpretation

A positive test is one in which pain is elicited in the leg as the fingers press in the popliteal space, indicating a pressure or tension on the sciatic nerve.

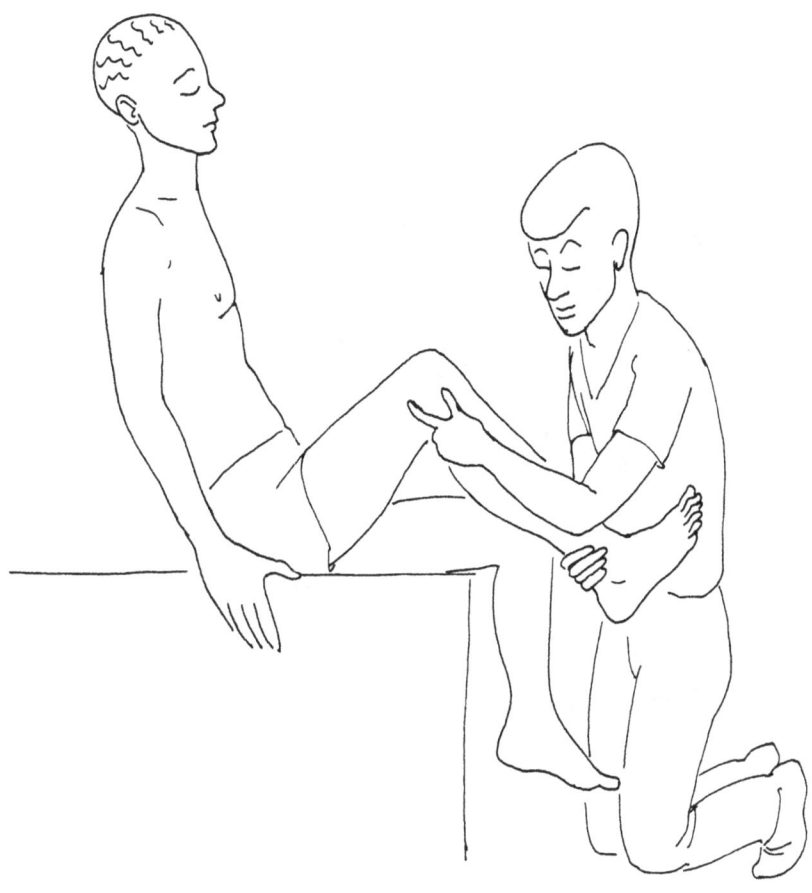

Bowstring/Cram Test

Description

The patient lies supine. The examiner performs a passive straight leg raise test. If there is pain with straight leg raise, pain is reduced by flexing the knee to about 20°. The examiner then applies pressure to the popliteal area with the thumb.

Interpretation

A positive test is one in which painful radicular symptoms are reproduced with pressure at the popliteal area, indicating tension or pressure on the sciatic nerve.

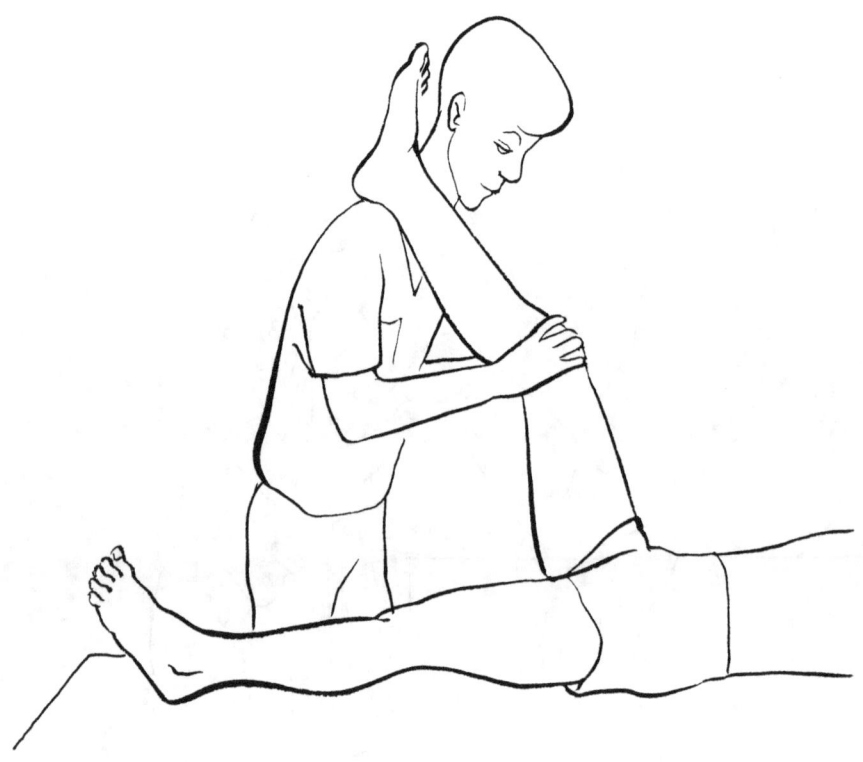

Sciatic Nerve Test

Description

The patient lies on the uninvolved side with the involved hip and knee flexed to about 90°. The examiner holds the patient's pelvis with one hand. With the other hand the examiner palpates the patient's greater trochanter and ischial tuberosity and then presses firmly with the thumb into the soft tissue at the midpoint between the greater trochanter and the ischial tuberosity.

Interpretation

A positive test is one which causes discomfort/tenderness when the pressure is applied, indicating inflammation of the sciatic nerve.

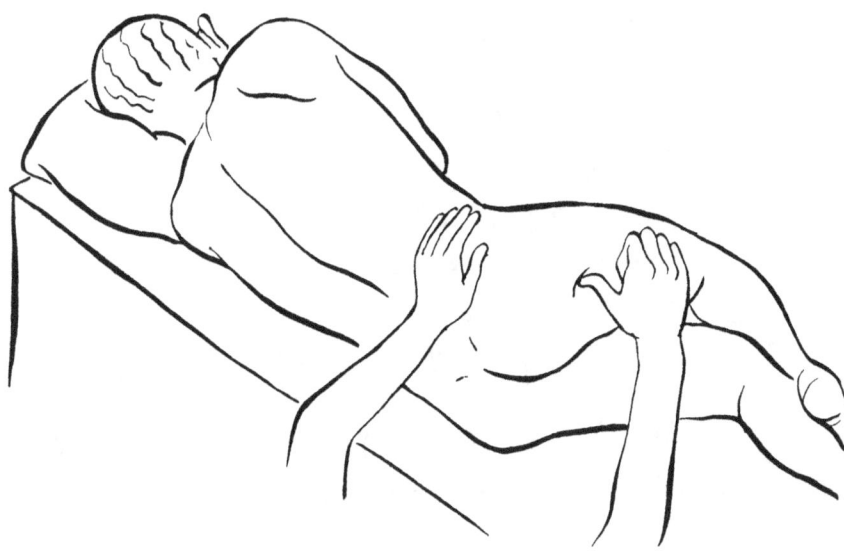

Nachlas Test

Description

The patient lies prone. The examiner holds the patient's distal tibiofibula and passively flexes the patient's knee to full range of motion.

Interpretation

A positive test is one in which pain is elicited in the lumbar area, indicating a lumbar disc disease. Pain in the buttock indicates a sacroiliac joint dysfunction.

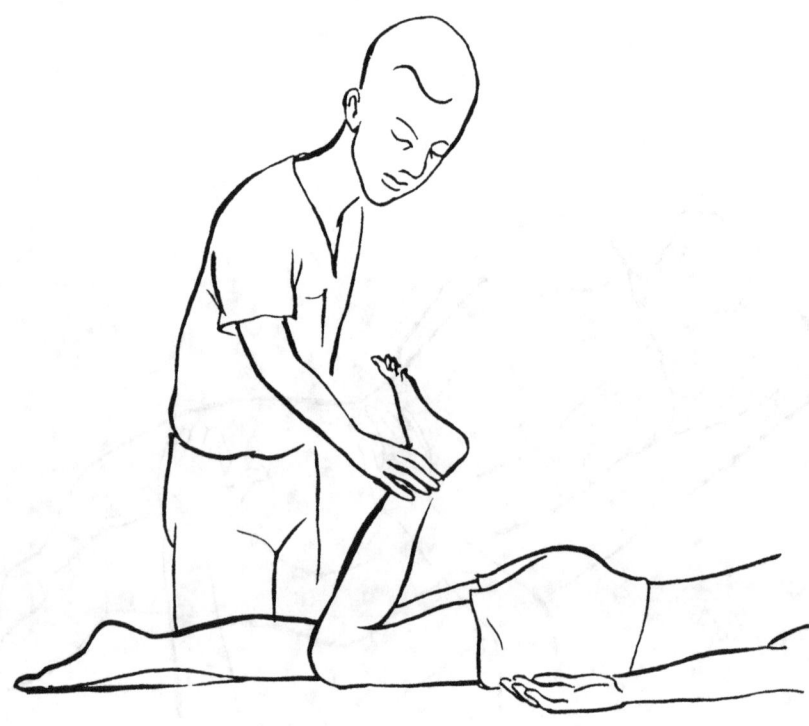

Straight Leg Raising Test

Description

The patient lies supine. The examiner raises the patient's leg upward by supporting the foot around the calcaneus while keeping the knee extended.

Interpretation

A positive test is one in which pain is produced in the lower back and extends all the way down the leg, indicating sciatic nerve irritation.

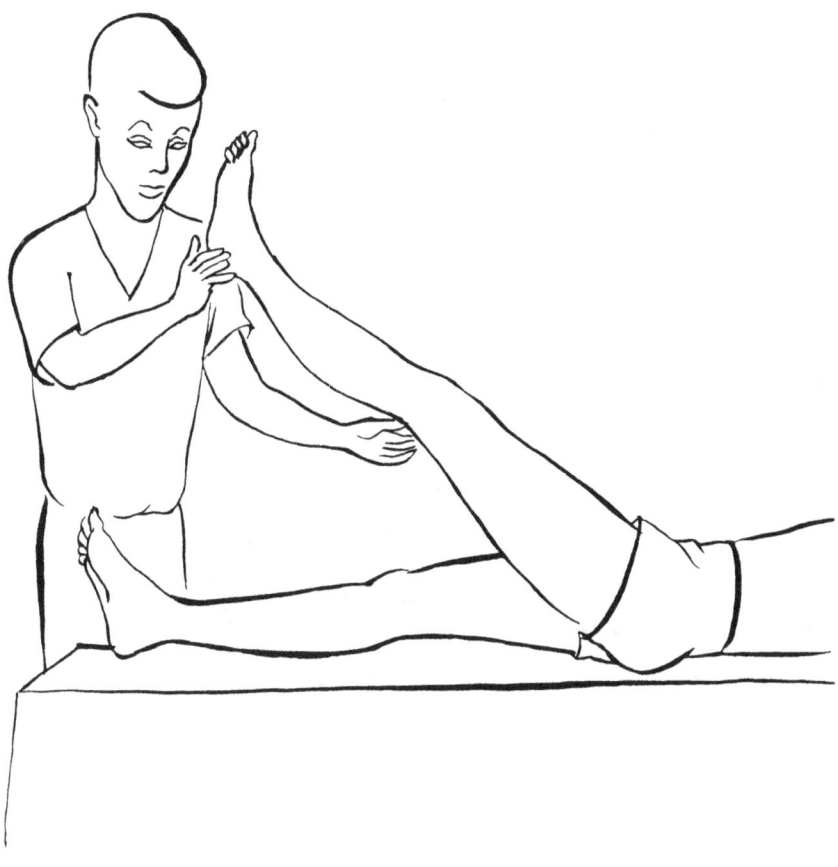

Well Leg Straight Leg Raising Test

Description

The patient lies supine. The examiner raises the patient's uninvolved leg upward by supporting the foot around the calcaneus while keeping the knee extended.

Interpretation

A positive test is one which causes low back and radiating leg pain on the involved side, indicating a nerve root compression or a herniated disc in the lumbar spine.

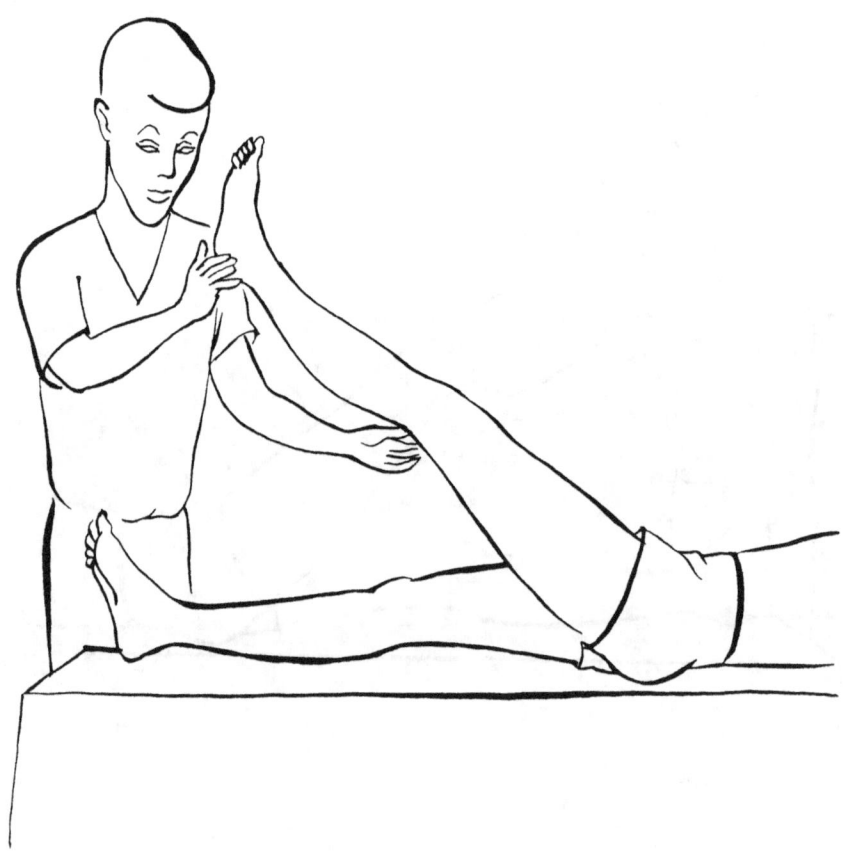

Sitting Straight Leg Raising Test

Description

The patient sits on the edge of the table with knees and hips flexed to 90°. The examiner holds the patient's foot and then extends the patient's knee.

Interpretation

A positive test is one in which pain is produced in the lower back and extends down the leg, indicating sciatic nerve irritation.

Comments

This test confirms the straight leg raising test. If the sitting straight leg raising is pain free and the supine straight leg raising causes considerably more reaction, the patient is probably exaggerating the symptoms.

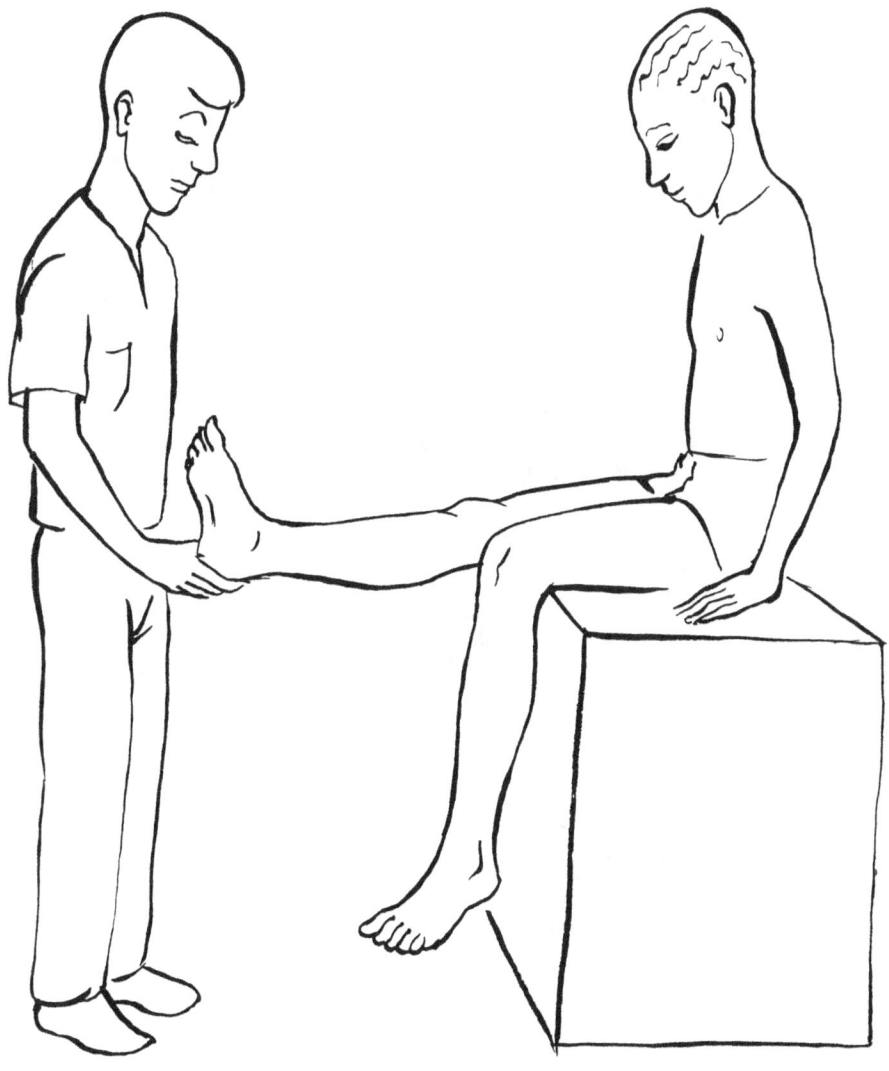

Lasegue Test

Description

The patient lies supine. The examiner grasps the patient's distal tibiofibula with one hand and supports the distal femur with the other hand. The examiner flexes the patient's hip and knee to 90° and then extends the knee.

Interpretation

A positive test is one in which pain is produced in the sciatic nerve distribution when the knee is extended less than about 70°, indicating sciatic nerve irritation.

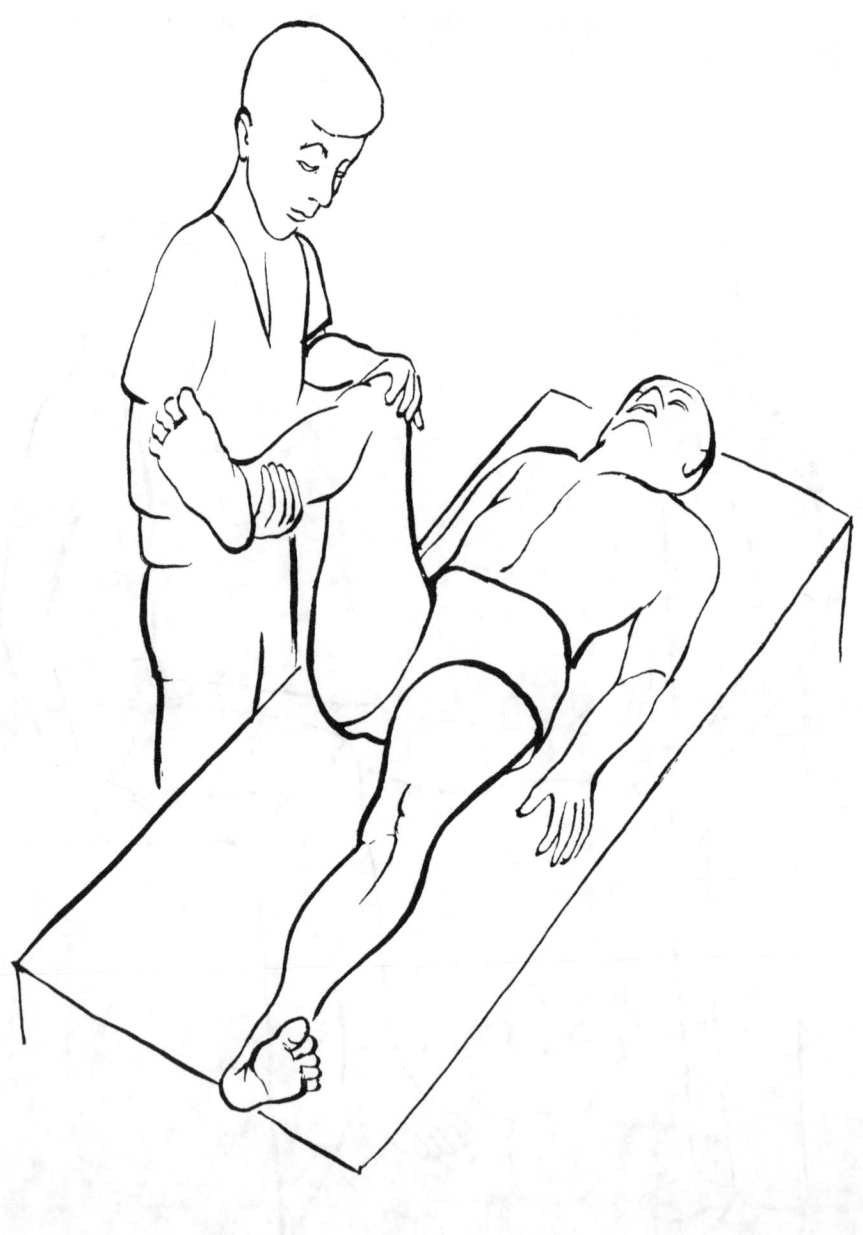

Braggard Test

Description

The patient lies supine. The examiner holds the patient's distal tibiofibula with one hand and raises the patient's leg passively to the point of pain, then lowers the leg about 5° and dorsiflexes the foot with the other hand.

Interpretation

A positive test is one in which pain is elicited in the thigh and/or the leg, indicating sciatic radiculopathy.

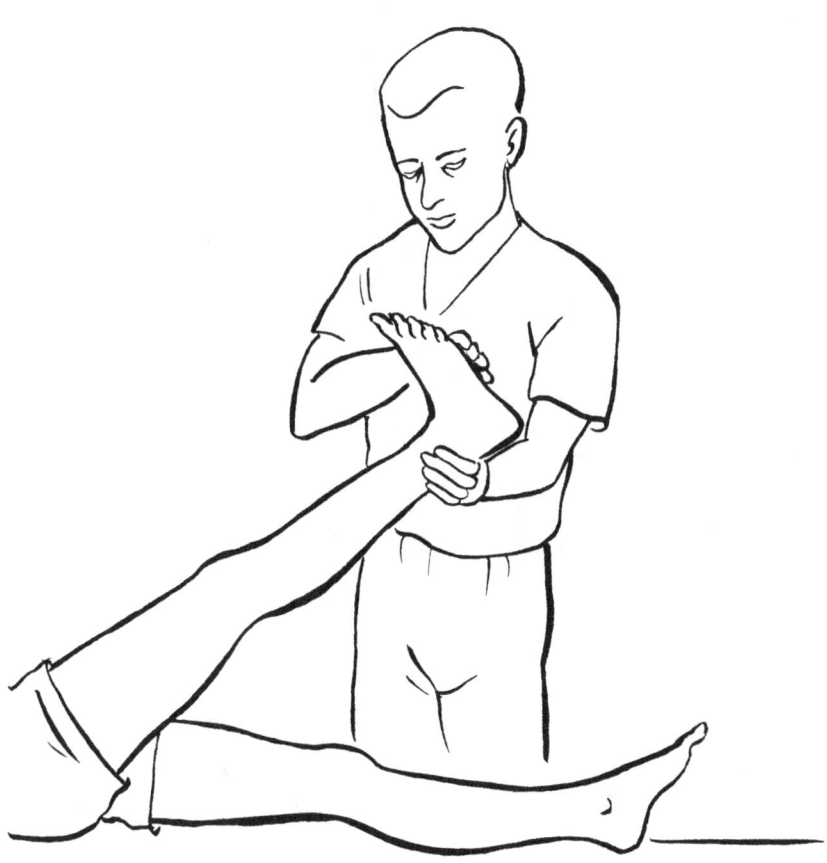

Buckling Test

Description
The patient lies supine. The patient is instructed to actively flex the hip at least to 70° with the knee held in the extended position.

Interpretation
A positive test is one in which the patient flexes the knee to flex the hip to 70°, indicating sciatic radiculopathy.

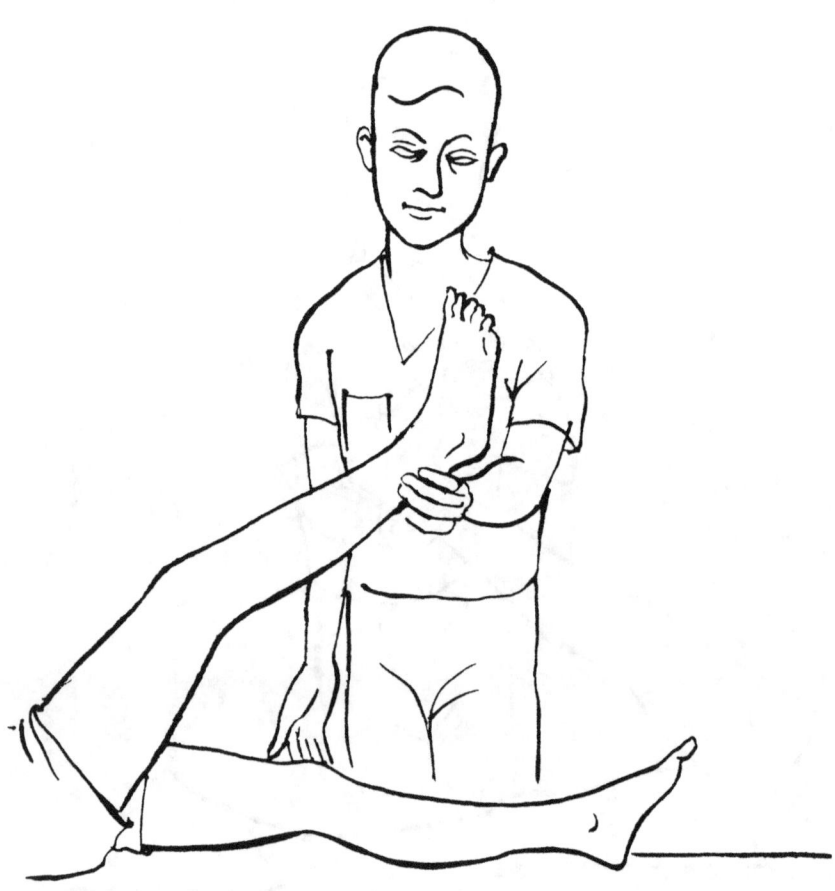

Goldthwaith Test

Description

The patient lies supine. The examiner places one hand under the patient's lumbar spine with each finger under an interspinous space. With the other hand, the examiner grasps the patient's distal tibiofibula and raises the leg straight like performing a straight leg raising test.

Interpretation

A positive test is one in which pain is elicited before fanning out of the lumbar vertebra, indicating a sacroiliac joint dysfunction. Elicitation of radiating pain during lumbar fanning indicates sciatic radiculopathy.

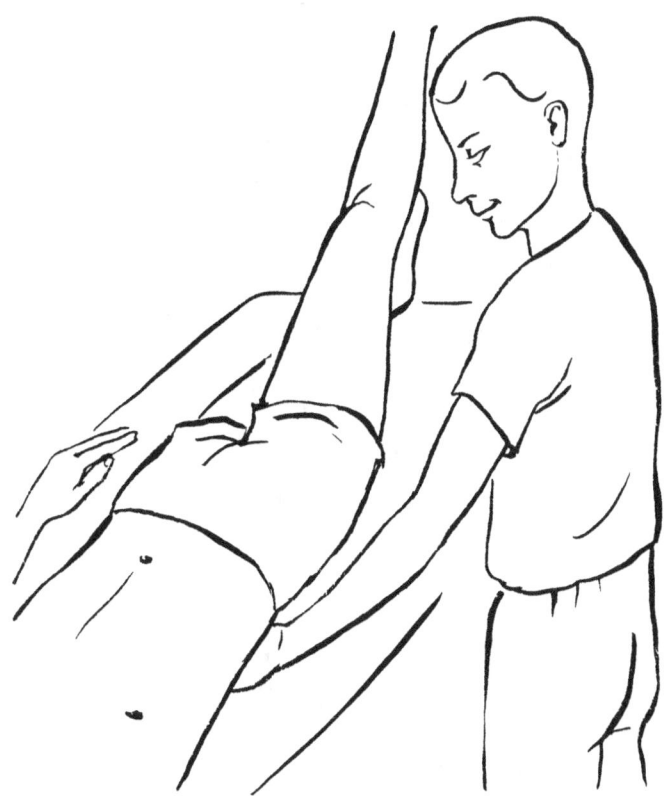

Minor Test

Description

The patient sits. The patient is then instructed to stand.

Interpretation

A positive test is one in which the patient supports himself/herself on the uninvolved side and keeps the involved leg flexed, indicating sciatic radiculopathy.

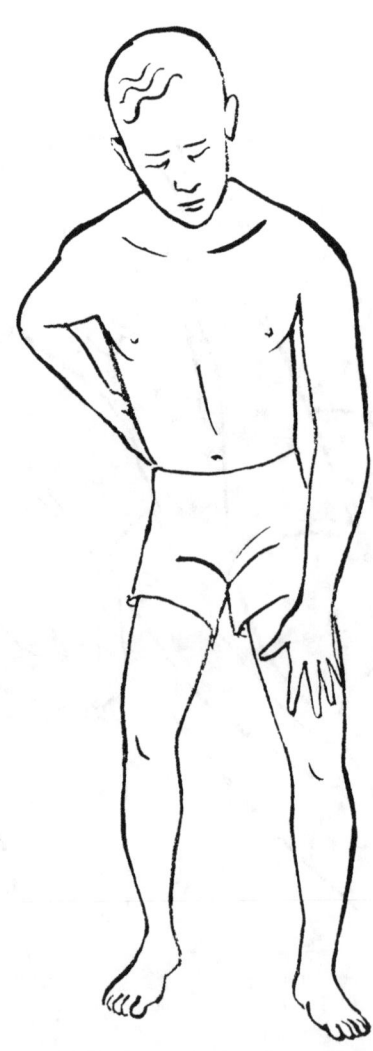

Turyn Test

Description

The patient lies supine with hips and knees extended. The examiner holds the patient's great toe and extends it.

Interpretation

A positive test is one in which pain is elicited in the gluteal region or radiates down the leg, indicating sciatic radiculopathy.

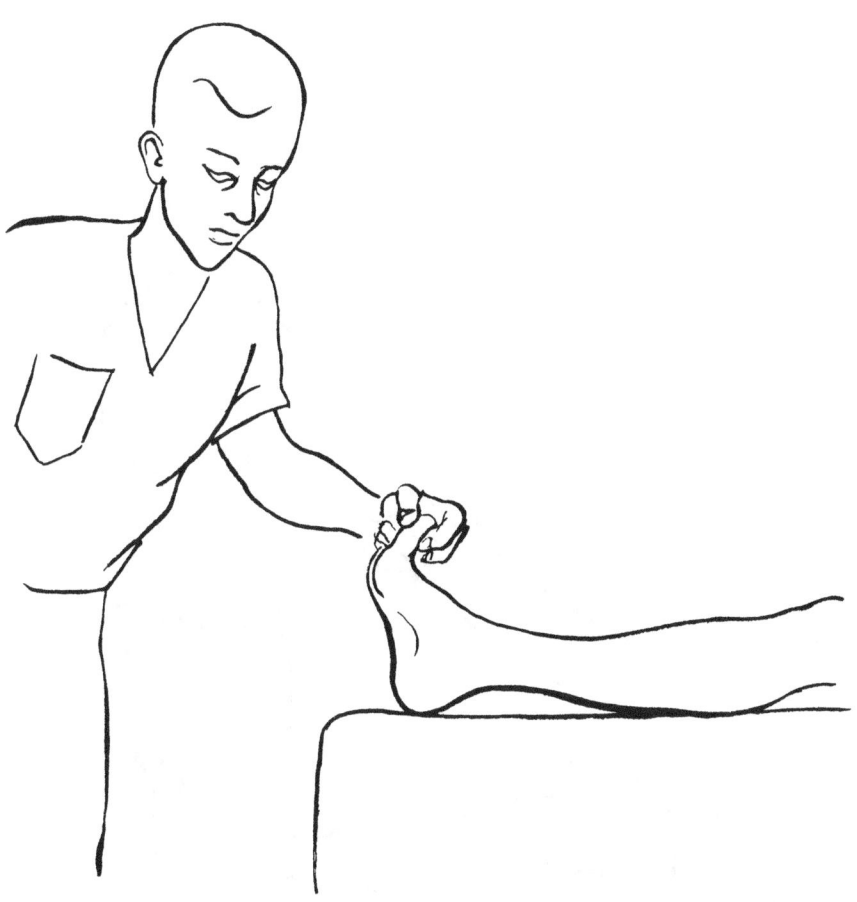

Sicard Test

Description

The patient lies supine with hips and knees extended. The examiner holds the patient's distal tibiofibula with one hand and raises the patient's leg passively to the point of pain, then lowers the leg about 5° and extends the great toe with the other hand.

Interpretation

A positive test is one in which pain is elicited in the thigh and/or the leg, indicating sciatic radiculopathy.

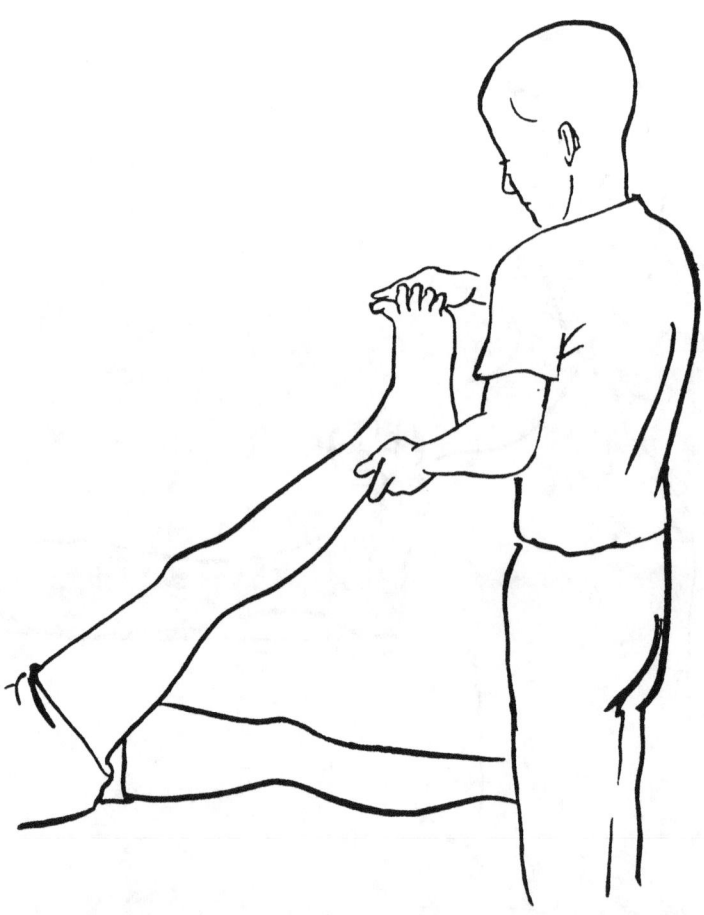

Hoover Test

Description

The patient lies supine. The examiner puts one hand under the patient's heel on the involved side and the other hand under the heel of the uninvolved side. The patient is then instructed to do a straight leg raise on the involved side.

Interpretation

A positive test is one in which the patient does not bear down as he/she attempts to raise the leg, indicating that the patient is probably not trying and is instead malingering.

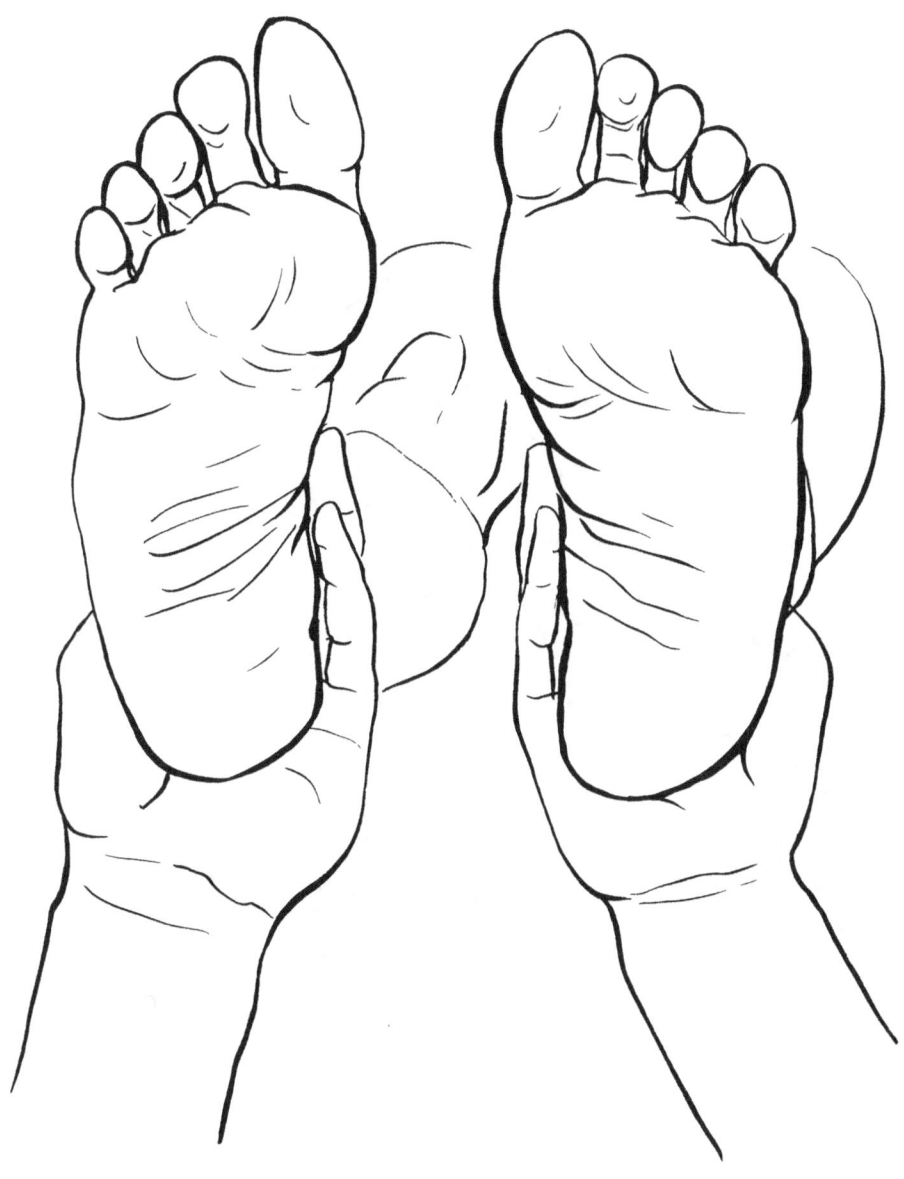

Fajersztajin Test

Description
The patient lies supine. The examiner holds the patient's distal tibiofibula with one hand, raises the patient's leg passively to 75° or to the point of pain, and dorsiflexes the foot with the other hand.

Interpretation
A positive test is one in which radicular pain is produced in the involved leg, indicating a possible ruptured disc in the lumbar spine.

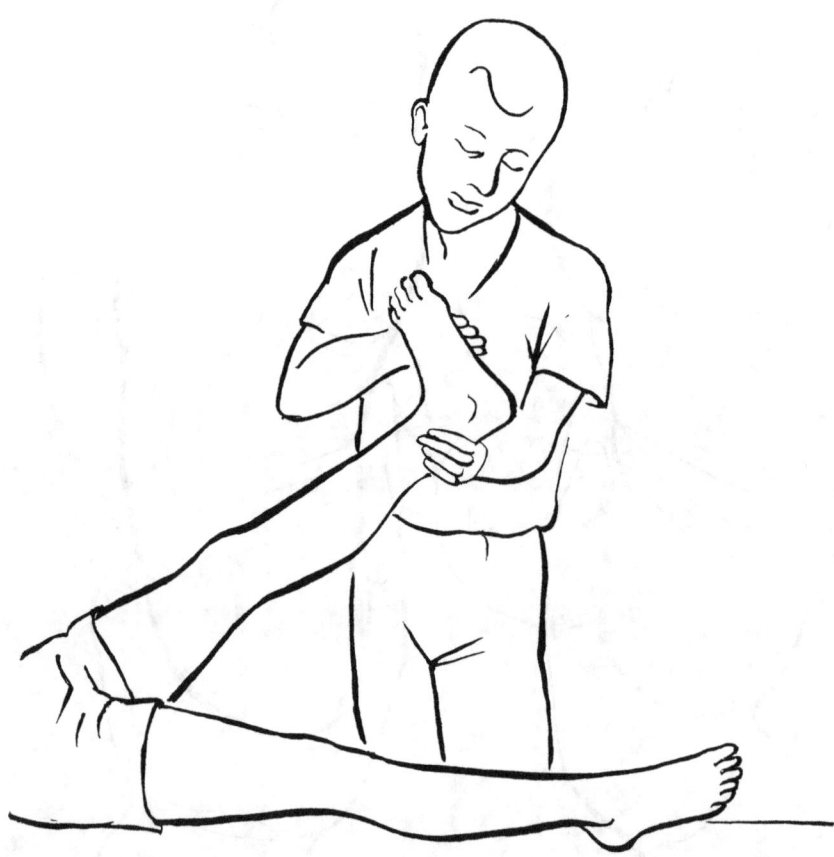

McKenzie Side Glide Test

Description

The patient stands. The examiner stands next to the patient and grasps the patient's pelvis with both hands. The examiner places one shoulder against the patient's thorax to block its movement. The examiner then pulls the patient's body toward the examiner and holds this position for 10-15 seconds. The test is then repeated on the other side.

Interpretation

A positive test is one which causes increased pain and associated symptoms on the involved side, indicating possible disc lesion in the lumbar spine.

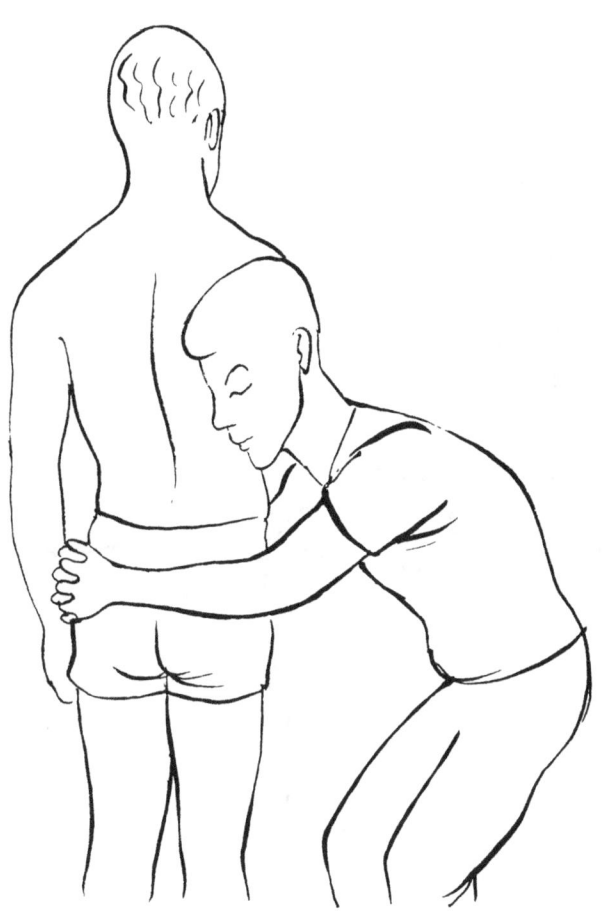

Bechterew Test

Description

The patient sits on the edge of the table with both legs hanging over the edge. The patient is then instructed to extend one knee at a time, alternating. If pain is not elicited, then the patient is instructed to extend both knees together.

Interpretation

A positive test is one in which pain is elicited in the thigh and/or the leg when both the knees are extended, or the patient leans back and then extends the knees, indicating disk involvement in the lumbar spine.

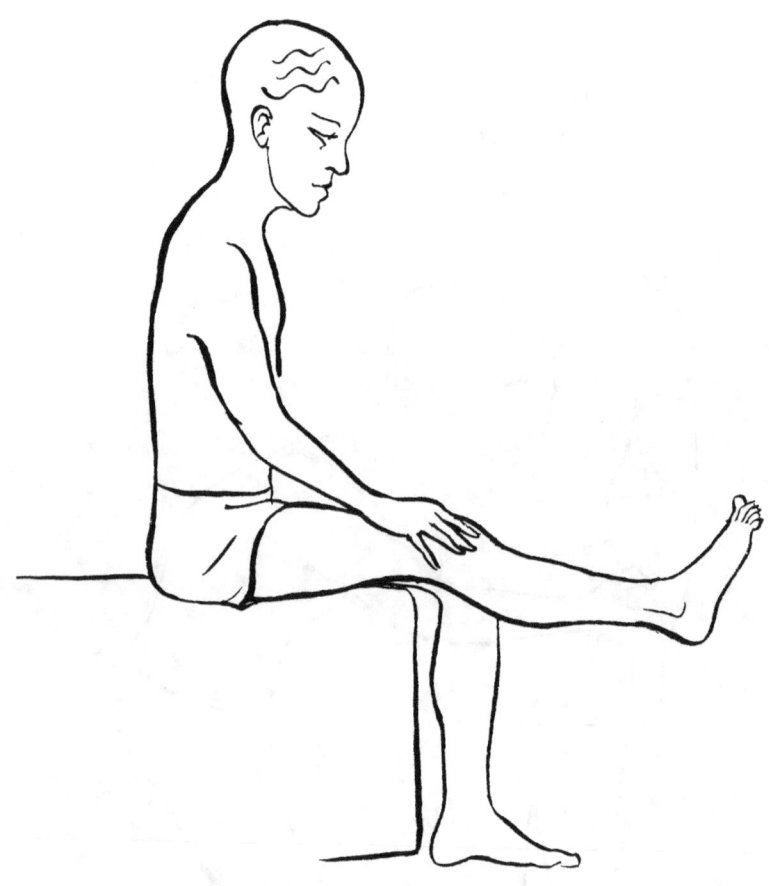

Compression Test

Description

The patient sits in a chair. The examiner stands behind the patient and presses inferiorly on both of the patient's shoulders.

Interpretation

A positive test is one in which there is an increase in pain in either the lumbar spine or the lower extremities, indicating a narrowing of the neural foramina or pressure on the facet joints.

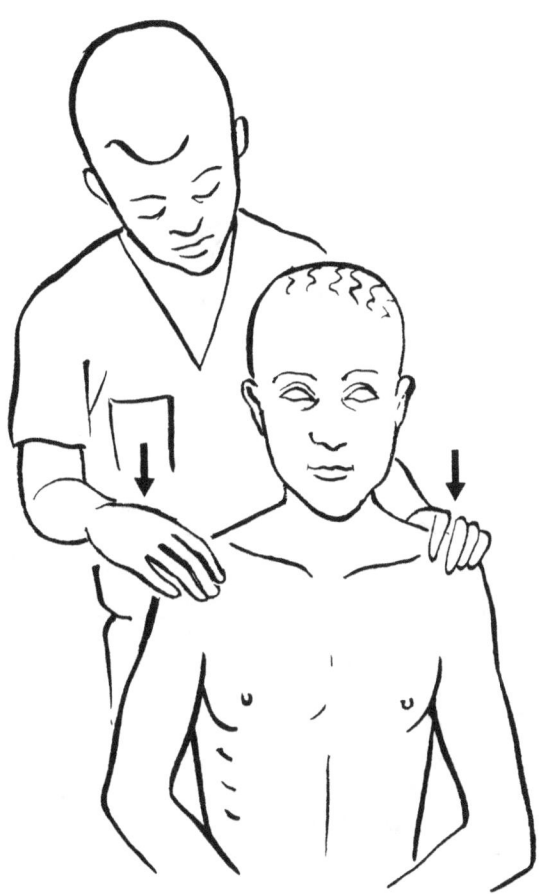

Valsalva Test

Description
The patient sits in a chair with the feet resting on the floor. The patient is then instructed to bear down as if the patient were trying to move the bowel.

Interpretation
A positive test is one in which bearing down causes pain in the lumbar spine or down the legs, indicating thecal or intrathecal pathology.

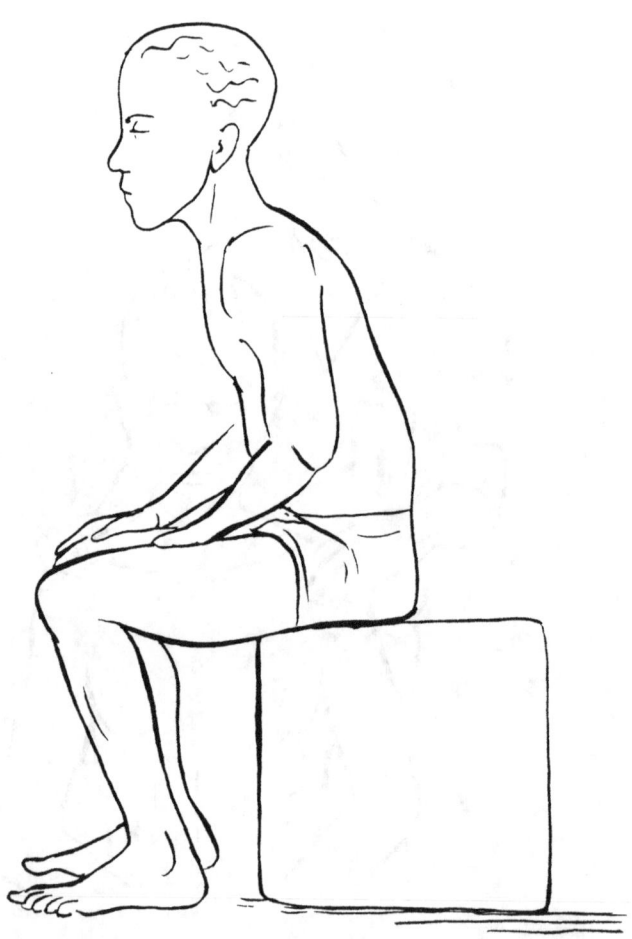

Distraction Test

Description

The patient sits. The examiner stands behind the patient. The patient is instructed to cross the arms across the chest. The examiner reaches from behind and grasps both of the patient's arms and applies an upward traction on the spine.

Interpretation

A positive test is one in which pain and other symptoms are relieved, indicating spinal nerve root impingement.

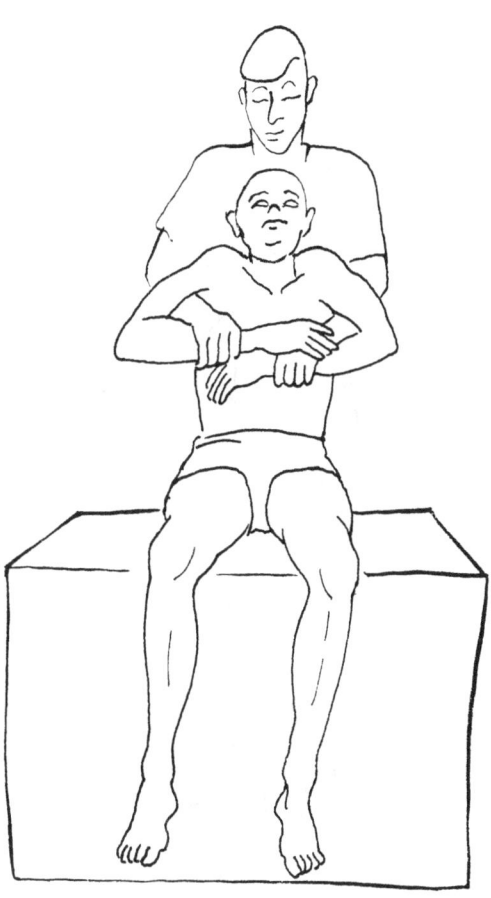

Heel Walking Test

Description
The patient stands. The patient is then instructed to walk on the heels.

Interpretation
A positive test is one in which the patient is unable to walk on the heels, indicating involvement of L4-L5 nerve roots.

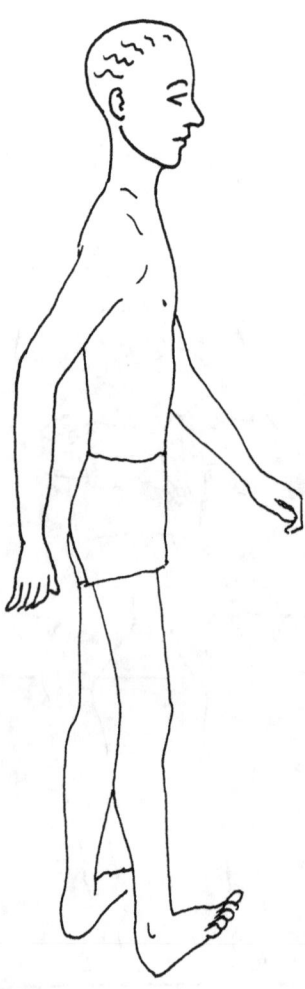

Toe Walking Test

Description

The patient stands. The patient is then instructed to walk on the toes.

Interpretation

A positive test is one in which the patient is unable to walk on the toes, indicating involvement of S1-S2 nerve roots.

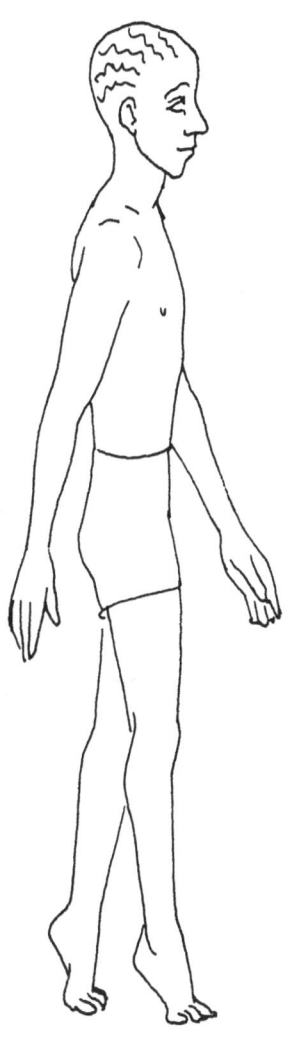

Piriformis Test

Description

The patient lies on the uninvolved side. The examiner fully flexes the patient's knee and flexes the hip to 90°. The examiner stabilizes the patient's pelvis with one hand and with the other hand pushes the knee downward.

Interpretation

A positive test is one which produces pain in the buttock, indicating piriformis syndrome.

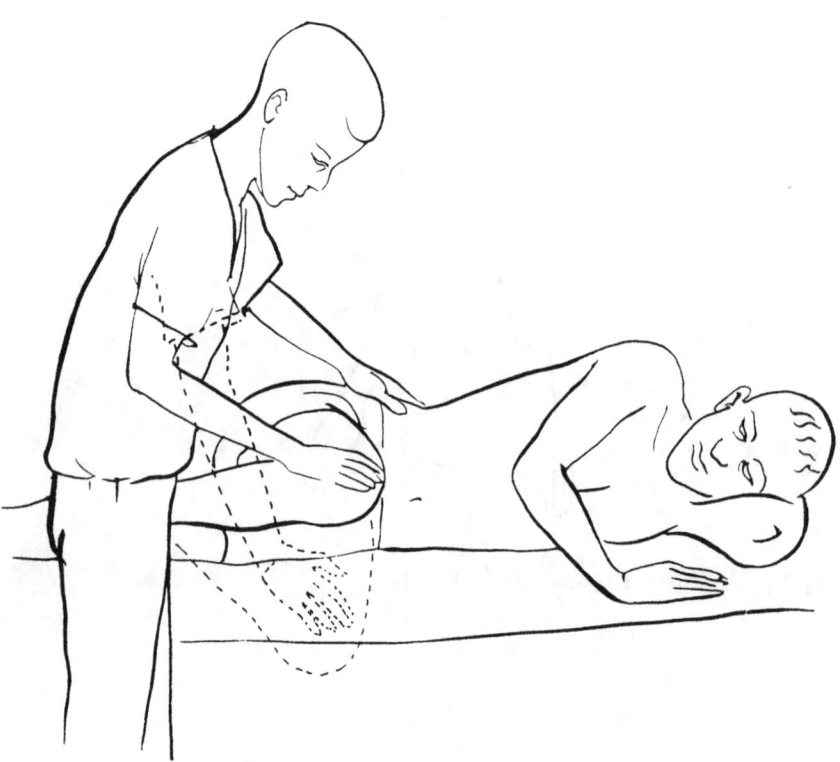

Freiberg Test

Description

The patient lies prone. The examiner grasps the patient's distal tibiofibula and flexes the patient's knee to approximately 90°, then internally rotates the hip.

Interpretation

A positive test is one which produces tenderness at the sacroiliac notch on the belly of the piriformis muscle, indicating piriformis syndrome.

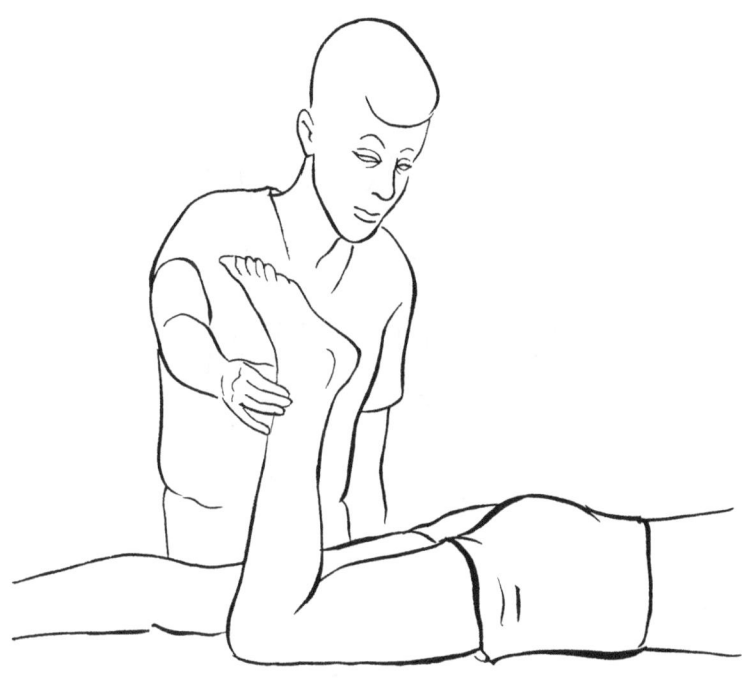

Piriformis Tightness Test

Description

The patient sits on the edge of the table with the legs hanging downward and the hips in adducted position. The examiner holds the patient's distal tibiofibula and externally rotates the hip.

Interpretation

A positive test is one in which external rotation of the hip is restricted, indicating tightness of the piriformis muscles.

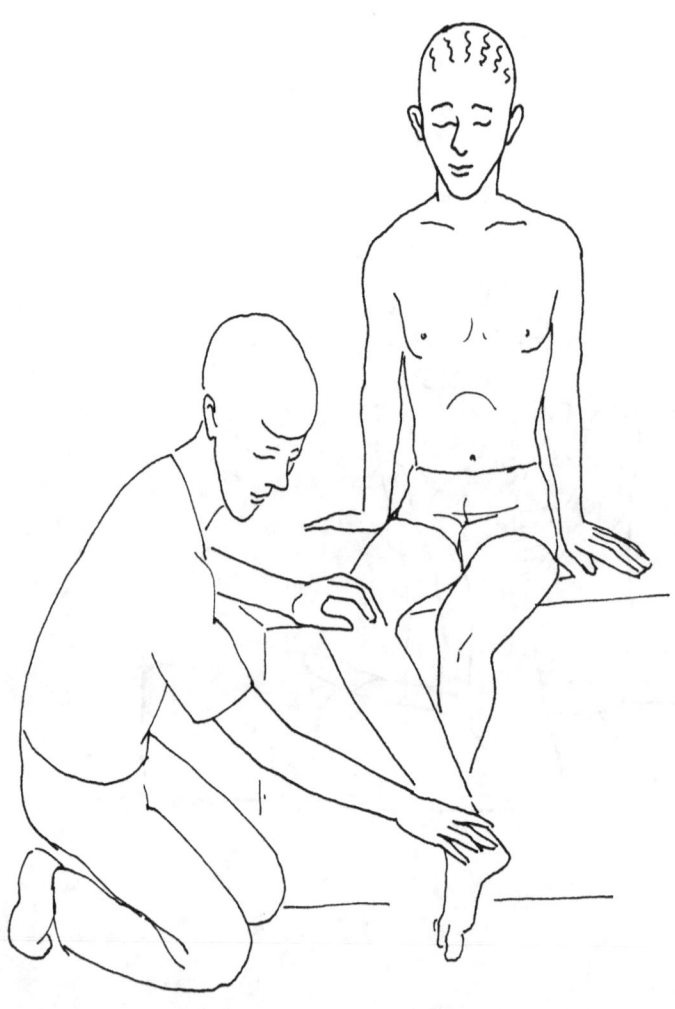

Pace Test

Description

The patient sits on the table with hips and knees flexed. The examiner places the hands on the lateral aspects of the knees and asks the patient to push the hands apart.

Interpretation

A positive test is one which produces pain and shows weakness on the involved side, indicating piriformis syndrome.

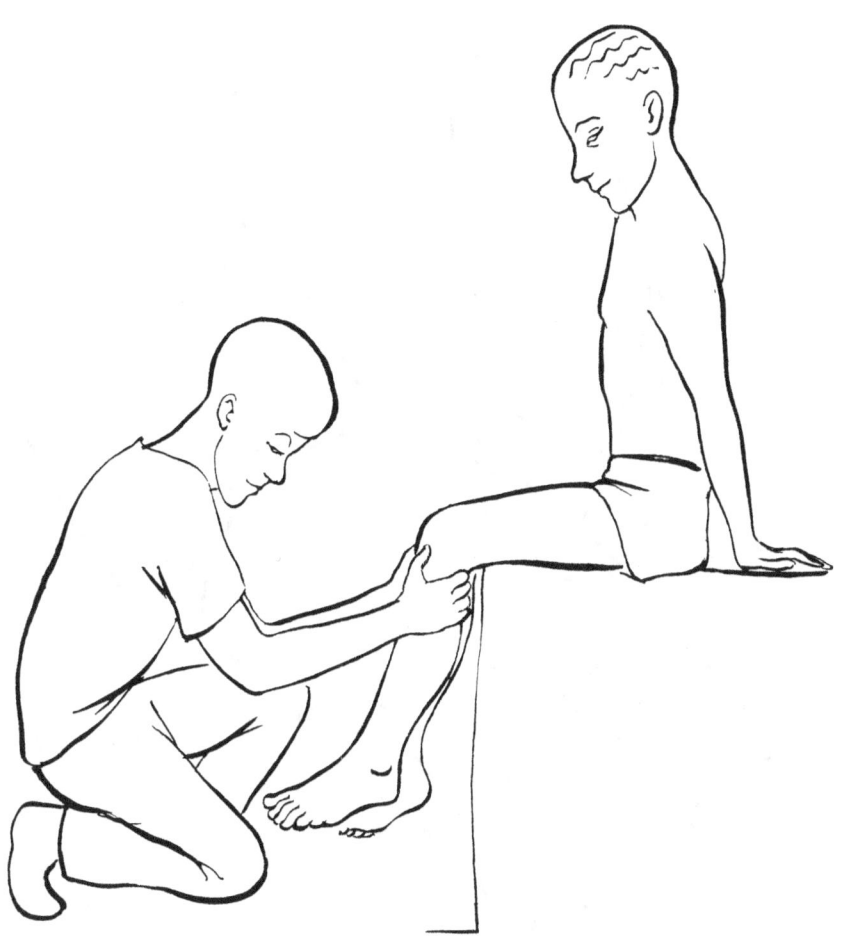

Abdominal Reflex Test

Description

The patient lies supine. The examiner strikes each quadrant of the patient's abdomen with the sharp end of a reflex hammer.

Interpretation

A positive test is one in which the umbilicus does not move, indicating an upper motor neuron lesion. An absence of either upper or lower quadrant reflex indicates a lower motor neuron lesion at T7-T10 and T10-L1, respectively.

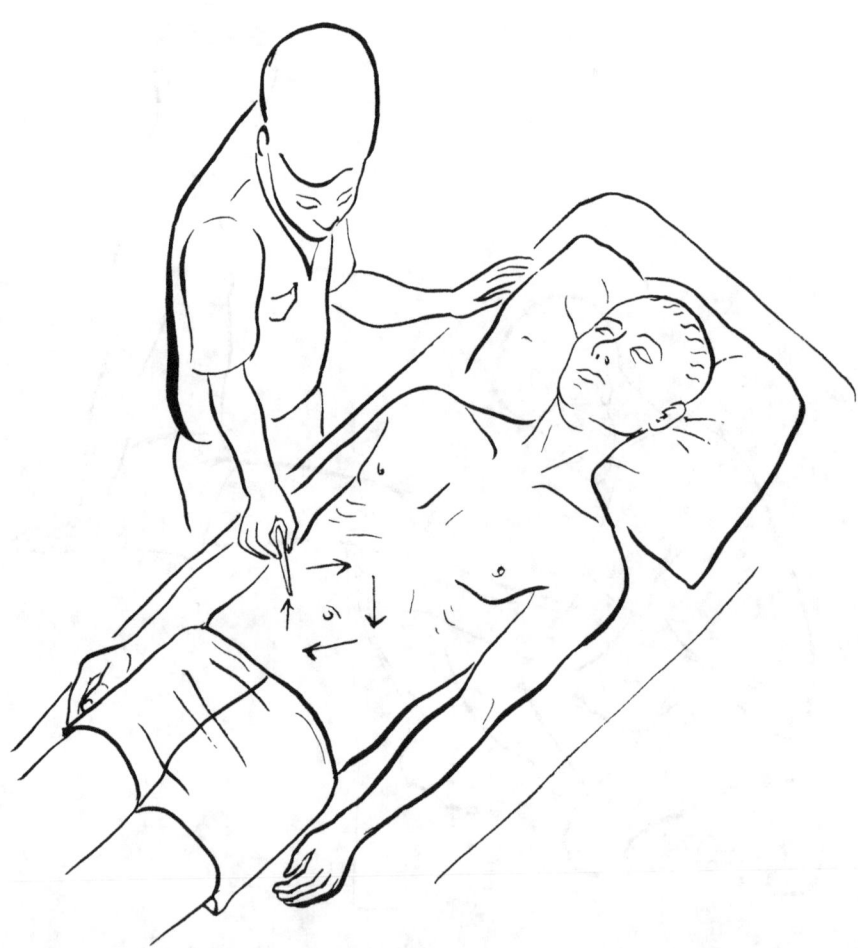

Cremasteric Reflex Test

Description

The patient lies supine. The examiner strikes the inner side of the patient's upper thigh with the sharp end of a reflex hammer. The test is then repeated on the opposite side.

Interpretation

A positive test is one in which the scrotal sac does not pull upward as the cremaster muscle contracts, indicating an upper motor neuron lesion. A unilateral absence of the reflex indicates a lower motor neuron lesion between L1 and L2.

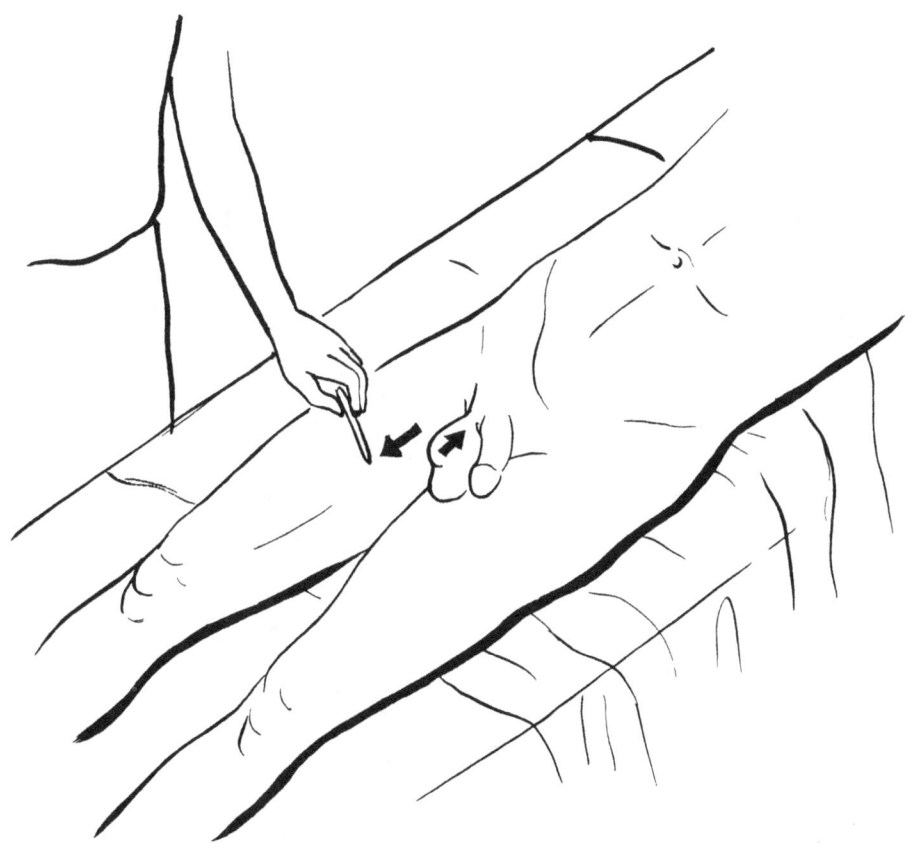

Knee Reflex Test

Description
The patient sits on the edge of the table with legs dangling free. When the patient's leg is totally relaxed, the examiner taps the infrapatellar tendon at the level of the knee joint. The reflex is compared to that of the opposite side. The reflex is noted as either normal, hypo, hyper, or absent.

Interpretation
A positive test is one in which the reflex is either hypo, hyper, or absent, indicating an L4 neurologic level dysfunction.

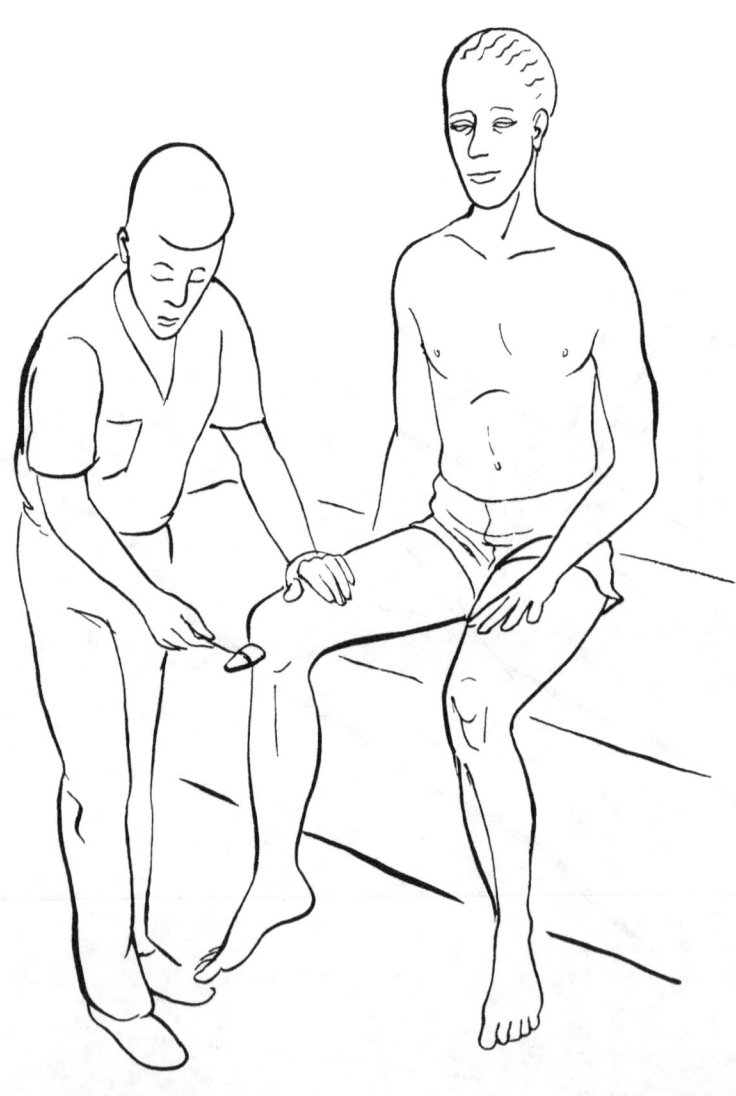

Ankle Reflex Test

Description

The patient sits with legs hanging over the table or kneels on a chair. The gastrocnemius muscle is relaxed. The examiner slightly dorsiflexes the patient's ankle and then taps the Achilles tendon with a reflex hammer. The reflex is tested on the opposite side. The reflex is noted as either normal, hypo, hyper, or absent.

Interpretation

A positive test is one in which the reflex is either hypo, hyper, or absent, indicating an S1 neurologic level dysfunction.

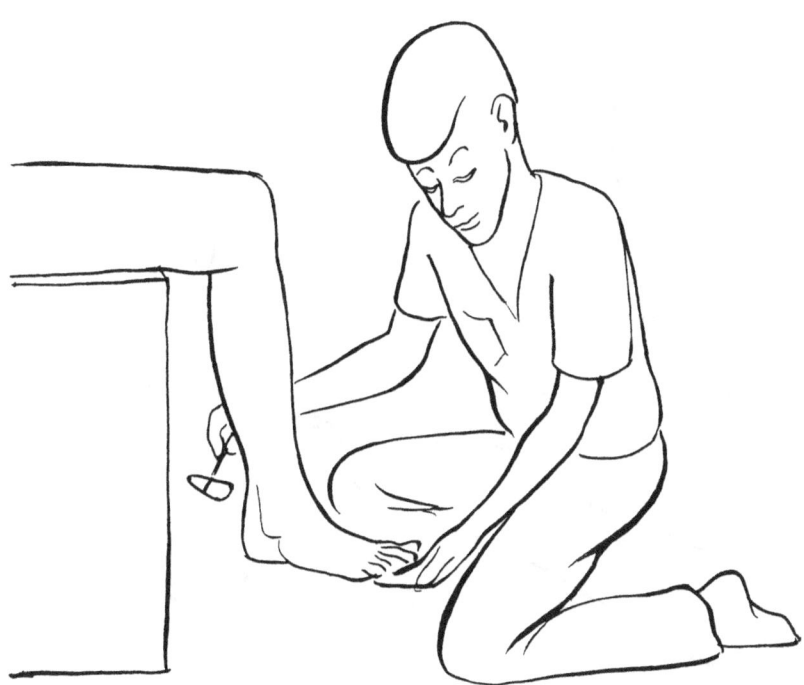

Babinski Reflex Test

Description
The patient lies supine. The examiner uses a blunt instrument and draws across the sole of the foot, starting at the heel, moving along the lateral aspect, and crossing the ball of the foot.

Interpretation
A positive test is one which consists of extension of the great toe, usually associated with fanning of the other toes, indicating an upper motor neuron lesion.

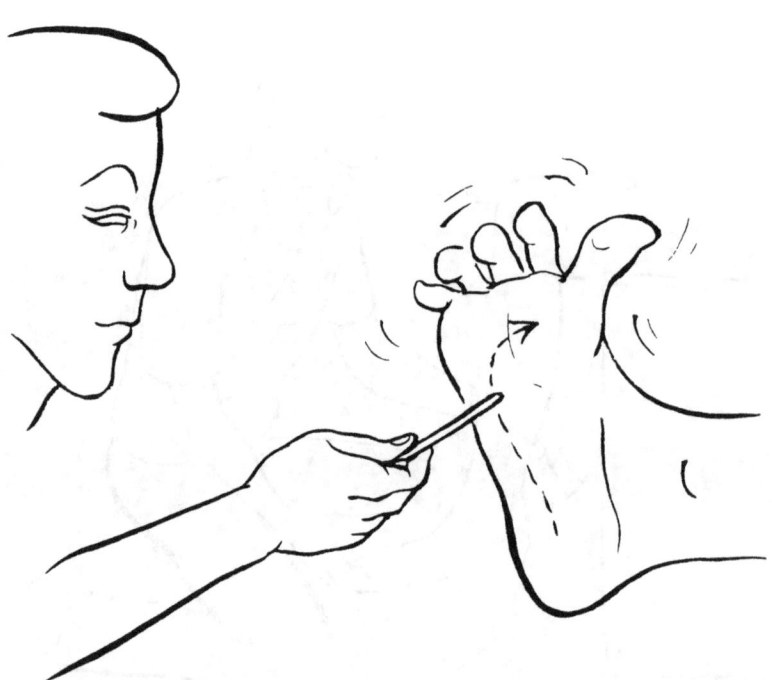

Chaddock Test

Description

The patient lies supine. The examiner uses a blunt instrument and draws across the lateral aspect of the foot beneath the lateral malleolus.

Interpretation

A positive test is one which causes extension of the great toe, usually associated with fanning of the other toes, indicating an upper motor neuron lesion.

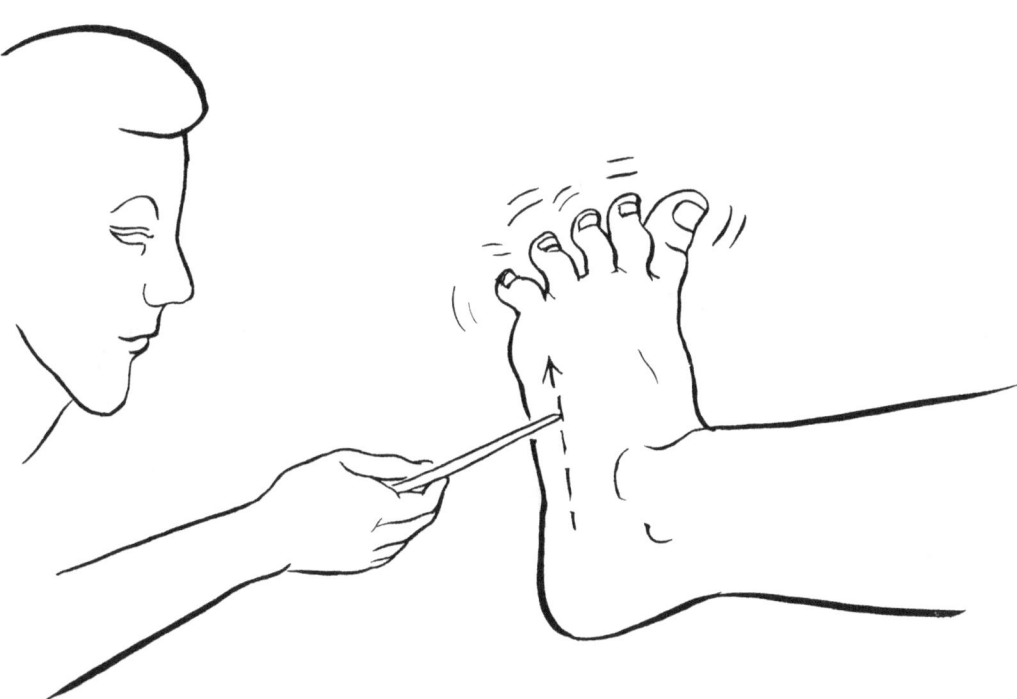

Rossolimo Test

Description
The patient lies supine. The examiner taps on the patient's ball of the foot on the plantar surface of the great toe.

Interpretation
A positive test is one which causes extension of the toes, indicating an upper motor neuron lesion.

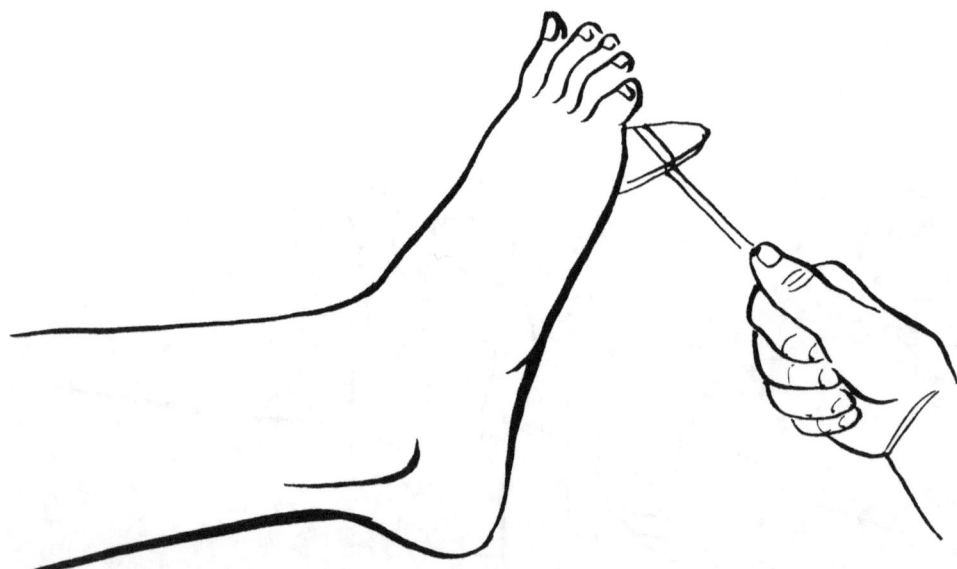

Oppenheim Test

Description

The patient lies supine. The examiner uses a blunt instrument and draws along the crest of the tibia.

Interpretation

A positive test is one which causes extension of the great toe, usually associated with fanning of the other toes, indicating an upper motor neuron lesion.

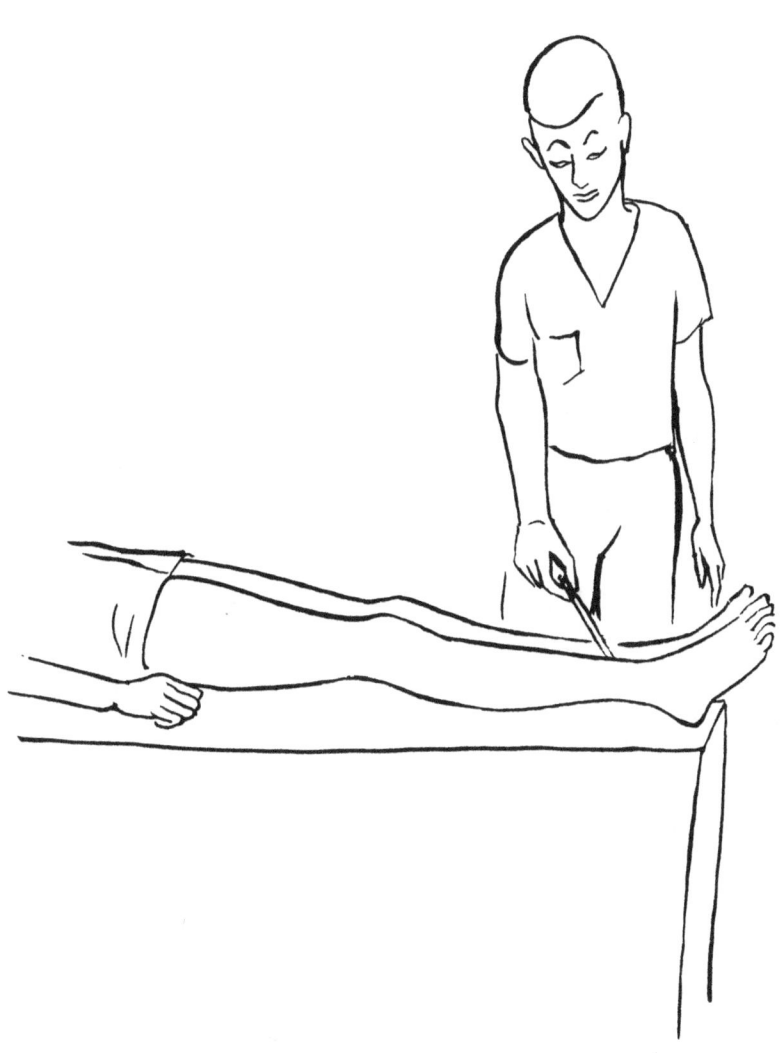

Section 11
Sacrum and Pelvis

Fabere/Patrick Test

Description

The patient lies supine. The examiner stabilizes the patient's pelvis with one hand. With the other hand, the examiner places the foot of the patient's involved side on the opposite knee. In this way, the hip joint is flexed, abducted, and externally rotated. The examiner then slowly lowers the involved leg toward the table.

Interpretation

A positive test is one in which pain is produced in the posterior and lateral sides of the hip, indicating sacroiliac joint and low lumbar dysfunction. Pain in the anterior hip indicates hip dysfunction.

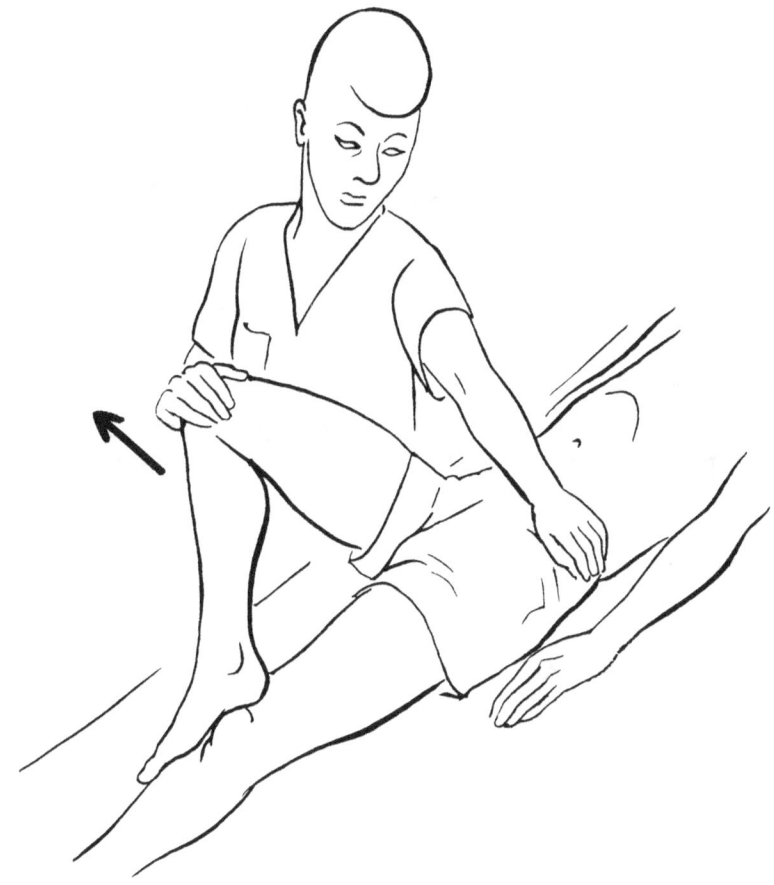

FADIR Test

Description

The patient lies supine. The examiner flexes the patient's hip, adducts it, and then internally rotates the hip.

Interpretation

A positive test is one which causes pain in the posterior and lateral side of the pelvis, indicating sacroiliac joint and/or lumbar dysfunction, while anterior pain indicates hip dysfunction.

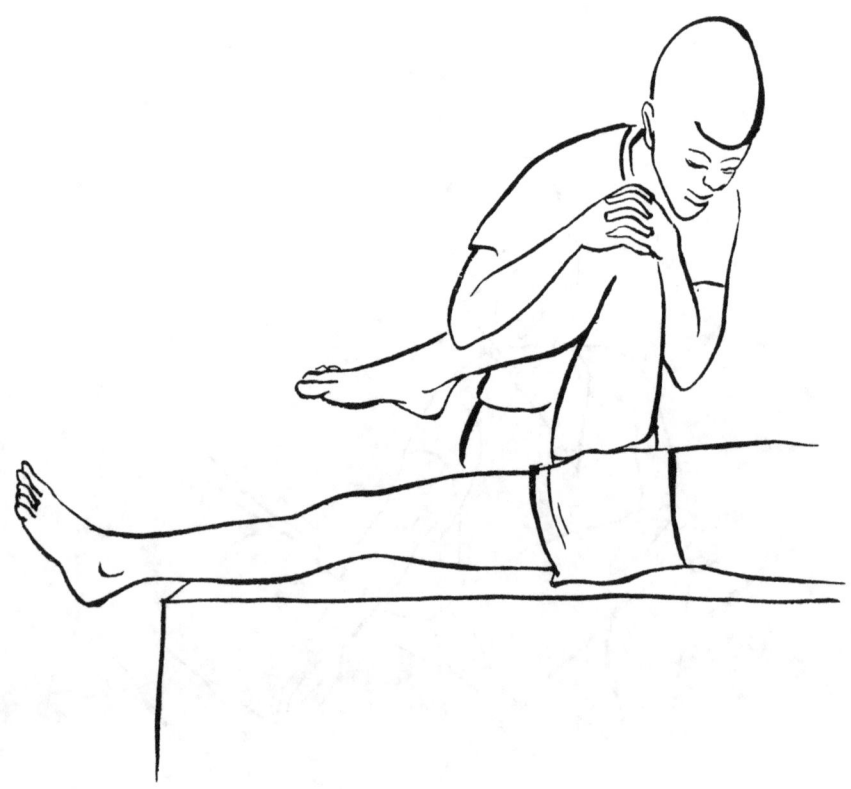

Toe Walking Test

Description

The patient stands. The patient is then instructed to walk on the toes.

Interpretation

A positive test is one in which the patient is unable to walk on the toes, indicating involvement of S1-S2 nerve roots.

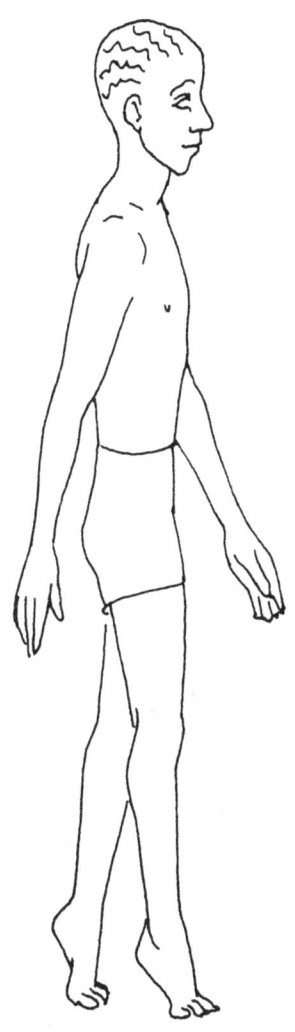

Hibb Test

Description

The patient lies prone. The examiner passively flexes the patient's knee beyond 90° and then internally rotates the hip.

Interpretation

A positive test is one in which pain is elicited in the sacroiliac joint, indicating a sacroiliac joint dysfunction. Pain in the hip joint indicates a hip joint dysfunction.

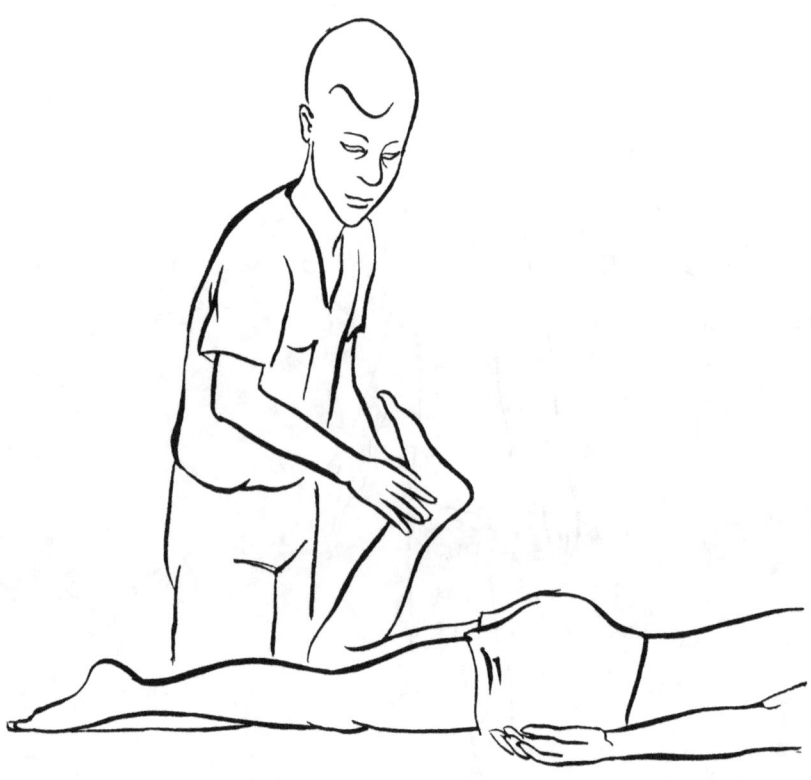

Nachlas Test

Description
The patient lies prone. The examiner passively flexes the patient's knee to full range of motion.

Interpretation
A positive test is one in which pain is elicited in the buttock, indicating a sacroiliac joint dysfunction. Pain in the lumbar area indicates a lumbar disc disease.

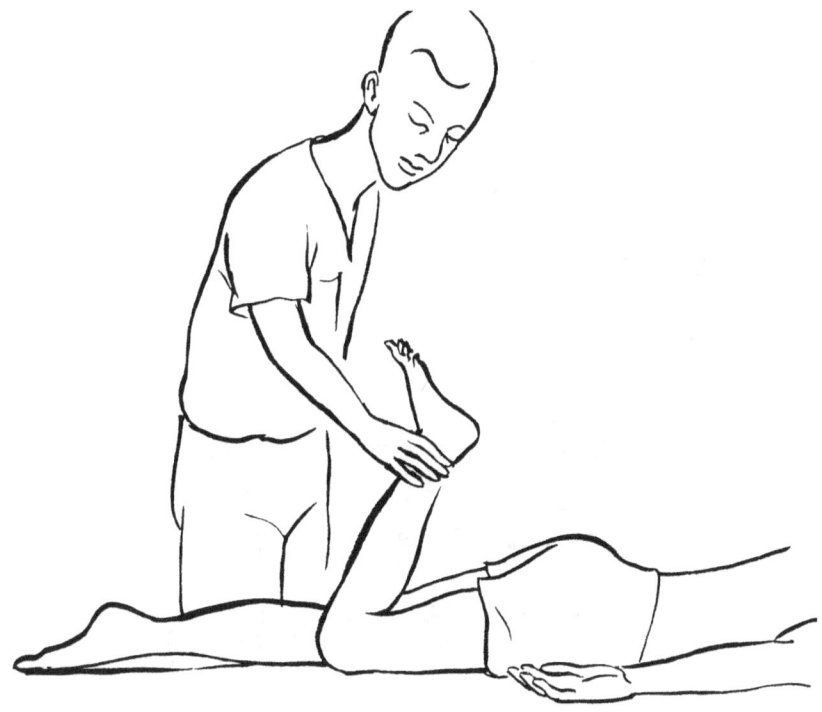

Resisted Abduction Test

Description

The patient lies on the uninvolved side with the uninvolved knee slightly flexed. The examiner stands behind the patient. The examiner instructs the patient to abduct the involved hip to about 45° and to maintain this position while the examiner applies a downward pressure.

Interpretation

A positive test is one which elicits pain in the sacroiliac joint, indicating a sacroiliac joint sprain.

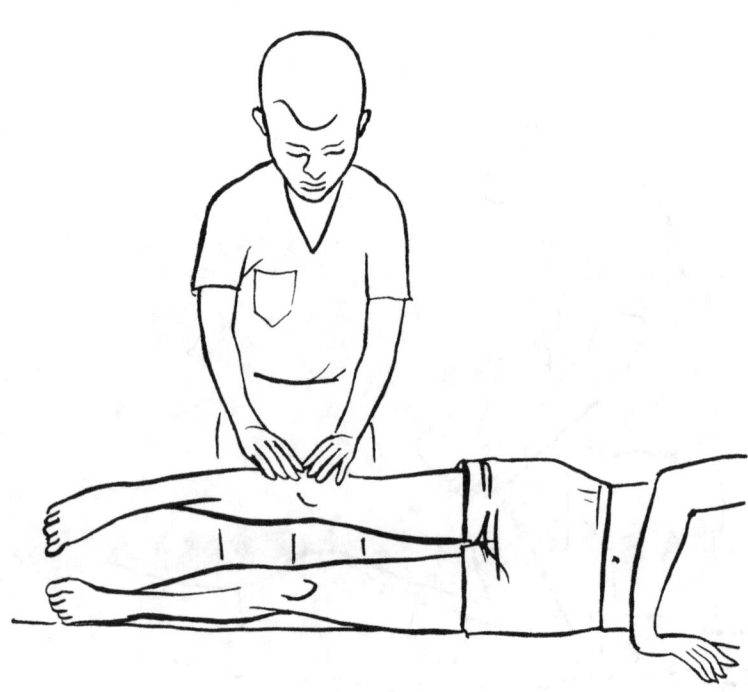

Standing Iliac Crest Levels Test

Description
The patient stands with feet approximately 12 inches apart. The examiner squats behind the patient and places the radial border of the index finger and web spaces of the hands at the patient's waist on each side. The examiner then moves hands down on the iliac crests to gently push the soft tissue away. The examiner assesses the level of the iliac crests in relation to each other.

Interpretation
A positive test is one in which one iliac crest is higher than the other, indicating apparent leg length discrepancy.

Comments
If the test is positive, use a lift to correct the discrepancy before proceeding to further standing mobility tests.

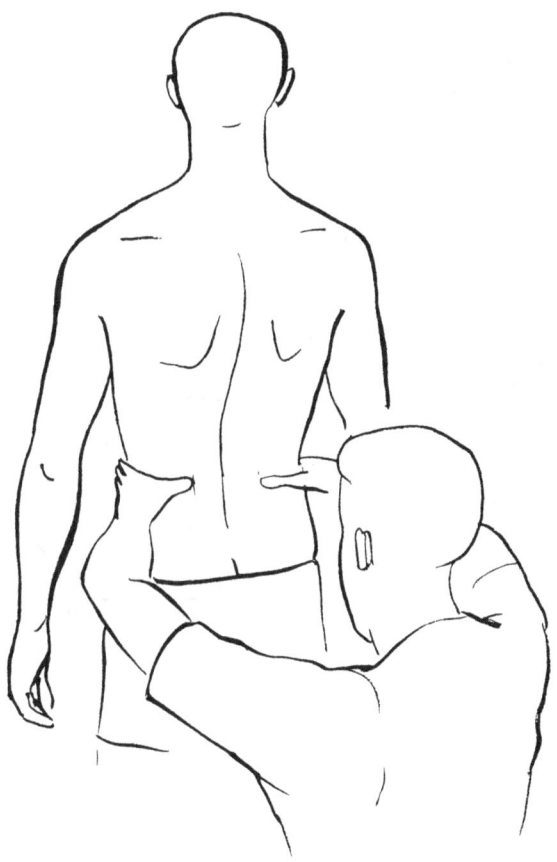

Lewin-Gaenslen Test

Description

The patient lies on the uninvolved side with the uninvolved knee and hip slightly flexed. The examiner stands behind the patient and stabilizes the patient's pelvis with one hand. The examiner holds the patient's knee joint and extends the hip.

Interpretation

A positive test is one which elicits pain in the sacroiliac joint, indicating a sacroiliac joint dysfunction.

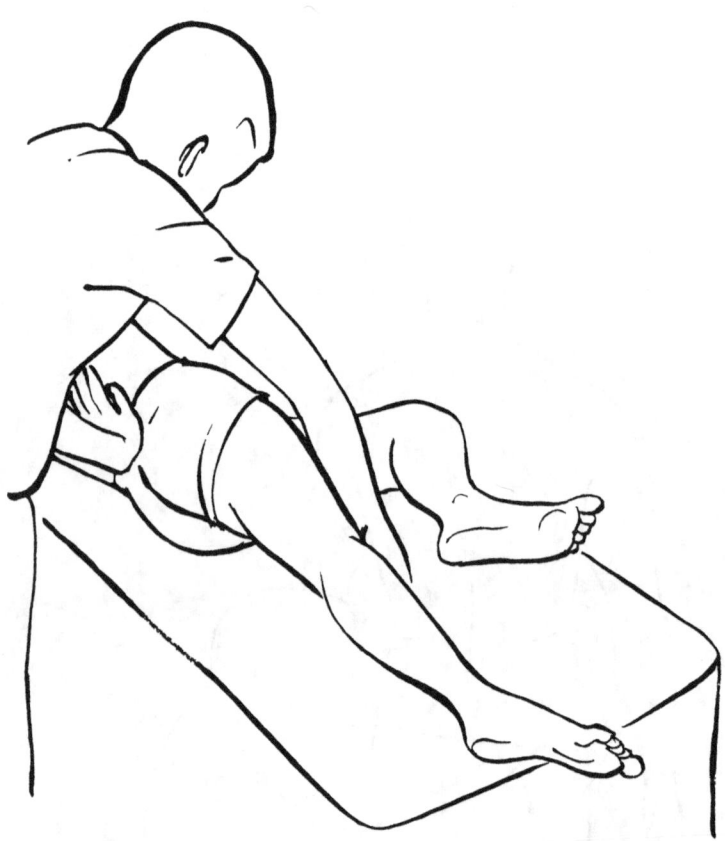

Standing Anterior Superior Iliac Spine Test

Description

The patient stands with feet approximately 12 inches apart. The examiner squats in front of the patient at eye level with the anterior superior iliac spine (ASIS). The examiner then palpates the ASIS with the thumbs and assesses the relative superoinferior relationships in positions.

Interpretation

A positive test is one in which the ASIS positions are not level in relation to each other, indicating sacroiliac joint dysfunction.

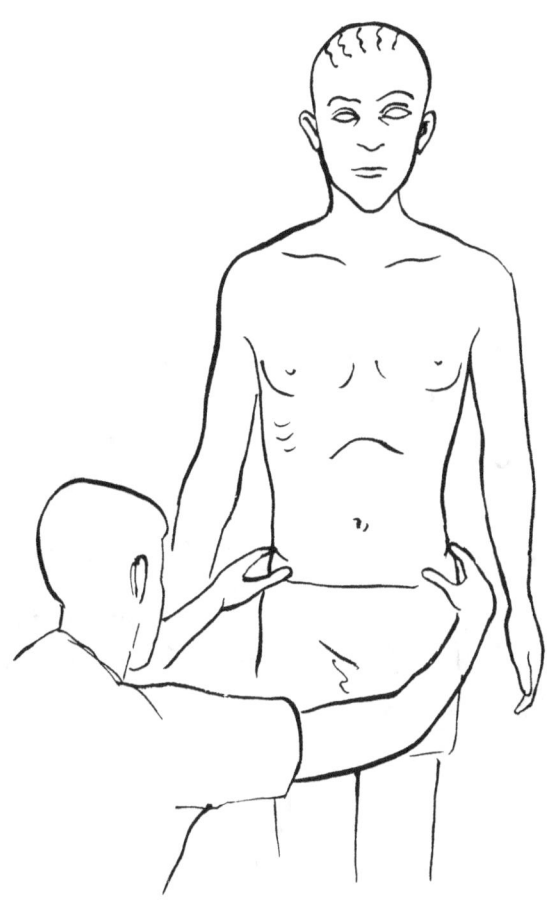

Standing Posterior Superior Iliac Spine Test

Description

The patient stands with feet approximately 12 inches apart. The examiner squats behind the patient at eye level with the posterior superior iliac spine (PSIS). The examiner then palpates the PSIS with the ulnar borders of the thumbs and assesses the relative superoinferior relationships in positions.

Interpretation

A positive test is one in which the PSIS positions are not level in relation to each other, indicating sacroiliac joint dysfunction.

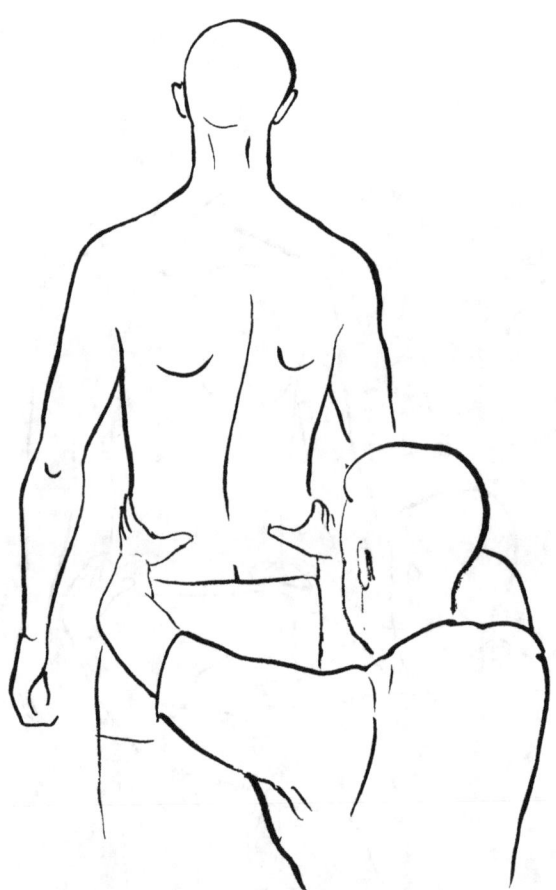

Standing Flexion Test

Description

The patient stands with feet approximately 12 inches apart. The examiner stands behind the patient and places the thumbs directly under each posterior superior iliac spine (PSIS). The patient is instructed to bend forward as far as possible while keeping the knees extended. The examiner observes the amount of cranial movement of each PSIS.

Interpretation

A positive test is one in which one PSIS moves farther in a cranial direction than the other, indicating sacroiliac dysfunction. The side with the greater movement is the side of articular restriction.

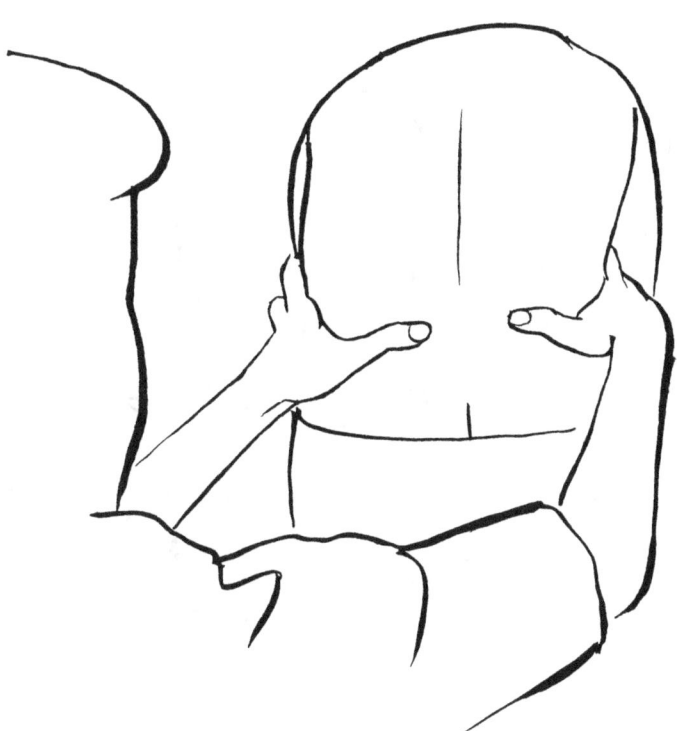

Sitting Iliac Crest Levels Test

Description
The patient sits erect on a flat surface. The examiner squats behind the patient and places the radial border of the index finger and web spaces of the hands at the patient's waist on each side. The examiner then moves hands down on the iliac crests to gently push the soft tissue away. The examiner assesses the level of the iliac crests in relation to each other.

Interpretation
A positive test is one in which one iliac crest is higher than the other, indicating sacroiliac joint dysfunction.

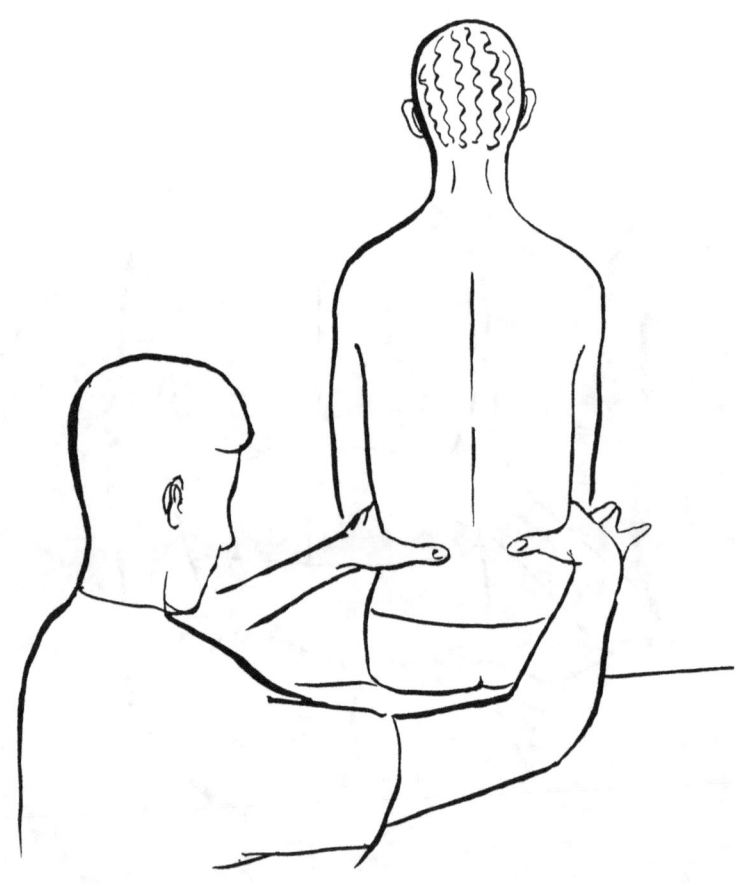

Sitting Anterior Superior Iliac Spine Test

Description

The patient sits erect on a flat surface. The examiner squats in front of the patient at eye level with the anterior superior iliac spine (ASIS). The examiner palpates the ASIS with the thumbs and assesses the relative superoinferior relationships in positions.

Interpretation

A positive test is one in which the ASIS positions are not level in relation to each other, indicating sacroiliac joint dysfunction.

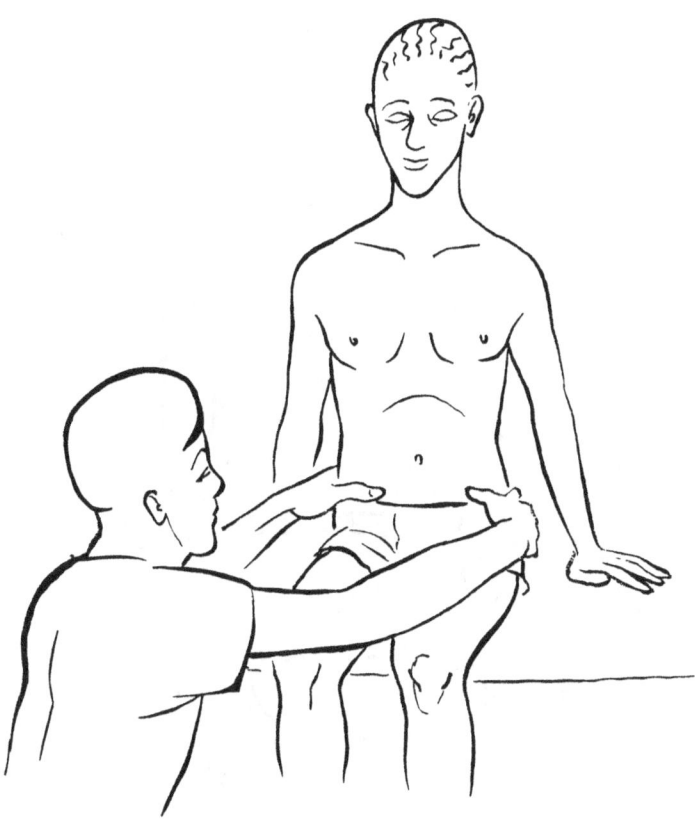

Sitting Posterior Superior Iliac Spine Test

Description

The patient sits erect on a flat surface. The examiner squats behind the patient at eye level with the posterior superior iliac spine (PSIS). The examiner then palpates the PSIS with the ulnar borders of the thumbs and assesses the relative superoinferior relationships in positions.

Interpretation

A positive test is one in which the PSIS positions are not level in relation to each other, indicating sacroiliac joint dysfunction.

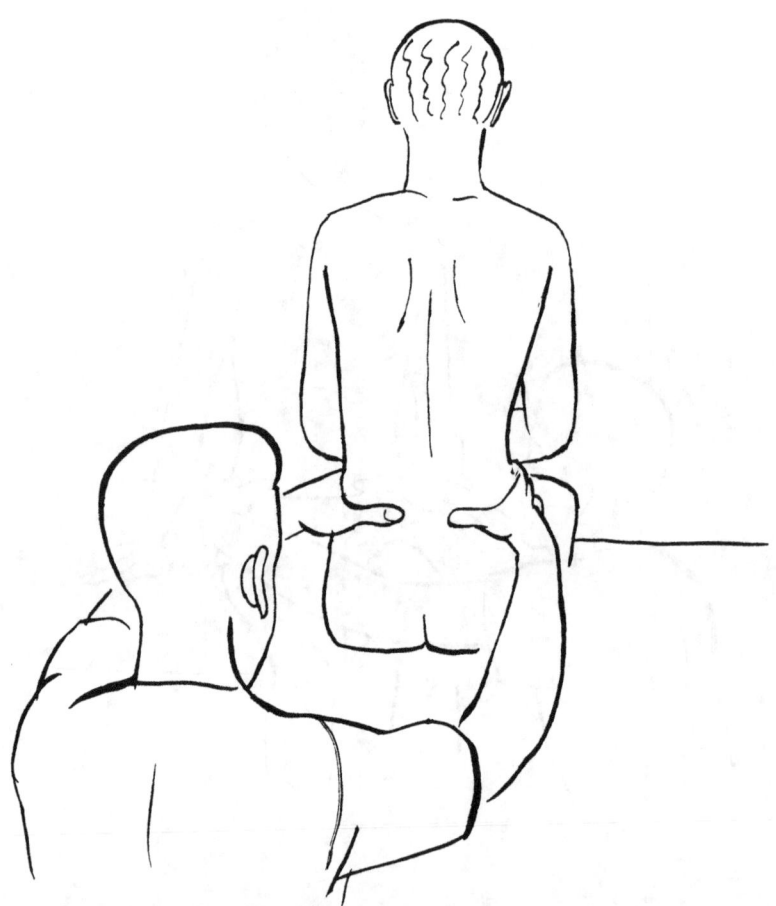

Sitting Flexion Test

Description

The patient sits in a chair sideways with feet flat on the floor and knees flexed to 90°. The patient's legs are sufficiently apart to allow the shoulders to come between them when forward bending the spine. The examiner squats behind the patient and places a thumb directly under each posterior superior iliac spine (PSIS). The patient is then instructed to bend forward as far as possible between the knees and to reach the hands toward the floor.

Interpretation

A positive test is one in which one PSIS moves more superiorly than the other, indicating sacroiliac joint dysfunction. The side with greater movement indicates articular restriction.

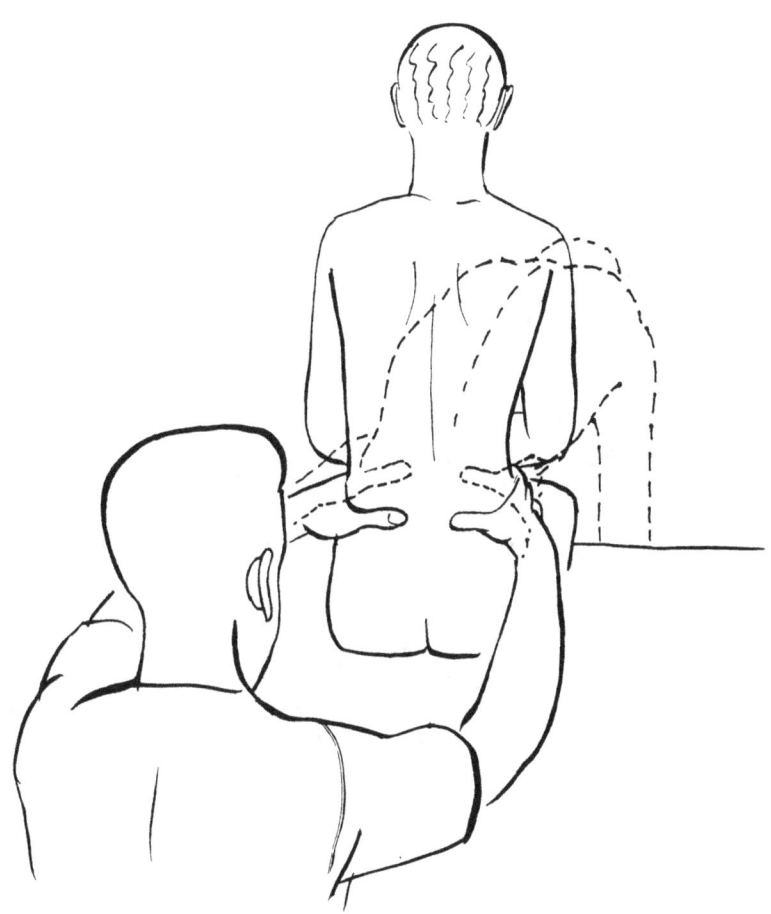

Long Sitting Test

Description

The patient lies supine. The examiner places his/her thumbs on the inferior borders of the medial malleoli to outline the position of the malleoli. The patient is then instructed to sit up. The examiner notes any changes in the relationship of the malleoli.

Interpretation

A positive test is one in which one leg appears to lengthen in relationship to the other when the patient comes to sitting position from supine, indicating posterior innominate rotation on that side. Conversely, one leg appearing to shorten in relationship to the other indicates an anterior innominate rotation on that side. One leg remaining consistently shorter or longer in relationship to the other indicates an anatomical leg-length difference.

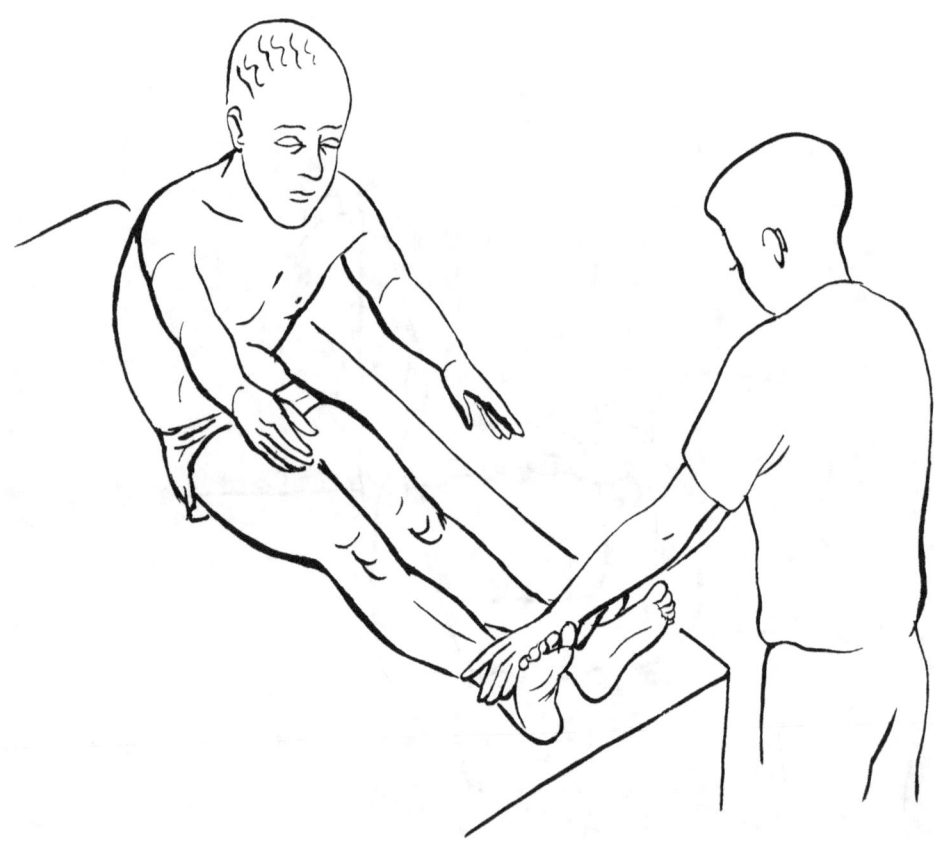

Spring Test

Description
The patient lies on the uninvolved side. The examiner places one hand over the anterolateral rim of the ilium and applies a downward thrust.

Interpretation
A positive test is one which elicits pain in the sacroiliac joint on the side of thrust, indicating sacroiliac joint dysfunction.

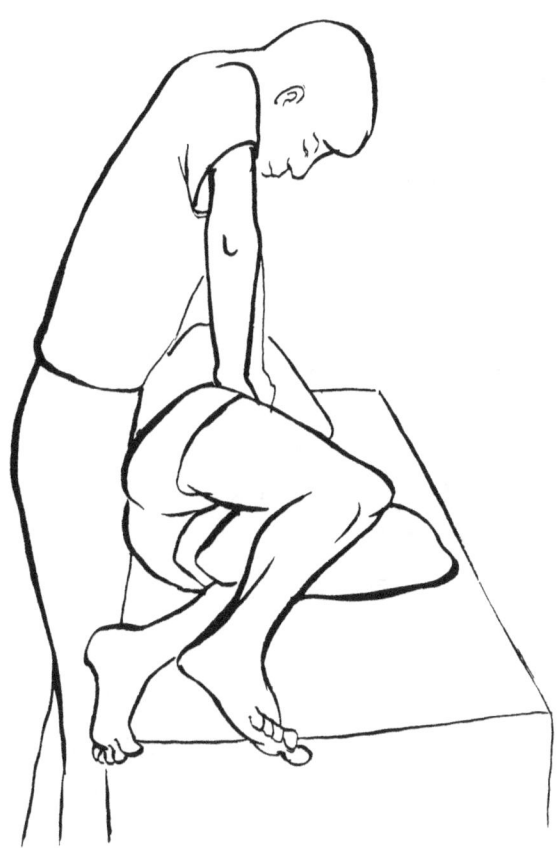

Compression Test

Description

The patient lies supine. The examiner crosses the arms and places the heels of the hands on the anterior superior iliac spine (ASIS) of the ilia. The examiner then applies pressure downward and laterally on the ASIS to take up any slack and then gives a sudden, sharp spring to the ASIS. Excessive motion of the pelvis is avoided to minimize the movement of the lumbar spine.

Interpretation

A positive test is one in which the patient complains of reproduction of pain in the gluteal or posterior crural areas when the pressure is applied, indicating sacroiliac joint dysfunction.

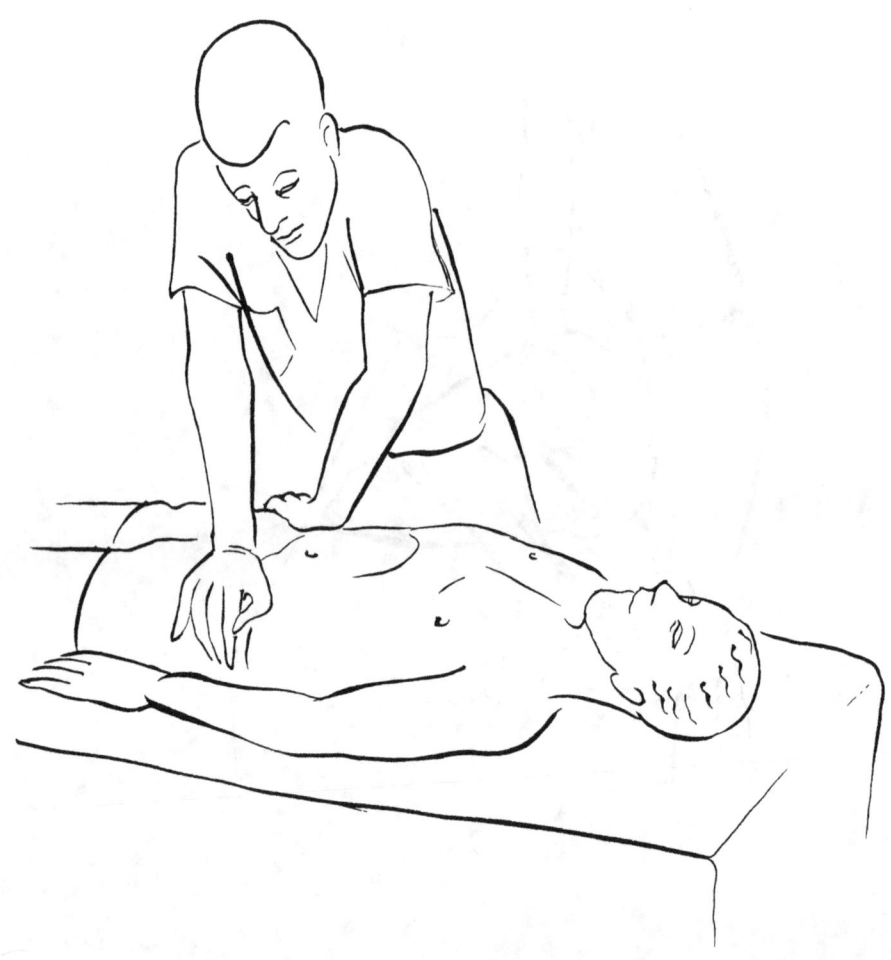

Distraction Test

Description

The patient lies supine. The examiner places the heels of the hands on the lateral iliac wings. The examiner then applies inward pressure on the iliac wings.

Interpretation

A positive test is one in which the patient complains of reproduction of pain in the gluteal or posterior crural areas when the pressure is applied, indicating sacroiliac joint dysfunction.

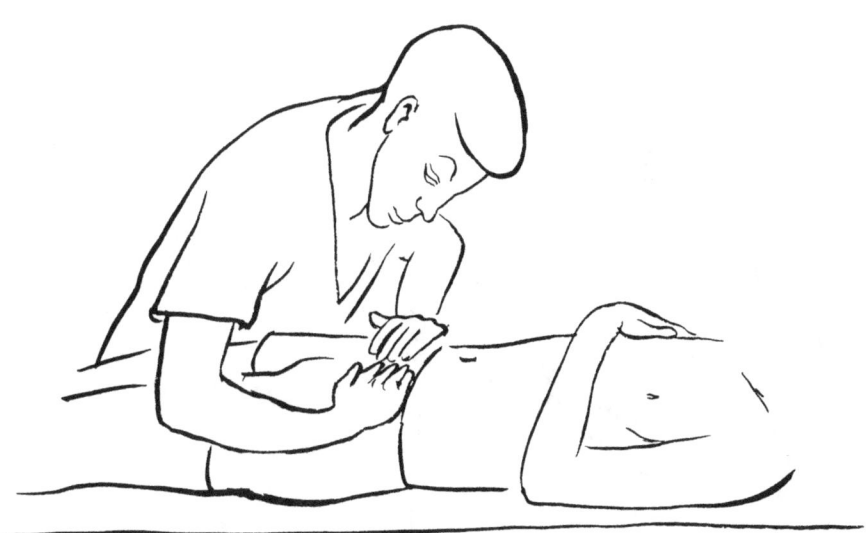

Prone Knee Flexion Test

Description

The patient lies prone. The examiner stands at the end of the table and grasps the patient's feet so that the examiner's thumbs pass along the distal end of the calcaneus. The examiner maintains the index fingers just posterior to the lateral malleoli and distal fibula shafts and holds the feet in the same degree of pronation-supination and slight external rotation. The feet are placed next to each other. The examiner notes the apparent leg length by observing the position of the heels in relationship to each other. The examiner then passively flexes the patient's knees to 90°. The examiner notes any change in the relationship of the heel positions to each other as the patient's knees are passively flexed.

Interpretation

A positive test is one in which one leg (the leg that appears shorter in relationship to the other at the initial approximation of the feet) appears to lengthen in relationship to the other as the test is performed, indicating posterior innominate rotation on that side. If this leg remains apparently shorter or becomes even shorter in relationship to the other leg, that side has an anterior innominate rotation.

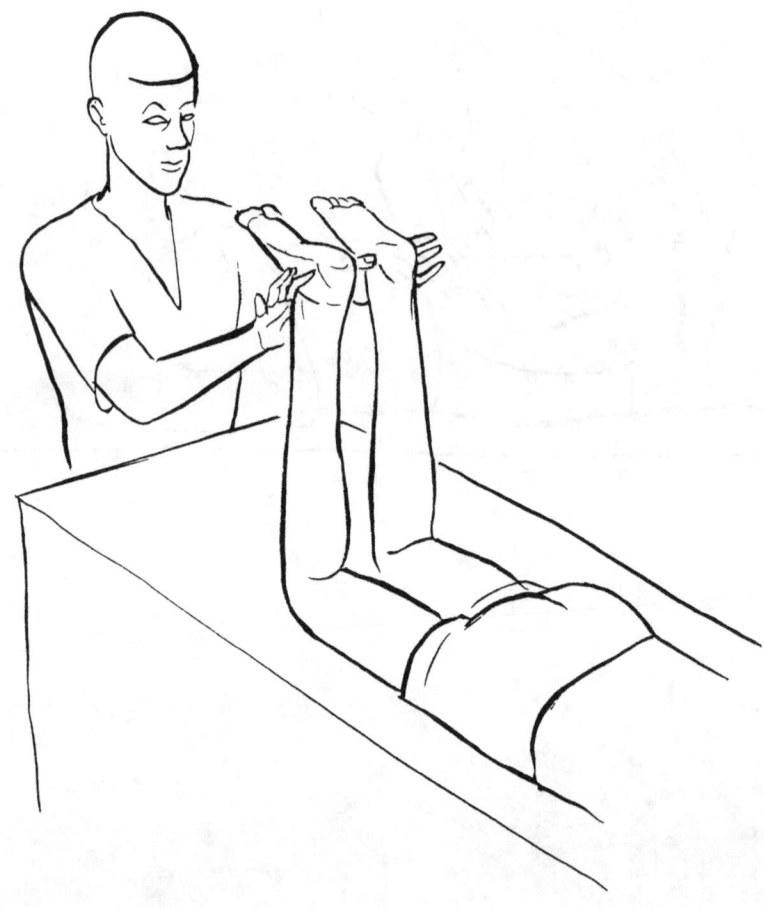

Yeoman Test

Description

The patient lies prone. The examiner stabilizes the patient's pelvis with one hand and with the other hand flexes the patient's knee. The examiner grasps the bent knee and then hyperextends the hip. The test is repeated on the other leg.

Interpretation

A positive test is one in which pain is produced in the sacroiliac joint, indicating sprain of the anterior sacroiliac ligaments.

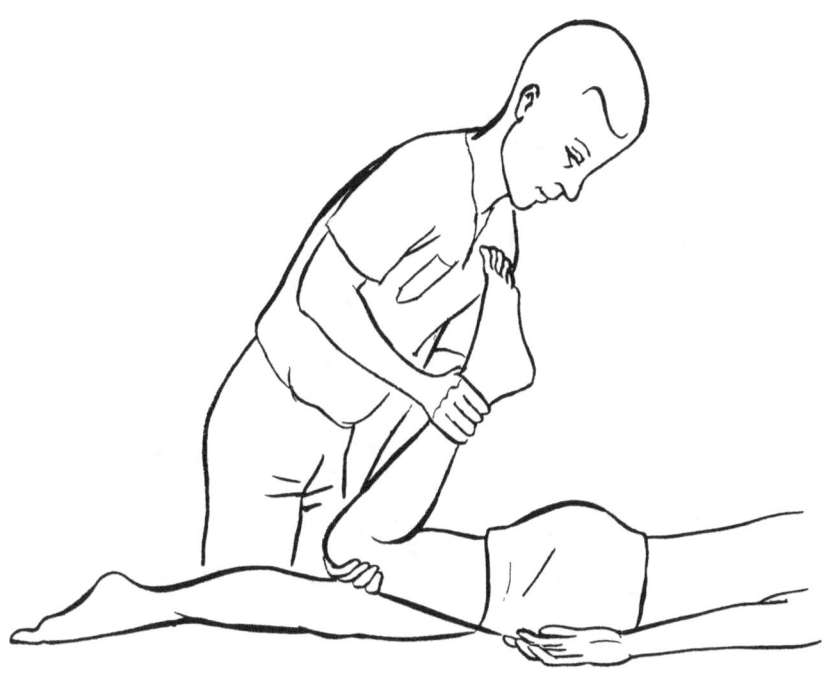

Hip Extension Test

Description

The patient lies prone. The examiner stabilizes the patient's pelvis with one hand and with the other hand holds the distal femur and then hyperextends the hip. The test is repeated on the other side and the results compared.

Interpretation

A positive test is one in which the leg feels heavier and the range is restricted, indicating hypomobility in the sacroiliac joint or sacroiliac joint dysfunction on that side.

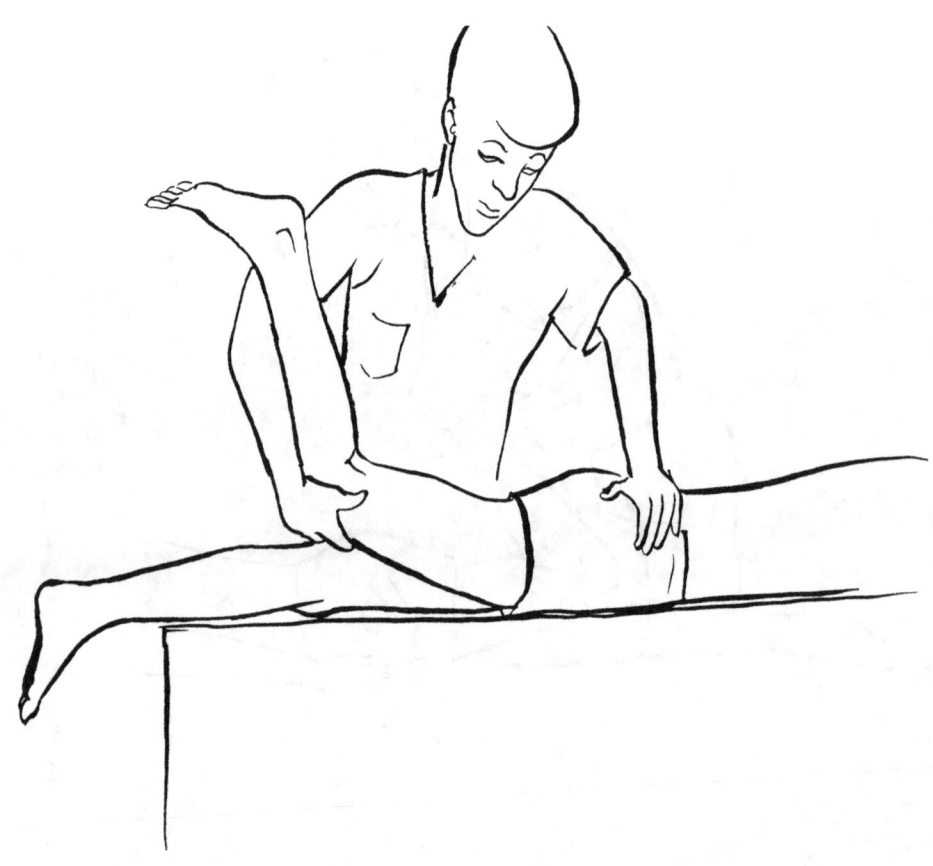

Sacral Apex Pressure Test

Description

The patient lies prone. The examiner places the base of one hand at the apex of the patient's sacrum and then applies a downward pressure to the apex of the sacrum.

Interpretation

A positive test is one which elicits pain over the joint, indicating a sacroiliac joint dysfunction on that side.

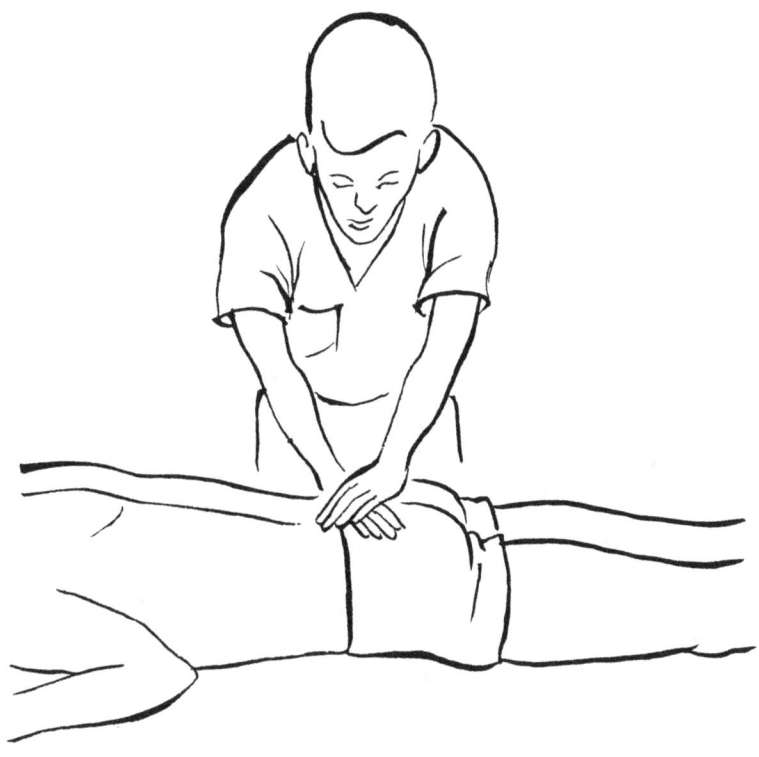

Backward Bending Test

Description
The patient stands. The examiner places his/her thumbs on the patient's sacral sulci and instructs the patient to bend backward.

Interpretation
A positive test is one in which the sulcus does not deepen, indicating a hypomobile sacroiliac joint on that side.

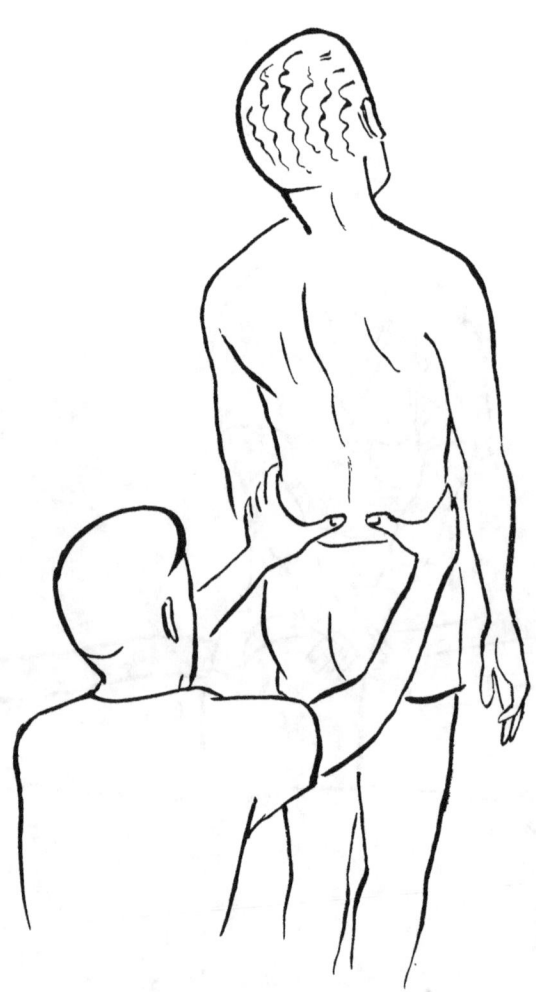

Gillet Test

Description

The patient stands with feet approximately 12 inches apart. The examiner stands behind the patient and places one thumb directly under one posterior superior iliac spine (PSIS) and the other thumb at the S2 tubercle at the level of PSIS. The patient is then instructed to stand on one leg and to flex the other hip and knee toward the chest. The examiner palpates the PSIS on the side being flexed. The test is then repeated on the other side.

Interpretation

A positive test is one in which the palpated PSIS does not dip down as the motion is completed at the hip joint, indicating sacroiliac joint dysfunction.

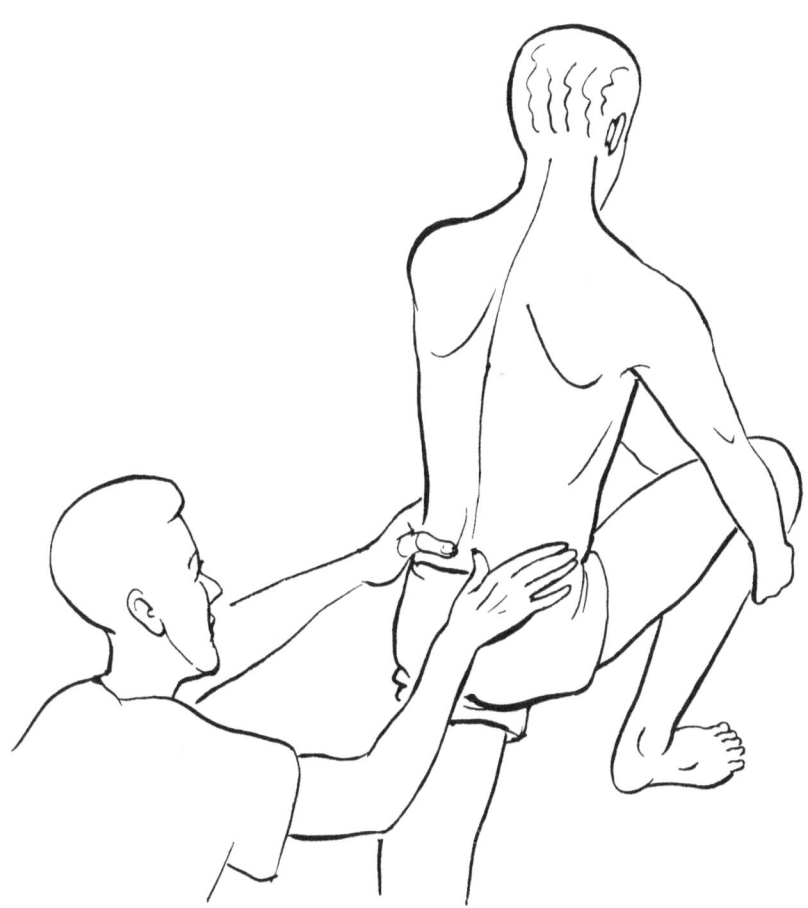

Gaenslen Test

Description

The patient lies supine. The patient is then instructed to draw both legs onto the chest. The examiner shifts the patient to the side of the table so that one buttock extends over the edge of the table. The patient is then allowed to drop the unsupported leg over the table while continuing to support the opposite leg in the flexed position.

Interpretation

A positive test is one in which pain is increased in the area of the sacroiliac joint, indicating sacroiliac joint pathology.

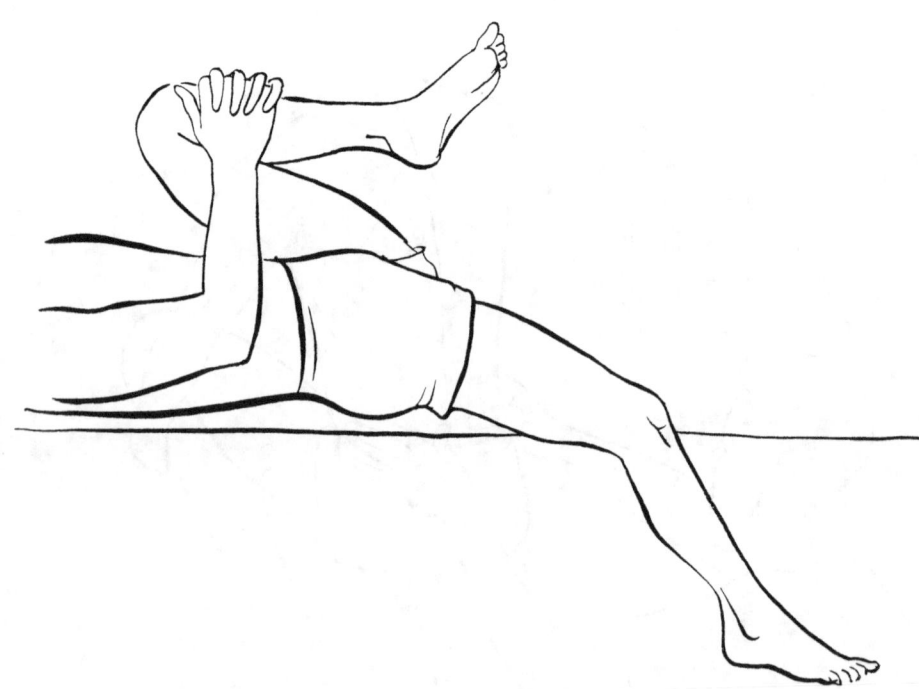

Sphinx Test

Description

The patient lies prone. The examiner palpates the sacral sulci and notes the relative depth of the sacral sulci. The examiner then palpates the inferior lateral angles (ILAs) and notes the relative position of the ILAs. The patient is then instructed to rise from the prone position onto elbows and to rest chin in hands. The examiner again palpates the sacral sulci and ILAs, and notes the relative positions.

Interpretation

A positive test is one in which: (1) the sacral sulcus remains shallow on the side that is blocked, indicating a sacral-iliac dysfunction; (2) the ILA opposite to the deep sacral sulcus becomes more posterior, indicating forward sacral torsion.

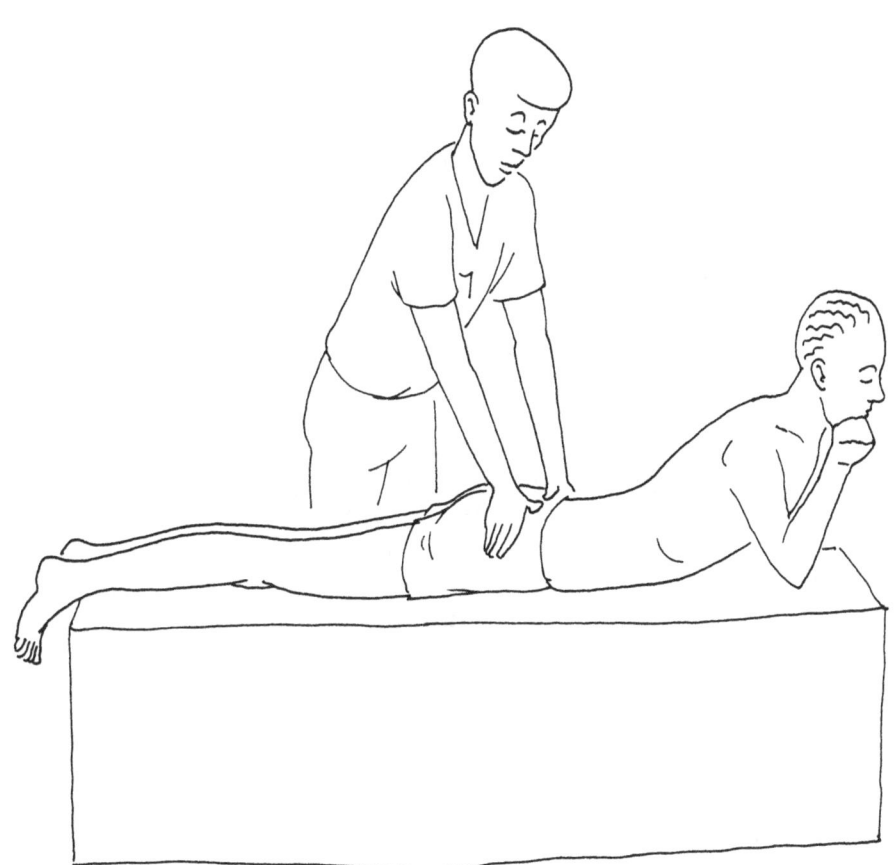

March Test

Description

The patient stands. The examiner palpates and places the thumbs just below the posterior iliac crest. The patient is then instructed to flex the hip on one side to about 90°. The test is then repeated on the other side.

Interpretation

A positive test is one in which one posterior superior iliac crest moves downward either slowly, indicating a hypomobile sacroiliac joint, or quickly, indicating a hypermobile sacroiliac joint.

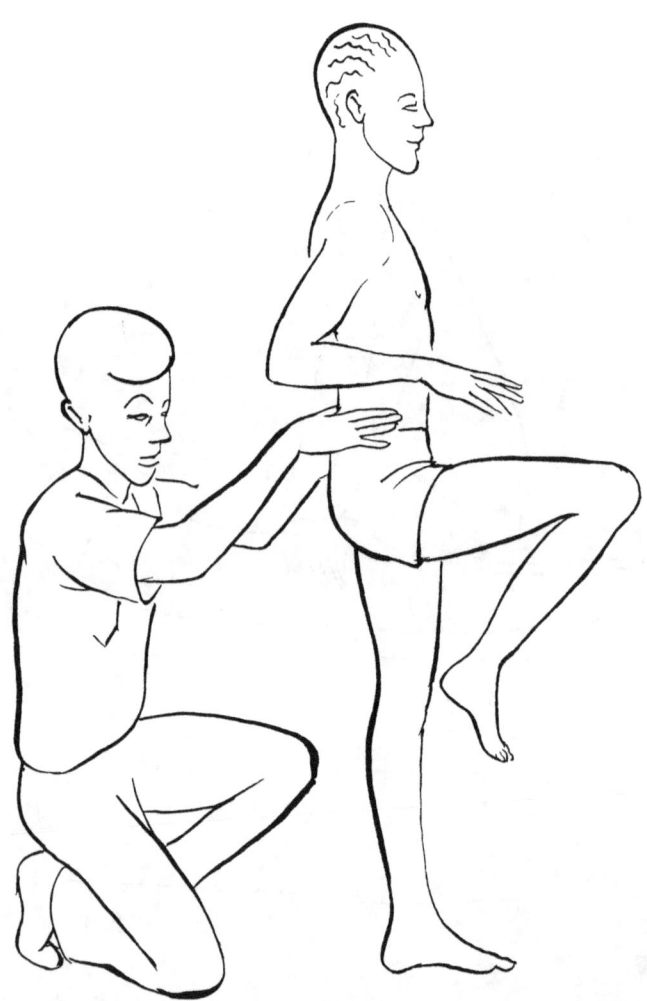

Flamingo Test

Description

The patient stands. The patient is instructed to stand on one leg. The patient is then instructed to hop on one leg. The test is then repeated on the other leg.

Interpretation

A positive test is one in which pain is produced in the sacroiliac joint or symphysis pubis, indicating dysfunction in the sacroiliac joint or symphysis pubis. The pain may be increased during hopping.

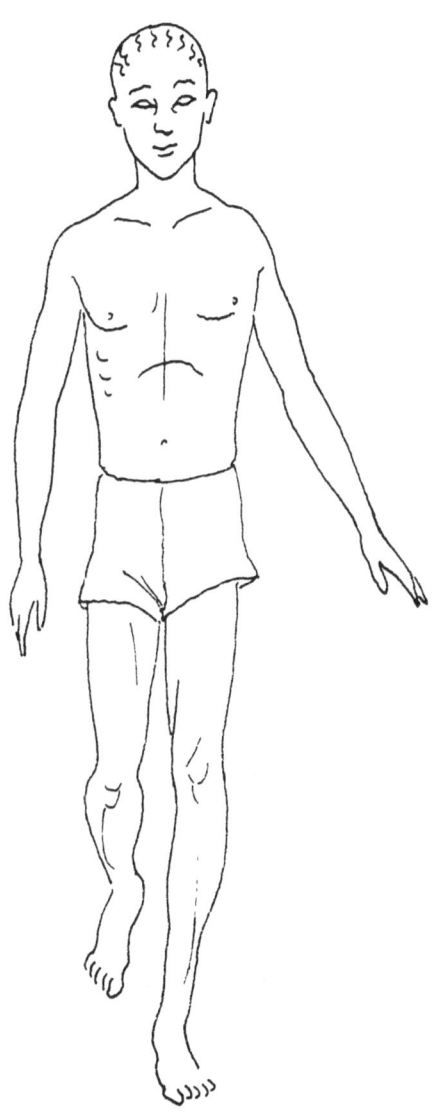

Bibliography

Beetham, W. P., H. F. Polley, C. H. Slocum, and W. F. Weaver. 1985. *Physical examination of the joints*. Philadelphia: W. B. Saunders.

Cailliet, R. 1975. *Hand pain and impairment*. Philadelphia: F. A. Davis.

Cross, M. J., and K. J. Crichton. 1987. *Clinical examination of the injured knee*. New York: Gower Medical Publishing.

D'Ambrosia, R. D. 1977. *Musculoskeletal disorders: Regional examination and differential diagnosis*. 3d edition. Philadelphia: J. B. Lippincott.

Donatelli, R., and M. J. Wooden, eds. 1989. *Orthopedic physical therapy*. New York: Churchill Livingstone.

Gould, J. A., ed. 1990. *Orthopaedic and sports physical therapy*. 2d edition. Philadelphia: C. V. Mosby Company.

Hoppenfeld, S. 1976. *Physical examination of the spine and extremities*. New York: Appleton-Century-Crofts.

Kelikian, H., and A. S. Kelikian. 1985. *Disorders of the foot*. Philadelphia: W. B. Saunders.

Kennedy, J. C. 1979. *The injured adolescent knee*. Baltimore: Williams and Wilkins.

Kessler, R. M., and D. Hertling. 1983. *Management of common musculoskeletal disorders: Physical therapy principles and methods*. Philadelphia: Harper and Row.

Kulund, D. N. 1988. *The injured athlete*. 2d edition. New York: Lippincott.

Magee, D. J. 1992. *Orthopedic physical assessment*. 2d edition. Philadelphia: W. B. Saunders.

Mangine, R. E., ed. 1988. *Clinics in physical therapy: Physical therapy of the knee*. New York: Churchill Livingstone.

McRae, R. 1990. *Clinical orthopaedic examination*. 3d edition. New York: Churchill Livingstone.

O'Donoghue, D. H. 1984. *Treatment of injuries to athletes*. 4th edition. Philadelphia: W. B. Saunders.

Post, M. 1986. *Physical examination of the musculoskeletal system*. Chicago: Year Book Medical Publishers.

Saunders, H. D. 1985. *Evaluation, treatment and prevention of musculoskeletal disorders*. Minneapolis: H. D. Saunders.

Schamber, D. 1984. *Simply performed tests on the hand*. New York: Vantage Press.

Turek, S. L. 1984. *Orthopaedic principles and their applications*. 4th edition. Philadelphia: J. B. Lippincott.

Sectional Index

Shoulder, 1
- Adson Test, 35
- Allen Test, 36
- Anterior Apprehension Test, 4
- Anterior Drawer Test, 10
- Anterior Instability Test, 6
- Bicipital Tendonitis Test, 28
- Capsular Laxity Test, 18
- Clunk Test, 19
- Costoclavicular Test, 40
- Dawbarn Test, 26
- Drop Arm Test, 21
- Dugas Test, 24
- Feagin Test, 17
- Fulcrum Test, 9
- Gilcrest Test, 32
- Glenohumeral Joint Stability Test, 3
- Halstead Test, 41
- Heuter Test, 34
- Hyperabduction Test, 39
- Impingement Test, 22
- Jerk Test, 14
- Lippman Test, 30
- Ludington Test, 33
- Norwood Test, 13
- Painful Arc Test, 23
- Posterior Apprehension Test, 11
- Posterior Drawer Test, 12
- Protzman Test, 5
- Push-Pull Test, 15
- Rockwood Test, 7
- Roos Test, 37
- Rowe Test, 8
- Speed Test, 31
- Subacromial Bursitis Test, 25
- Sulcus Test, 16
- Supraspinatus Tendonitis Test, 20
- Transverse Humeral Ligament Test, 27
- Wright Test, 38
- Yergason Test, 29

Elbow, 43
- Cozen Test, 47
- Elbow Flexion Test, 49
- Golfer Elbow Test, 48
- Ligamentous Stability Test, 45
- Pinch Grip Test, 50
- Pronator Teres Syndrome Test, 52
- Tennis Elbow Test, 46
- Tinel Test, 51

Wrist and Hand, 53
- Allen Test, 55
- Bunnel-Littler Test, 69
- Capsular Test, 66
- Egawa Test, 57
- Finkelstein Test, 64
- Flexor Digitorum Profundus Test, 68
- Flexor Digitorum Superficialis Test, 67
- Froment Test, 56
- Grind Test, 63
- Intrinsic Tightness Test, 70
- Linburg Test, 71
- Lunatotriquetral Ballottement Test, 61
- Murphy Test, 62
- Phalen Test, 58
- Retinacular/Capsular Test, 65
- Tinel Test, 59
- Watson Test, 60
- Weber Test, 73
- Wrinkle Test, 72

Hip, 75
- Allis Test, 99
- Barlow Test, 98
- Buttock Test, 79
- Craig Test, 90
- Ely Test, 83
- Fabere/Patrick Test, 77
- Femoral Nerve Stretch Test, 96
- Hibb Test, 78
- Ischial Bursitis Test, 92
- Leg Length Discrepancy Test, 91
- 90-90 Straight Leg Test, 85
- Noble Compression Test, 87
- Ober Test, 86
- Ortolani Click Test, 97
- Piriformis Test, 94
- Rectus Femoris Test, 82
- Sciatic Nerve Test, 95
- Scour Test, 89
- Telescoping Test, 100
- Thomas Test, 81
- Torque Test, 80
- Trendelenburg Test, 88
- Tripod Test, 84
- Trochanteric Bursitis Test, 93

Knee, 101
- Abduction Stress Test, 143
- Adduction Stress Test, 144
- Anterior Drawer Test, 138
- Apley Compression Test, 120
- Apley Distraction Test, 135
- Apprehension Test, 113
- Arcuate Spin Test, 152
- Bohler Test, 128
- Bounce Home Test, 119
- Bragard Test, 129
- Cabot Popliteal Test, 125
- Clarke Test, 110
- Cross-over Test, 150
- Dreyer Test, 115
- Dynamic Extension Test, 137
- Effusion Test, 104
- External Rotational Recurvatum Test, 140
- Fairbank Apprehension Test, 114
- Flexion Rotation Drawer Test, 141
- Fluctuation Test, 105
- Helfet Test, 132
- Hyperextension Recurvatum Test, 139
- Hyperflexion Meniscus Test, 124
- Jakob Test, 153
- Lachman Test, 136
- Losee Test, 149
- MacIntosh Test, 145
- Martens Test, 134
- McConnel Test, 108
- McMurray Test, 127
- Mediopatellar Plica Test, 116
- Nakajima Test, 133
- Noble Compression Test, 118
- O'Donoghue Test, 131
- Patella Femoral Grinding Test, 109
- Patellar Tap Test, 106
- Payr Test, 126
- Pivot Jerk Test, 146
- Pivot Shift Test, 151
- Plica "Stutter" Test, 117
- Posterior Drawer Test, 142
- Q-Angle (Patellofemoral Angle) Test, 154
- Retracting Meniscal Test, 130
- Slocum ALRI Test, 148
- Slocum Test, 147
- Spring Test, 122
- Steinmann Tenderness Displacement Test, 123
- Steinmann Test, 121
- Stroke Test, 103
- Tinel Test, 107
- Waldron Test, 111
- Wilson Test, 155
- Zohler Test, 112

Ankle and Foot, 157
- Anterior Drawer Test, 165
- Calf Compression Test, 162
- Eversion Stress Test, 167
- Homan Test, 161
- Hyperpronation Test, 171
- Inversion Stress Test, 164
- Kleiger Test, 168
- Modified Romberg Test, 159
- Posterior Drawer Test, 166
- Squeeze Test, 172
- Strunsky Test, 173
- Swing Test, 169
- Talar Tilt Test, 163
- Thompson Test, 160
- Tinel Test, 170

Temporomandibular, 175
- Chvostek Test, 178
- Jaw Reflex Test, 177
- Loading Test, 179
- Palpation Test, 180

Cervical, 181
- Adson Test, 190
- Alar Odontoid Integrity Test, 188
- Allen Test, 191
- Babinski Reflex Test, 214
- Biceps Reflex Test, 211
- Brachial Plexus Tension Test, 206
- Brachioradialis Reflex Test, 212
- Compression Test, 197
- Costoclavicular Test, 195
- Distraction Test, 210
- Dizziness Test, 186
- Foraminal Compression Test, 198
- Halstead Test, 196
- Hyperabduction Test, 194
- Jackson Compression Test, 199
- Kerning Test, 209
- Maximal Foraminal Compression Test, 200
- Milgram Test, 202
- Naffziger Test, 203
- O'Donoghue Test, 189
- Roos Test, 192
- Sharp-Purser Test, 187
- Shoulder Abduction Test, 207
- Shoulder Depression Test, 208
- Slump Test, 201
- Swallowing Test, 183

Temperature Test, 184
Triceps Reflex Test, 213
Upper Limb Tension Test, 205
Valsalva Test, 204
Vertebral Artery Test, 185
Wright Test, 193

Thoracic, 215
Abdominal Reflex Test, 217
Beevor Test, 220
First Thoracic Stretch Test, 219
Scapular Approximation Test, 218

Lumbar, 221
Abdominal Reflex Test, 268
Ankle Reflex Test, 271
Babinski Reflex Test, 272
Balance Test, 225
Bechterew Test, 258
Bowstring/Cram Test, 242
Braggard Test, 249
Brudzinski Test, 234
Buckling Test, 250
Chaddock Test, 273
Compression Test, 259
Cremasteric Reflex Test, 269
Distraction Test, 261
Fabere/Patrick Test, 223
FADIR Test, 224
Fajersztajin Test, 256
Femoral Nerve Stretch Test, 240
Flip Test, 233
Freiberg Test, 265
Goldthwaith Test, 251
Heel Walking Test, 262
Hoover Test, 255
Kerning Test, 238
Knee Reflex Test, 270
Lasegue Test, 248
McKenzie Side Glide Test, 257
Milgram Test, 237
Minor Test, 252
Nachlas Test, 244
Naffziger Test, 236
Oppenheim Test, 275
Pace Test, 267
Pheasant Test, 229
Piriformis Test, 264
Piriformis Tightness Test, 266
Prone Knee-Bending Test, 239
Rossolimo Test, 274
Schober Test, 231

Sciatic Nerve Test, 243
Sciatic Tension Test, 241
Sicard Test, 254
Sitting Straight Leg Raising Test, 247
Skin Rolling Test, 230
Slump Test, 235
Squat Test, 227
Straight Leg Raising Test, 245
Thomas Test, 226
Toe Walking Test, 263
Turyn Test, 253
Valsalva Test, 260
Weight Shift Test, 232
Well Leg Straight Leg Raising Test, 246
Yeoman Test, 228

Sacrum and Pelvis, 277
Backward Bending Test, 302
Compression Test, 296
Distraction Test, 297
Fabere/Patrick Test, 279
FADIR Test, 280
Flamingo Test, 307
Gaenslen Test, 304
Gillet Test, 303
Hibb Test, 282
Hip Extension Test, 300
Lewin-Gaenslen Test, 286
Long Sitting Test, 294
March Test, 306
Nachlas Test, 283
Prone Knee Flexion Test, 298
Resisted Abduction Test, 284
Sacral Apex Pressure Test, 301
Sitting Anterior Superior Iliac Spine Test, 291
Sitting Flexion Test, 293
Sitting Iliac Crest Levels Test, 290
Sitting Posterior Superior Iliac Spine Test, 292
Sphinx Test, 305
Spring Test, 295
Standing Anterior Superior Iliac Spine Test, 287
Standing Flexion Test, 289
Standing Iliac Crest Levels Test, 285
Standing Posterior Superior Iliac Spine Test, 288
Toe Walking Test, 281
Yeoman Test, 299

Alphabetical Index

Abdominal Reflex Test, 217, 268
Abduction Stress Test, 143
Adduction Stress Test, 144
Adson Test, 35, 190
Alar Odontoid Integrity Test, 188
Allen Test, 36, 55, 191
Allis Test, 99
Ankle Reflex Test, 271
Anterior Apprehension Test, 4
Anterior Drawer Test, 10, 138, 165
Anterior Instability Test, 6
Apley Compression Test, 120
Apley Distraction Test, 135
Apprehension Test, 113
Arcuate Spin Test, 152

Babinski Reflex Test, 214, 272
Backward Bending Test, 302
Balance Test, 225
Barlow Test, 98
Bechterew Test, 258
Beevor Test, 220
Biceps Reflex Test, 211
Bicipital Tendonitis Test, 28
Bohler Test, 128
Bounce Home Test, 119
Bowstring/Cram Test, 242
Brachial Plexus Tension Test, 206
Brachioradialis Reflex Test, 212
Bragard Test, 129
Braggard Test, 249
Brudzinski Test, 234
Buckling Test, 250
Bunnel-Littler Test, 69
Buttock Test, 79

Cabot Popliteal Test, 125
Calf Compression Test, 162
Capsular Laxity Test, 18
Capsular Test, 66
Chaddock Test, 273
Chvostek Test, 178
Clarke Test, 110
Clunk Test, 19
Compression Test, 197, 259, 296
Costoclavicular Test, 40, 195
Cozen Test, 47
Craig Test, 90
Cremasteric Reflex Test, 269
Cross-over Test, 150

Dawbarn Test, 26
Distraction Test, 210, 261, 297
Dizziness Test, 186
Dreyer Test, 115
Drop Arm Test, 21
Dugas Test, 24
Dynamic Extension Test, 137

Effusion Test, 104
Egawa Test, 57
Elbow Flexion Test, 49
Ely Test, 83
Eversion Stress Test, 167
External Rotational Recurvatum
   Test, 140

Fabere/Patrick Test, 77, 223, 279
FADIR Test, 224, 280
Fairbank Apprehension Test, 114
Fajersztajin Test, 256
Feagin Test, 17
Femoral Nerve Stretch Test, 96, 240
Finkelstein Test, 64
First Thoracic Stretch Test, 219
Flamingo Test, 307
Flexion Rotation Drawer Test, 141
Flexor Digitorum Profundus Test, 68
Flexor Digitorum Superficialis Test, 67
Flip Test, 233
Fluctuation Test, 105
Foraminal Compression Test, 198
Freiberg Test, 265
Froment Test, 56
Fulcrum Test, 9

Gaenslen Test, 304
Gilcrest Test, 32
Gillet Test, 303
Glenohumeral Joint Stability Test, 3
Goldthwaith Test, 251
Golfer Elbow Test, 48
Grind Test, 63

Halstead Test, 41, 196
Heel Walking Test, 262
Helfet Test, 132
Heuter Test, 34
Hibb Test, 78, 282
Hip Extension Test, 300
Homan Test, 161

Hoover Test, 255
Hyperabduction Test, 39, 194
Hyperextension Recurvatum Test, 139
Hyperflexion Meniscus Test, 124
Hyperpronation Test, 171

Impingement Test, 22
Intrinsic Tightness Test, 70
Inversion Stress Test, 164
Ischial Bursitis Test, 92

Jackson Compression Test, 199
Jakob Test, 153
Jaw Reflex Test, 177
Jerk Test, 14

Kerning Test, 209, 238
Kleiger Test, 168
Knee Reflex Test, 270

Lachman Test, 136
Lasegue Test, 248
Leg Length Discrepancy Test, 91
Lewin-Gaenslen Test, 286
Ligamentous Stability Test, 45
Linburg Test, 71
Lippman Test, 30
Loading Test, 179
Long Sitting Test, 294
Losee Test, 149
Ludington Test, 33
Lunatotriquetral Ballottement Test, 61

MacIntosh Test, 145
March Test, 306
Martens Test, 134
Maximal Foraminal Compression Test, 200
McConnel Test, 108
McKenzie Side Glide Test, 257
McMurray Test, 127
Mediopatellar Plica Test, 116
Milgram Test, 202, 237
Minor Test, 252
Modified Romberg Test, 159
Murphy Test, 62

Nachlas Test, 244, 283
Naffziger Test, 203, 236
Nakajima Test, 133
90-90 Straight Leg Test, 85
Noble Compression Test, 87, 118
Norwood Test, 13

O'Donoghue Test, 131, 189
Ober Test, 86
Oppenheim Test, 275
Ortolani Click Test, 97

Pace Test, 267
Painful Arc Test, 23
Palpation Test, 180
Patella Femoral Grinding Test, 109
Patellar Tap Test, 106
Payr Test, 126
Phalen Test, 58
Pheasant Test, 229
Pinch Grip Test, 50
Piriformis Test, 94, 264
Piriformis Tightness Test, 266
Pivot Jerk Test, 146
Pivot Shift Test, 151
Plica "Stutter" Test, 117
Posterior Apprehension Test, 11
Posterior Drawer Test, 12, 142, 166
Pronator Teres Syndrome Test, 52
Prone Knee-Bending Test, 239
Prone Knee Flexion Test, 298
Protzman Test, 5
Push-Pull Test, 15

Q-Angle (Patellofemoral Angle) Test, 154

Rectus Femoris Test, 82
Resisted Abduction Test, 284
Retinacular/Capsular Test, 65
Retracting Meniscal Test, 130
Rockwood Test, 7
Roos Test, 37, 192
Rossolimo Test, 274
Rowe Test, 8

Sacral Apex Pressure Test, 301
Scapular Approximation Test, 218
Schober Test, 231
Sciatic Nerve Test, 95, 243
Sciatic Tension Test, 241
Scour Test, 89
Sharp-Purser Test, 187
Shoulder Abduction Test, 207
Shoulder Depression Test, 208
Sicard Test, 254
Sitting Anterior Superior Iliac Spine Test, 291
Sitting Flexion Test, 293
Sitting Iliac Crest Levels Test, 290
Sitting Posterior Superior Iliac Spine Test, 292

Sitting Straight Leg Raising Test, 247
Skin Rolling Test, 230
Slocum ALRI Test, 148
Slocum Test, 147
Slump Test, 201, 235
Speed Test, 31
Sphinx Test, 305
Spring Test, 122, 295
Squat Test, 227
Squeeze Test, 172
Standing Anterior Superior Iliac Spine Test, 287
Standing Flexion Test, 289
Standing Iliac Crest Levels Test, 285
Standing Posterior Superior Iliac Spine Test, 288
Steinmann Tenderness Displacement Test, 123
Steinmann Test, 121
Straight Leg Raising Test, 245
Stroke Test, 103
Strunsky Test, 173
Subacromial Bursitis Test, 25
Sulcus Test, 16
Supraspinatus Tendonitis Test, 20
Swallowing Test, 183
Swing Test, 169

Talar Tilt Test, 163
Telescoping Test, 100
Temperature Test, 184

Tennis Elbow Test, 46
Thomas Test, 81, 226
Thompson Test, 160
Tinel Test, 51, 59, 107, 170
Toe Walking Test, 263, 281
Torque Test, 80
Transverse Humeral Ligament Test, 27
Trendelenburg Test, 88
Triceps Reflex Test, 213
Tripod Test, 84
Trochanteric Bursitis Test, 93
Turyn Test, 253

Upper Limb Tension Test, 205

Valsalva Test, 204, 260
Vertebral Artery Test, 185

Waldron Test, 111
Watson Test, 60
Weber Test, 73
Weight Shift Test, 232
Well Leg Straight Leg Raising Test, 246
Wilson Test, 155
Wright Test, 38, 193
Wrinkle Test, 72

Yeoman Test, 228, 299
Yergason Test, 29

Zohler Test, 112

www.ingramcontent.com/pod-product-compliance
Lightning Source LLC
Chambersburg PA
CBHW080235180526
45167CB00006B/2282